GROWING UP TOBACCO FREE

PREVENTING NICOTINE ADDICTION IN CHILDREN AND YOUTHS

Barbara S. Lynch and Richard J. Bonnie, *Editors*

Committee on Preventing Nicotine Addiction
in Children and Youths

Division of Biobehavioral Sciences and Mental Disorders

Institute of Medicine

NATIONAL ACADEMY PRESS
Washington, D.C.   1994

NATIONAL ACADEMY PRESS • 2101 Constitution Avenue, NW • Washington, DC 20418

NOTICE: The project that is the subject of this report was approved by the Governing Board of the National Research Council, whose members are drawn from the councils of the National Academy of Sciences, the National Academy of Engineering, and the Institute of Medicine. The members of the committee responsible for this report were chosen for their special competencies and with regard for appropriate balance.

This report has been reviewed by a group other than the authors according to procedures approved by a Report Review Committee consisting of members of the National Academy of Sciences, the National Academy of Engineering, and the Institute of Medicine.

The Institute of Medicine was chartered in 1970 by the National Academy of Sciences to enlist distinguished members of the appropriate professions in the examination of policy matters pertaining to the health of the public. In this, the Institute acts under both the Academy's 1863 congressional charter responsibility to be an adviser to the federal government and its own initiative in identifying issues of medical care, research, and education. Dr. Kenneth I. Shine is president of the Institute of Medicine.

This project was funded by the Robert Wood Johnson Foundation (Grant No. 20520-R); Metropolitan Life; the American Heart Association; by funds provided by the Cigarette and Tobacco Surtax Fund of the State of California through the Tobacco-Related Disease Research Program (Grant No. 3SP-0416); the Centers for Disease Control and Prevention and the National Institute on Drug Abuse (Grant No. M93-OSH-DASH); the Indian Health Service; the Center for Substance Abuse Prevention; and the National Cancer Institute, the Maternal and Child Health Bureau of the Health Resources and Services Administration, and the Agency for Health Care Policy and Research (Grant No. 1-R13-CA62355-01).

Library of Congress Cataloging-in-Publication Data

Growing up tobacco free : preventing nicotine addiction in children
and youths / Barbara S. Lynch and Richard J. Bonnie, editors ;
Committee on Preventing Nicotine Addiction in Children and Youths,
Institute of Medicine.

    p. cm.   First Printing, September 1994
    Includes bibliographical references and index.   Second Printing, January 1996
    ISBN 0-309-05129-0
    1. Children—Tobacco use—United States—Prevention. 2. Youth—
Tobacco use—United States—Prevention. I. Lynch, Barbara S.
II. Bonnie, Richard J. III. Institute of Medicine (U.S.).
Committee on Preventing Nicotine Addiction in Children and Youths.
HV5745.G75   1994
362.29'67'083—dc20   94-31455
                                          CIP

COMMITTEE ON PREVENTING NICOTINE
ADDICTION IN CHILDREN AND YOUTHS

Paul R. Torrens, M.D., M.P.H. (Chair)
Professor of Health Services Administration
Department of Health Services
School of Public Health
University of California, Los Angeles

Albert Bandura, Ph.D.
David Starr Jordan Professor of
Social Science in Psychology
Department of Psychology
Stanford University

Neal L. Benowitz, M.D.
Professor and Chief
Division of Clinical Pharmacology
Departments of Medicine, Pharmacy,
and Psychiatry
School of Medicine
University of California,
San Francisco

Richard J. Bonnie, LL.B.
John S. Battle Professor of Law
Director, Institute of Law, Psychiatry,
and Public Policy
University of Virginia School of Law

K. Michael Cummings, Ph.D.,
M.P.H.
Director, Smoking Control Program
Department of Cancer Control and
Epidemiology
Roswell Park Cancer Institute
Buffalo, New York

Donald R. Dexter, Jr., D.M.D.
Executive Director
Klamath Tribal Health and Family
Services
Klamath, Oregon

Ellen R. Gritz, Ph.D.
Professor and Chair
Department of Behavioral Science
M.D. Anderson Cancer Center
University of Texas, Houston

Gerardo Marín, Ph.D.
Professor of Psychology and
Associate Dean
College of Arts and Sciences
University of San Francisco

Mark Nichter, Ph.D., M.P.H.
Professor
Department of Anthropology
University of Arizona, Tucson

Peggy O'Hara, Ph.D.
Associate Professor and Director
of Graduate Programs in
Public Health
Department of Epidemiology and
Public Health
University of Miami School of
Medicine

Cheryl L. Perry, Ph.D.
Professor
Division of Epidemiology
School of Public Health
University of Minnesota

Thomas C. Schelling, Ph.D.
Distinguished Professor of Economics
and Public Affairs
School of Public Affairs
University of Maryland at
College Park

Herbert Severson, Ph.D.
Research Scientist
Oregon Research Institute and
Associate Professor
School of Psychology
University of Oregon

Sarah Moody Thomas, Ph.D.
Associate Director for Community
Education and Applications
Stanley S. Scott Cancer Center
Louisiana State University Medical
Center

Institute of Medicine Staff
Barbara S. Lynch, Ph.D., Study
Director
Robert Cook-Deegan, M.D., Director,
Division of Biomedical Sciences
and Mental Disorders
Sharon Russell, Project Assistant

PREFACE

In March 1991, the Institute of Medicine's Board on Biobehavioral Sciences and Mental Disorders identified the need for a study on preventing nicotine addiction in children and youths as one of its highest priorities, and directed the IOM staff to seek the resources required to conduct such a study. The Robert Wood Johnson Foundation generously took the lead in funding the project, joined by Metropolitan Life, the American Heart Association, the Tobacco-Related Disease Research Program (State of California), the Centers for Disease Control and Prevention, the National Institute on Drug Abuse, the National Cancer Institute, the Maternal and Child Health Bureau of the Health Resources and Services Administration, the Indian Health Service, the Center for Substance Abuse Prevention, and the Agency for Health Care Policy and Research. In April 1993, a committee of 14 individuals was appointed to conduct an 18-month study on the prevention of nicotine dependence among children and youths, addressing the following tasks:

- to review and evaluate the scientific literature on the epidemiology of nicotine dependence among children and youths;
- to review and evaluate the scientific literature on primary and secondary prevention of nicotine dependence among children and youths;
- to review and evaluate the scientific base of knowledge about the causes of nicotine addiction, including physiological, social, psychological, educational, and environmental factors; product advertising and promotion tactics; and public policy;
- to review important "grass roots" programs on tobacco use and youths; and
- to outline a research agenda that makes practical, science-based policy

recommendations that will contribute to accomplishing the Healthy People 2000 Goals of reducing nicotine dependence among children and youths.

The Committee met five times over the course of the study. It invited presentations and written submissions from experts in the field of tobacco control. The Committee also held six focus groups with adolescents in different geographical regions. In a cooperative effort with the Coalition for America's Children, the Committee conducted a survey of 250 organizations that have youth memberships or that serve youths. To assess the level of tobacco-related research relevant to youths, the Committee contacted federal research agencies and private foundations to solicit information about their activities related to youth tobacco use. In addition, the Committee carefully reviewed the extensive research literature on nicotine addiction and youths as well as the comprehensive summary and analysis of this literature compiled by the surgeon general in the 1994 report on smoking and health.[1]

The relation between scientific knowledge and social policy is often complex and controversial. In this study, however, the Committee's task was immensely simplified by the clarity of the nation's public health objectives in relation to tobacco use. The premises of this report, as discussed in chapter 1, are that the nation has a compelling interest in reducing the morbidity and mortality caused by nicotine addiction, and that nicotine addiction can be most efficiently reduced in the long run by preventing children and youths from using tobacco products and from becoming addicted to them. The question is not whether society should try to prevent tobacco consumption by children and youths, but rather how this objective should be accomplished. The disputed issues, in short, relate to means, not ends.

Within this framework, the Committee has sought to conduct a rigorous and open-minded inquiry. The Committee has identified the menu of social interventions that might be undertaken to prevent nicotine addiction among children and youths and reached a common view regarding the policies and programs that are likely to be most effective in achieving this goal. These issues are largely, though not exclusively, scientific ones. The main questions are whether and to what extent a given policy or program can be expected to reduce the onset of tobacco use and addiction among children and youths. Informed judgments on these questions provide an essential foundation for prudent policymaking and priority-setting.

The Committee could have confined itself to scientific judgments about the efficacy of various policies and programs, leaving to policymakers the evaluative task of weighing the costs of these interventions against anticipated public health gains. However, the Committee was charged with the additional responsibility of making "practical science-based policy recommendations that will contribute to accomplishing the Year 2000 goals of reducing nicotine dependence among children and youths." The Committee has tried to respond to this challenge.

The material in this report is organized as a blueprint for policymaking. In the context of each type of intervention, the Committee has summarized the pertinent empirical evidence and sought to demonstrate why, in our opinion, the recommended policies or programs are justified. The Committee did not think it necessary to duplicate in this report all the information on the etiology of smoking by children and youths appearing in the surgeon general's recent report. Instead, the Committee presents the information bearing most directly on the potential effects of policies and programs designed to reduce nicotine addiction among children and youths.

In conducting its study and writing this report, the Committee has benefitted immensely from the path-breaking efforts of researchers and policymakers in other countries, especially Canada, Australia, New Zealand, and Finland, and from information provided by the World Health Organization and the International Union Against Cancer. This debt can be partially repaid if the proposals made in the report provide a useful model for reformers in other parts of the globe.

Tobacco use is a worldwide epidemic, and every nation is confronted by a challenge similar to the one faced in the United States. During the 1990s in developed countries, tobacco will cause approximately 30% of all deaths among persons 35-69 years of age, making it the largest single cause of premature death in the developed world.[2] The global health burden of tobacco use is likely to increase geometrically in the coming decades. It also seems likely that aggressive marketing by the international tobacco companies will require an aggressive response by public health officials in the developing world and in the countries of Central and Eastern Europe and the former Soviet Union. The Committee was not charged to address international tobacco control. In the course of its deliberations, however, the Committee unanimously reached the conclusion that decisive actions taken here at home to promote a youth-centered strategy to prevent tobacco-related disease and death should be accompanied by an unequivocal commitment to help other nations achieve similar aspirations.

REFERENCES

1. Centers for Disease Control and Prevention. *Preventing Tobacco Use Among Young People: A Report of the Surgeon General.* Washington, D.C.: U.S. Department of Health and Human Services, 1994.

2. Peto, Richard, Alan D. Lopez, Jillian Boreham, Michael Thun, and Clark Heath, Jr. "Mortality from Tobacco in Developed Countries: Indirect Estimation from National Vital Statistics." *The Lancet* 339 (1992): 1268, 1274-1275.

ACKNOWLEDGMENTS

The Committee on Preventing Nicotine Addiction in Children and Youths expresses its appreciation to the co-funders of this 18-month study: the Robert Wood Johnson Foundation, Metropolitan Life, the American Heart Association, the Tobacco-Related Disease Research Program of California, the Centers for Disease Control and Prevention, the National Institute on Drug Abuse, the National Cancer Institute, the Maternal and Child Health Bureau of the Health Resources and Services Administration, the Indian Health Service, the Center for Substance Abuse Prevention, and the Agency for Health Care Policy and Research.

The Institute of Medicine thanks each of the institutions with which the Committee members are affiliated for the time and support services involved in the work of the Committee members and in the preparation of the report. The IOM extends special appreciation to Cornell University School of Law for its assistance to Richard Bonnie, who was a visiting professor at Cornell during the year of the Committee's work.

Many persons outside of the Committee contributed to this study in various ways. The Committee gratefully acknowledges the assistance of the reviewers of the report, as well as the coordinator and monitor of the review process, all of whom made valuable suggestions for improving the report. Numerous other individuals provided technical information by sending materials, by engaging in telephone discussions, by making presentations to the Committee, and by writing background papers. The following consultants made presentations at Committee meetings:

Ron Davis, M.D., Chief Medical Officer, Michigan Department of Health;

Cliff Douglas, Manager, Government Relations, American Cancer Society, Washington, D.C.;

Gary Giovino, Ph.D., Chief, Epidemiology Branch, Office of Smoking and Health, Centers for Disease Control and Prevention;

Larry Gruder, Ph.D., Director, Tobacco-Related Disease Research Program, University of California, Berkeley;

Don Shopland, Coordinator, Smoking and Tobacco Control Program, National Cancer Institute, Bethesda, Maryland;

John Slade, M.D., Associate Professor of Medicine, St. Peter's Medical Center, New Brunswick, New Jersey;

Larry Wallack, Dr. P.H., Professor, School of Public Health, University of California, Berkeley.

The following consultants presented commissioned background papers to the Committee:

Judy Butler, Research Associate, Stanford Center for Research in Disease Prevention, Stanford University;

Anthony Comerford, New Hope Foundation, Inc., and John Slade, M.D., St. Peter's Medical Center, New Brunswick, New Jersey;

John Pierce, Ph.D., Associate Professor and Head, Cancer Prevention and Control, University of California, San Diego.

The following research assistants were especially helpful in providing information and assistance to the Committee:

Laura Akers, Oregon Research Institute, Eugene, Oregon;
Peter Christianns, University of Miami, Department of Public Health;
Elizabeth Davidson, University of Virginia, School of Law.

Finally, numerous individuals helped expedite preparation of the report by providing assistance on a temporary or as-needed basis. The Committee thanks Karen Autrey, Jay Ball, Claudia Carl, Holly Dawkins, Mike Edington, Linda Humphrey, Brian Huse, Lynn Leet, Constance Pechura, Zoe Schneider, Gail Spears, Nina Spruill, Sally Stanfield, and Mike Stoto.

During the course of the study, the Committee, in conjunction with the Coalition for America's Children, conducted a survey of the coalition's 250 member organizations to determine whether they have policies and programs for tobacco control. The survey provided information about the potential role of organizations that serve young people. As a means of providing input to the Committee from experts in the field of substance abuse prevention, the Institute for Health Promotion and Disease Prevention Research of the University of Southern California planned a prevention conference to dovetail with a meeting of the Committee. The presentations and recommendations that were generated at that meeting were considered by the Committee in its deliberations. As a means of assessing the level and type of research funding that is invested in nicotine addiction and tobacco control, the IOM staff conducted a search of all relevant government agencies and foundations for abstracts describing funded research on nicotine prevention in youths since 1990. A summary of those projects and funds is included in chapter 9. The Committee appreciates the efforts of all persons who made the above surveys and conference possible.

CONTENTS

XIII

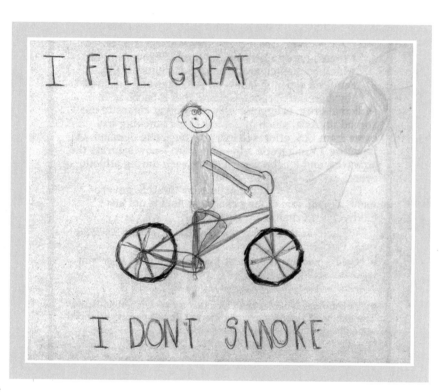

Craig Perrino, P.S. 50, Staten Island

CONTENTS

1 TOWARD A YOUTH-CENTERED PREVENTION POLICY

THE NEED FOR A YOUTH-CENTERED TOBACCO CONTROL POLICY

Use of tobacco products is the nation's deadliest addiction. Smoking cigarettes is the leading cause of avoidable death in the United States. More than 400,000 people die prematurely each year from diseases attributable to tobacco use.[1] The toll of deaths attributable to tobacco use is greater than the combined toll of deaths from AIDS, car accidents, alcohol, suicides, homicides, fires, and illegal drugs (figure 1-1). Smoking is the main cause of 87% of deaths from lung cancer, 30% of all cancer deaths, 82% of deaths from pulmonary disease, and 21% of deaths from chronic heart disease.[2] Use of smokeless tobacco* is a cause of oral cancer.[3] In a study of women who did not smoke but did use snuff chronically, the risk for oral cancers was 50 times greater than for nonusers.[4]

According to a recent estimate by the Office of Technology Assessment, each smoker who died in 1990 as a result of his or her smoking, on average, would have lived at least 15 additional years if a nonsmoker. (This assumes that individuals who die from smoking-related causes would have experienced the life expectancy of the total population—that is, smokers and nonsmokers combined—had they not died prematurely.) For the population at large, this premature mortality translates into 6 million years of potential life lost each year.[5]

It is difficult, of course, to calculate a dollar value for the human costs of

---

*The term "smokeless tobacco" is used in this report to comprise all forms of nasal snuff, oral snuff, and chewing (spitting) tobacco.

3

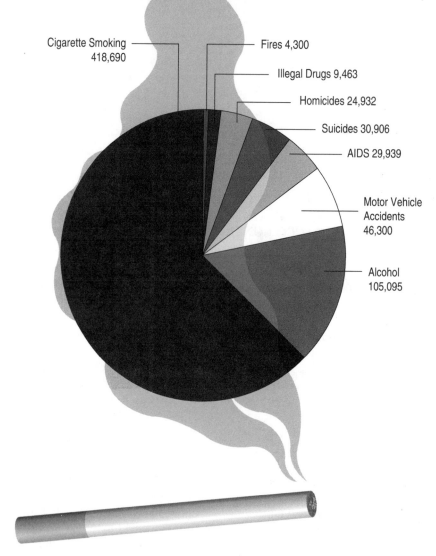

Cigarettes kill more Americans than AIDS, alcohol, car accidents, murders, suicides, drugs, and fires combined.

Cigarette Smoking 418,690
Fires 4,300
Illegal Drugs 9,463
Homicides 24,932
Suicides 30,906
AIDS 29,939
Motor Vehicle Accidents 46,300
Alcohol 105,095

FIGURE 1-1 Number of deaths per year, 1990. Source: Office on Smoking and Health. Centers for Disease Control and Prevention.

tobacco-related diseases. The suffering of patients and families resulting from tobacco-related morbidity and mortality is unquantifiable. Lost productivity and health care expenditures can be quantified, but the magnitude of the estimates depends on a variety of theoretical and technical questions, including whether the costs of health care should be offset by the "savings" in social security expenditures and health care costs not incurred because people died prematurely.[6] The Office of Technology Assessment put the social cost of smoking in 1990 at $68 billion. This high-end estimate includes $20.8 billion in direct health costs, $6.9 billion in lost productivity attributable to smoking-related disability, and $40.3 billion in lost productivity attributable to smoking-related premature deaths.[7] Whatever its total magnitude, the social cost of smoking is substantial. Even based on conservative assumptions, expected lifetime medical expenditures of the average smoker exceed those of the average nonsmoker by 28% for men and 21% for women. Each year, decisions by more than 1 million youths to become regular smokers commit the health care system to $8.2 billion in extra medical expenditures over their lifetimes.[8] (These figures, which are in 1990 dollars discounted at 3%, reflect the average experience in the population of persons who become smokers and take into account variations in the number of years of smoking.)

The nation has a compelling interest in reducing the social burden of tobacco use. This can be accomplished by preventing people from starting to use tobacco and by getting users to quit. The premise of this report is that, in the long run, tobacco use can be most efficiently reduced through a youth-centered policy aimed at preventing children and adolescents from initiating tobacco use. Moreover, because the prevalence of tobacco use among youths has remained stubbornly constant for 10 years, and may even be rising, a youth-centered prevention policy must be aggressively implemented if tobacco-related morbidity and mortality are to be significantly reduced.

Tobacco Use: Addictive and Mostly Initiated During Childhood and Adolescence

In 1988, the surgeon general issued a major report demonstrating that cigarettes and other forms of tobacco are addicting, that most tobacco users use tobacco regularly because they are addicted to nicotine, and that most tobacco users find it difficult to quit because they are addicted to nicotine. Tobacco use is not a choice like jogging or a habit like eating chocolate; it is an addiction that is fueled by nicotine.

Most smokers begin smoking during childhood and adolescence, and nicotine addiction begins during the first few years of tobacco use. Moreover, decades of experience in tracking tobacco use show that if people do not begin to use tobacco as youngsters, they are highly unlikely to initiate use as adults. For any cross section of adults who smoke daily, 89% began using cigarettes and

Tobacco use begins early.
Adults who are daily smokers
began smoking:

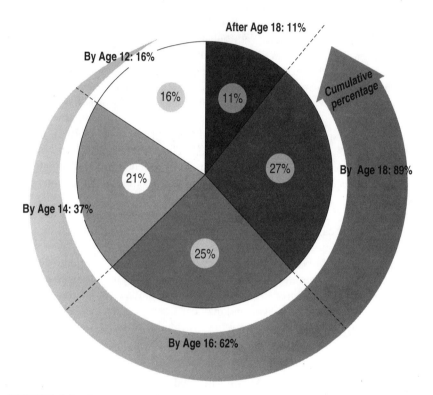

FIGURE 1-2   Source: Data from the National Household Surveys on Drug Abuse, United States, 1991.   Office on Smoking and Health. Centers for Disease Control and Prevention.

71% began smoking daily by or at age 18 (figure 1-2).[9] In short, decisions by youths about whether to use tobacco have lifelong consequences. On the one hand, if a person reaches the age of 18 without being a user of tobacco products, he or she is highly unlikely to become a tobacco user during adulthood. On the other hand, most children and youths who initiate regular tobacco use become addicted and their addiction persists for many years thereafter, perhaps throughout their lives. This is why a youth-centered prevention policy is an essential part of any coherent strategy for countering tobacco-related disease and death.

Tobacco Use by Children and Youths: No Longer Declining

Since 1964, when the surgeon general called the nation's attention to the health hazards of cigarettes, the prevalence of smoking has declined substantially—from 40.4% of the adult population in 1965 to 25.7% in 1991. This trend accelerated between 1987 and 1990, when the rate of smoking among adults dropped by 1.1% per year, more than double the rate of decrease in the preceding 20 years. Among adults, the number of former smokers (43 million) is now nearly that of current smokers (46 million). In fact, among men alive today, more are former smokers than current smokers.[10]

Despite these impressive successes, the nation's progress toward eliminating tobacco-related disease is in jeopardy. The estimated prevalence of smoking among adults appears to have leveled off in 1990 at around 26% (figure 1-3).

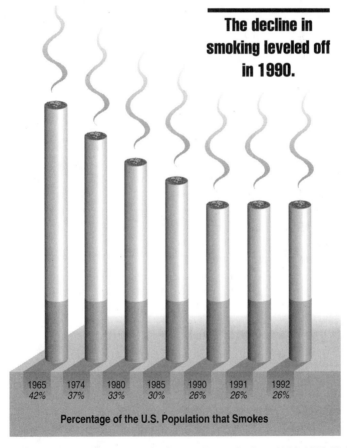

The decline in smoking leveled off in 1990.

| 1965 | 1974 | 1980 | 1985 | 1990 | 1991 | 1992 |
| 42% | 37% | 33% | 30% | 26% | 26% | 26% |

Percentage of the U.S. Population that Smokes

FIGURE 1-3   Source: Data from Monitoring the Future Project, 1976–1993, University of Michigan, 1994.

The use of smokeless tobacco, especially snuff, continues to increase, having tripled between 1972 and 1991. The estimated prevalence of use of smokeless tobacco by adults was 2.9% in 1991—5.6% among men and 0.6% among women. Among 18- to 24-year-old men, the rate was 8.2%.[11] Unless these current trends are reversed, the nation will fall far short of two key Year 2000 Health Objectives—a 15% prevalence of regular smoking among adults and a reduction of smokeless tobacco use by males ages 12-24 to a prevalence of no more than 4%.[12]

Why has the momentum toward reducing tobacco use been stalled? The answer lies in the replenishment of the tobacco-using population with new recruits. Despite the marked decline in adult smoking prevalence and the intensifying social disapproval of smoking, it has been estimated that 3,000 young people become *regular* smokers every day.[13] According to 1993 data from the University of Michigan's Monitoring the Future Study, 29.9% of the nation's high school seniors were current smokers (that is, they smoked within the past 30 days) and 19% smoked daily. Among eighth grade students in 1993, 16.7% were current smokers and 8.3% smoked daily.[14] Estimates of the number of cigarettes consumed annually by about 3 million children and youths in the United States has been estimated conservatively at 516 million packs.[15] According to the Monitoring the Future Study, in 1993, 10.7% of high school seniors were using smokeless tobacco and 3.3% were doing so daily.[16] It has been estimated that children and youths consume 26 million containers of smokeless tobacco annually.[17]

The prevalence of smoking by youths has remained basically unchanged since 1980. Among high school seniors, the prevalence of regular smokers (i.e., those who have smoked in the past 30 days) was 30.5% in 1980 and 29.9% in 1993; the prevalence of daily smokers was 21.3% in 1980 and 19.0% in 1993 (figures 1-4 and 1-5). Small increases and decreases occurred in the rates over the years, but a statistically significant increase of 1.8% in daily smoking from 1992-1993 has concerned public health officials.[18] Although little use of smokeless tobacco was seen among adolescents before 1970, the prevalence of its use among older teens (16-19 years old) increased nearly 10-fold between 1970 and 1985,[19] and overall appears to have remained constant since then.[20] As these trends clearly show, the forces that have been reducing tobacco use by adults—especially getting adults to quit—have not been as effective in reducing the onset of tobacco use among children and youths.

Beneath these aggregate prevalence figures lies an intriguing reminder of the ethnic diversity of American society. Since 1980, while daily smoking prevalence has remained stubbornly high among non-Hispanic white youths who are high school seniors (22% in 1980, 20% in 1992, and 23% in 1993), there has been a dramatic decline in daily smoking among African-American youths (16% in 1980, to 3.7% in 1992, and 4.4% in 1993).[21] Public health officials are uncertain about the reasons for these divergent trends among ethnic subgroups of American youths, and the research needed to clarify those reasons has not yet

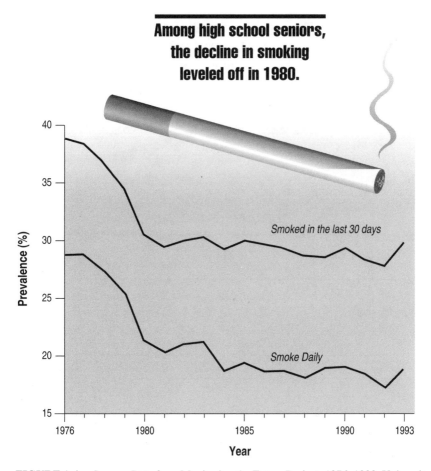

Among high school seniors, the decline in smoking leveled off in 1980.

FIGURE 1-4   Source: Data from Monitoring the Future Project, 1976–1993, University of Michigan. Courtesy of Office on Smoking and Health, Centers for Disease Control and Prevention.

been done. However, the Committee is hopeful that a tobacco-free norm may have taken root among African-American youths. The key questions are whether this trend will be sustained in the African-American population and whether well-crafted public policies can extend it to the U.S. population as a whole. In any case, the decline in smoking among African-American youths is a bright spot in an otherwise dim picture.

The Emerging Public Health Consensus

There seems to be general agreement among public health officials that

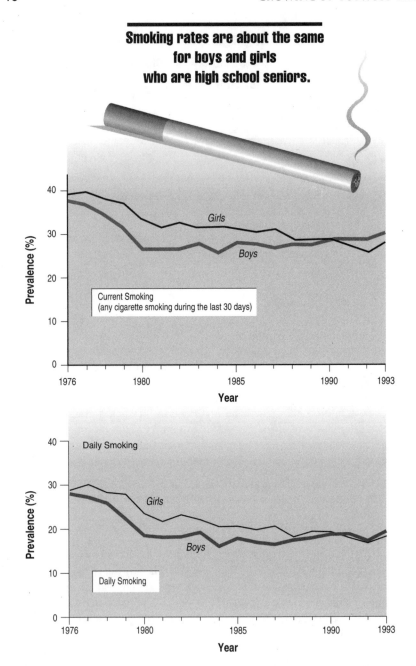

FIGURE 1-5   Source: Data from Monitoring the Future Project, 1976–1993, University of Michigan. Courtesy of Office on Smoking and Health, Centers for Disease Control and Prevention.

aggressive measures will be needed to make a substantial and enduring reduction in the prevalence of tobacco use by America's children and youths. Indeed, public health officials are worried that the incidence of youthful consumption will rise unless decisive steps are taken to prevent it. These concerns are rooted in the economics of the tobacco market. Because of the overall decline in adult consumption, and a significant increase in tobacco taxes over the last few years, the tobacco companies have been competing for shares of a shrinking market. Declining demand has led to the introduction of generic brands, discount pricing, and other forms of price competition. It has also led to a remarkable increase in expenditures for advertising and promotion. Collectively, the tobacco industry spent more than $4.6 billion in 1991 to advertise and promote tobacco products, a 13% increase over 1990 expenditures.[22] The population of the United States is exposed to this massive array of pro-tobacco messages every day. Inevitably, these messages "promote" tobacco use to children and youths as well as adults, and to impressionable nonusers of tobacco products as well as users.

The surgeon general has observed that "clearly, young people are being indoctrinated with tobacco promotion at a susceptible time in their lives."[23] Many public health officials and observers are convinced that the tobacco industry has purposely targeted its promotional activities on youth. The Committee is not in a position to assess the intentions of tobacco advertisers and producers, but the ubiquitous display of messages promoting tobacco use clearly fosters an environment in which experimentation by youths is expected, if not implicitly encouraged. This social environment is inimical to the health and well-being of the nation's children and, ultimately, to the health of American society. It should be changed. The justification for such a change does not depend on proving that makers and sellers of tobacco products intend to induce nicotine addiction among the nation's young people; it is enough that their promotional activities make tobacco use seem attractive and have a natural tendency to trigger a chain of events that has disastrous public health consequences in the long run.

In sum, two trends have raised widespread concern among public health officials regarding the present status of tobacco control efforts. First, the prevalence of smoking and smokeless tobacco use by youths has remained stubbornly high while the prevalence of tobacco use by adults has declined. Second, aggressive marketing by the tobacco companies has increased the volume of pro-tobacco messages at the same time that public health advances seem to have slowed, or even come to a halt. These combined concerns have led to a consensus among public health experts that tobacco control efforts must focus more heavily on preventing children and youths from using tobacco products and becoming dependent on them. A vigorous effort to prevent initiation of tobacco use by children and youths must be the centerpiece of the nation's tobacco control policy and should be among its highest public health priorities.

Public Support for a Youth-Centered Tobacco Control Policy

A youth-centered tobacco control strategy has broad public support. In a national survey of adults, a majority (73%) favored an increase in the tax on cigarettes as a measure to help finance health care reform. Those who were opposed to the tax on cigarettes were asked how their support would change if the money were used for various other purposes. A majority of that group (73%) said that they would be more likely to support a tax if the money were used to *discourage smoking among young people*. Of the entire population surveyed, 62% believe that increasing the cigarette tax would discourage young people from starting to smoke, and 76% favor restrictions of cigarette advertising that appeals to children.[24] Another poll, of U.S. voters, found that the most popular restriction on the sales of tobacco products would be a ban on cigarette vending machines: 73% (including 66% of all smokers) said they favor banning cigarette machines "in order to make it more difficult for kids to obtain cigarettes."[25] Two-thirds of voters favor banning smoking in all public places, such as restaurants, stores, and government buildings—policies that would promote a tobacco-free social norm for youths. About two-thirds of the voters surveyed agree with the assertion that tobacco companies "do everything they can to get teenagers and young people to take up smoking."[26] In a third poll of smokers, 70% were concerned that their children would eventually start smoking because they see them smoking, 93% agreed that more should be done to educate kids about the dangers of cigarettes, and only 17% believed that tobacco manufacturers should be allowed to advertise their products to high school students or to children (7%).[27]

Growing public support for youth-centered tobacco control measures is also reflected in the activity of local advocacy coalitions and in grassroots political action. Hundreds of localities have enacted local ordinances banning vending machines, establishing smoke-free environments in public places, and otherwise promoting a tobacco-free norm.[28] Unfortunately, strong grassroots support for tobacco control policies at the local level has too often been neutralized through powerful lobbying by the tobacco industry at the state level, resulting in weak state legislation that preempts more restrictive local measures. Legislative initiatives at local and state levels relating to advertising and promotion have also been stymied by a preemptive provision of federal law that precludes "any requirement or prohibition based on smoking and health." As discussed below, this preemption must be repealed in order to enable state and local governments to implement youth-centered tobacco control initiatives and thereby carry out the public will.

Ethical Foundation of a Youth-Centered Tobacco Control Policy

A youth-centered tobacco control policy has a firm ethical foundation. American society ordinarily values and respects the prerogative of adults to decide how to live their own lives as long as they do not endanger anyone else. If adequately informed, adults are assumed to be capable of making rational and voluntary choices that involve weighing the risks and benefits of a particular behavior in light of their own preferences and values. The applicability of the informed choice model to tobacco use has been a subject of ongoing controversy in the literature of applied moral philosophy.[29] Although some writers[30] have accepted the possibility of a rational and voluntary choice to use tobacco by adequately informed (and unaddicted) adults, others have pointed out that the onset of addiction compromises the voluntariness of subsequent choices, even by adults.[31] As a practical matter, however, arguments about the rationality of choices by adults to initiate tobacco use are beside the point because at least 70% of adult daily smokers already became daily smokers, and presumably were addicted, by the time they were 18 years old. Thus, the critical issue is whether children and adolescents are in a position to make informed and rational choices about whether to become tobacco users.

No one argues that preteens have the necessary abilities to make rational choices about tobacco use. Yet, as shown in chapter 2, a significant proportion of adult smokers begin using tobacco before becoming teenagers. Data from the 1990 Youth Risk Behavior Survey indicate that 56% of youths have tried smoking and 9% have become regular smokers *by age 13*.[32]

Some researchers have suggested that adequately informed adolescents (over age 13) exhibit cognitive decision-making skills similar to those used by young adults (through age 25).[33] Others have claimed that adolescents are well informed about the health risks of tobacco use.[34] Even if these controversial assertions were accepted, they do not show that adolescents are in a position to make sound choices about tobacco use. One must also take into account other faulty beliefs held by adolescents regarding the consequences of tobacco use as well as adolescent tendencies to evaluate and weigh risks and benefits within a shortened time frame.

Adolescent decisions to engage in risky behaviors, including tobacco use, reflect a distinctive focus on short-term benefits and an accompanying tendency to discount long-term risks or dangers, and to believe that those risks can be controlled by personal choice. Decision-making deficiencies exhibited by children and youths who choose to use tobacco are most evident when their perceptions and reasoning are compared with the perceptions and reasoning of their peers who choose *not* to use tobacco.

Clearly, youths who choose to use tobacco perceive greater benefits relative to risks than youths who choose not to do so.[35] What is most striking, however, is the nature of the trade-off. When children and youths begin to use tobacco, they tend to do so for reasons that are transient in nature and closely linked to specific developmental tasks—for example, to assert independence and achieve perceived adult status, or to identify with and establish social bonds with peers who use tobacco (see chapters 2 and 3). Youths who smoke or intend to smoke tend to be heavily influenced by their perception of potential *social* benefits and risks of doing so. Compared with nonsmokers and youths who do not intend to smoke, smokers and likely smokers tend to exaggerate the social benefit (by overestimating its prevalence and popularity among peers and adults) and to underestimate the social risks (by underestimating the prevalence of negative attitudes toward smoking held by their peers).[36]

The evidence also shows a tendency among adolescents who have begun to smoke to discount long-term health risks. The issue is not one of general knowledge. Smokers seem to be aware of the link between tobacco use and various diseases, but data consistently show that young smokers, compared with nonsmokers, systematically give less weight to the long-term risks. For example, in 1989, only half of high school seniors who smoked (compared with three-fourths of nonsmokers) reported believing that smoking a pack or more per day is a serious health risk.[37]

Adolescent decision-making is plagued especially by the difficulty of envisioning long-term consequences and appreciating the personal relevance of these consequences. Abundant evidence demonstrates that youths who begin to use tobacco do not understand the nature of addiction and, as a result, believe they will be able to avoid the harmful consequences of tobacco use. They understand that a lifetime of smoking is dangerous, but they also tend to believe that smoking for a few years will *not* be harmful, a belief that is less common among nonsmokers.[38] Among 12- through 18-year-olds in the 1989 Teenage Attitudes and Practices Survey, 21% of smokers (compared with 3% of those who never smoked) said they believed that it is safe to smoke for only a year or two.[39] The key is that many youths who smoke do not expect to smoke over a lifetime and, in fact, expect to smoke only for a few years. They believe, in short, that they can escape the harmful consequences of an admittedly risky practice. What these youths do not appreciate, of course, is the grip of nicotine addiction.

Adolescents' failure to appreciate the long-term consequences of decisions to smoke is explicitly revealed by a longitudinal track of the University of Michigan's Monitoring the Future Study. As high school seniors, the subjects were asked "Do you think you will be smoking cigarettes 5 years from now?" Among respondents who were occasional smokers (less than one cigarette per day), 85% predicted that they probably or definitely would *not* be smoking in 5 years, as did 32% of those who smoked one pack per day. However, at follow-up 5-6 years later, of those who had smoked one pack per day as seniors, only 13% had quit and 70% still smoked one pack or more per day. Of those who smoked occasionally as seniors, only 58% had quit, but 37% had actually increased their cigarette consumption.[40]

If a youth decides to begin smoking at the age of 12 or 13, the deficit in his or her ability to appreciate the long-term risks of doing so is even more pronounced, and more disturbing, than it is at 16 or 17.[41] Indeed, it is clear that the grip of nicotine addiction is most powerful and most enduring for youths who begin smoking at the youngest ages. Unfortunately, the age of onset of tobacco use has decreased significantly over the past 20 years, especially for girls.[42]

Youths regret their choices to start smoking and report difficulty quitting *even during adolescence.* The 1989 Teenage Attitudes and Practices Survey data show that 74% of 12- through 18-year-old smokers reported that they had seriously thought about quitting, 64% had tried to quit, and 49% had tried to quit in the previous 6 months.[43] Among high school seniors (1985-1989), of those who had smoked at all in the past 30 days, 43% reported a desire to stop smoking. Of this group, and of the subgroup who smoked daily, 28% and 39%, respectively, stated that they had tried unsuccessfully to stop.[44] In the 1991 Youth Risk and Behavior Survey of over 12,000 adolescents in grades 9-12, a majority of self-reported smokers (54% of boys and 62% of girls) reported that they had tried to quit smoking in the previous 6 months.[45]

In sum, when children and adolescents begin to use tobacco, they are putting their health at risk without adequately appreciating the long-term consequences of their actions. The problem lies in the failure to appreciate the personal relevance of the long-term statistical risks of multiple diseases and a profound inability to understand the powerful grip of nicotine addiction. These deficiencies of risk perception (and the tendency also to exaggerate the perceived social benefits of using tobacco) justify concerted social action to prevent children and youths from starting to use tobacco.

THE ELEMENTS OF A YOUTH-CENTERED TOBACCO CONTROL POLICY

The U.S. Public Health Service has articulated its public health goals in *Healthy People 2000,* the result of a systematic planning process. Given that nearly one in five deaths in the United States is attributable to tobacco use,[46] reducing smoking would arguably have more impact on the nation's health than any other public health initiative. Since a lifetime of smoking generally commences with nicotine addiction in youth, one of the most important among the Healthy People 2000 objectives is number 3.5: "Reduce the initiation of cigarette smoking by children and youth so that no more than 15 percent have become regular cigarette smokers by age 20."[47] The baseline was 30% in 1987, so the goal was to reduce smoking initiation by half among children and youths. While the use of smokeless tobacco is not nearly as prevalent, the underlying addictive process is similar; therefore, the Committee believes that a natural corollary goal is to reduce youth initiation of smokeless tobacco use by half also. Prospects of achieving these goals, however, are extremely remote unless the nation commits itself to a major new initiative.

The traditional focus of primary prevention in tobacco policy has been school-based instruction. As discussed in chapter 5, these programs serve an important role, especially if they are part of broader community-wide initiatives.

However, model tobacco prevention programs have not been widely disseminated or adopted and, as a result, most school-based instruction appears to have only a modest impact. It is generally agreed by experts in the field that these programs cannot be expected to have an impact commensurate with the scope of the problem. More aggressive measures will be needed to counteract the social forces that continue to induce a quarter of the nation's young people to use tobacco products.

A successful strategy of preventing nicotine dependence in children and youths must encompass measures for reducing the accessibility of tobacco products to young people, and for increasing their cost; for strengthening the social factors tending to discourage consumption; and for erasing or mitigating social factors tending to encourage consumption. These devices typically require legislative or regulatory action. The body of this report summarizes what is known about the potential utility of various preventive measures and offers recommendations for action grounded in existing knowledge.

During the course of its study, the Committee reviewed a wide range of activities—federal efforts, state government programs, the actions of advocacy and health professional organizations, and policies of several foreign nations where tobacco control has been successfully pursued. Subsequent chapters deal with research and policy questions surrounding the addictive process, setting social norms, preventive and cessation interventions, advertising and promotion, pricing and taxation, diminishing youth access, and regulating tobacco products. Table 1-1 on pages 18-20 synthesizes the Committee's conclusions and recommendations.

During its deliberations, the committee assessed a variety of possible recommendations in terms of extent of potential impact, practicality of implementation, and likelihood of adoption. Model programs in Canada, Australia, New Zealand, California, and Massachusetts have implemented multiple program and policy components at the same time, rendering analysis of the impact of specific measures methodologically difficult. However, the composite effects have been substantial and there is strong reason to believe that a multi-pronged attack is far more likely to produce results than any single measure taken alone. Based on a review of results to date, the Committee concludes that several measures should be the subject of immediate attention at the state, federal, and local levels of government, and in the private sector. In addition, several other major initiatives will be required to sustain long-term progress.

Actions That Should Be Taken Immediately

Among the recommendations made throughout the report, several deserve emphasis as the most promising to achieve a pronounced impact on tobacco use by children and youths. The Committee believes that three recommendations should have top priority for immediate action:

> *Congress should enact a substantial increase in the federal excise tax on tobacco products to increase their price and to raise revenues for tobacco control, health care, and other uses.*

Data indicate that children and youths are more price-sensitive than adults, and that pricing has a strong and immediate impact on reducing sales of tobacco products overall. Increasing the price puts a higher barrier between youths and easy access (affordability) to the products, and therefore between youths and sustained tobacco use. This barrier will delay the initiation and reduce the number of new tobacco users. The Committee recommends that the federal excise tax be raised to a level comparable with that in other major industrialized countries. A reasonable target would be to increase the tax by $2.00 per pack of cigarettes, with proportional increases for smokeless tobacco products. This recommendation is discussed in chapter 6.

> *Congress should repeal the federal law that precludes state and local governments from regulating tobacco promotion and advertising occurring entirely within the state's borders.*

Many states and local governments have signaled a willingness to experiment with stronger measures to control the messages projected about tobacco use, particularly those to which children and youths are exposed. California, Massachusetts, and Maryland, for example, have strong anti-tobacco media programs in place. Yet, currently, state and local governments are impeded by federal law from regulating promotion and advertising of tobacco products in various visual media, including billboards, and at the point of sale. Federal preemption of this nature limits the ability of local communities to enact the public will and to restrict the pro-tobacco messages to which youths are regularly exposed. As a result, the effectiveness of public education and public health efforts in reducing tobacco use is also limited. This recommendation is discussed in chapter 4.

> *Congress should increase the capacity of state and local governments and coalitions of interested organizations to pursue youth-centered tobacco control policies.*

In recent years, major initiatives on tobacco control have taken place in states and in local communities. California, Massachusetts, and Michigan, for example, have implemented targeted programs that provide promising models for other states. Many local governments have established innovative programs to enforce youth access laws that have become models for other states and localities. The National Cancer Institute (NCI) has cultivated state initiatives in the 17 states participating in its pioneering American Stop Smoking Intervention Study

TABLE 1-1 Synthesis of key findings and recommendations

Chapter	Key findings	Selected policy recommendations	Research needs
2. The Nature of Nicotine Addiction	• Nicotine addiction is the cause of long-term tobacco use. • Once a person is addicted, cessation of tobacco use can be difficult. • Most smokers begin smoking during childhood or adolescence, and nicotine addiction becomes established in youthful smokers.	• See chapter 8.	• Determine factors that influence individual susceptibility to nicotine addiction. • Examine factors that predict nicotine addiction in its early stages. • Examine the relationship between characteristics of tobacco products and addiction.
3. Social Norms and the Acceptability of Tobacco Use	• A variety of social factors influence youths to experiment with tobacco. • Youths tend to overestimate the prevalence of tobacco use by adults and peers. • Communicating a tobacco-free norm is critical to discouraging youths from using tobacco.	• Parents should clearly and unequivocally express disapproval of tobacco use by their children. • Paid anti-tobacco advertising campaigns should be conducted to reverse the image appeal of pro-tobacco messages. • Tobacco-free policies should be adopted in all public locations.	• Elucidate the reasons for racial/ethnic group differences in tobacco use by teens. • Include youths in designing and evaluating health message campaigns.
4. Tobacco Advertising and Promotion	• The weight of evidence indicates that tobacco advertising and promotions encourage children and youths to use tobacco. • Some types of advertising and promotions especially appeal to children and youths. • Bans or restrictions on advertising and promotion appear to reduce tobacco consumption.	• Congress should repeal the law preempting states and localities from regulating cigarette advertising and promotion entirely within the states' borders. • States should ban tobacco ads or restrict them to a tombstone format. • Congress should adopt comprehensive restrictions on the advertising and promotion of tobacco products.	• Assess youths' responses by children and youths to tobacco advertising and promotional messages. • Determine differences in the responses to tobacco image advertising of various ethnic, gender, and social classes.

5. Prevention and Cessation of Tobacco Use: Research-Based Programs	• Refusal skills training and a comprehensive tobacco-free policy are essential elements of school-based tobacco prevention programs. • Most schools currently do not devote sufficient time or resources to teaching children about tobacco and its dangers. • School-based programs without a community-wide tobacco control effort will not have much impact on discouraging youth tobacco use.	• All schools should adopt the CDC guidelines to prevent tobacco use and addiction. • The federal government should develop a national child health policy that gives high priority to prevention of tobacco use. • Tobacco prevention should be integrated into existing drug prevention programs aimed at youths (e.g., DARE).	• Determine what schools currently are teaching about tobacco and what factors impede the adoption of the CDC guidelines. • Develop programs to help youths who are regular tobacco users to quit.
6. Tobacco Taxation in the United States	• Tobacco consumption is related to price. • Youths are more sensitive to price changes than are adults. • The United States has one of the lowest taxes on cigarettes of any industrialized country. • Higher taxes will reduce smoking.	• Congress should increase the federal tax on cigarettes by $2 per pack. • States should also consider increasing tobacco taxes as a way to reduce tobacco use. • Tobacco taxes should be increased periodically to account for inflation. • A portion of the excise tax revenue should be set aside for tobacco control programs.	• Assess the impact of tobacco price changes on consumption by youths. • Assess the effect of tax hikes on the use of alternative goods and smuggling.
7. Youth Access to Tobacco Products	• Nearly all youths report that it is easy to get tobacco products. • Among adolescent tobacco users, most buy their own tobacco despite laws prohibiting sales to minors. • Regular enforcement of youth access laws reduces illegal sales to minors and promotes a tobacco-free norm.	• States should eliminate tobacco vending machines. • States should license retailers, using fees to pay for enforcement. • Avenues of easy access to tobacco products should be eliminated, e.g., self-service displays, mail order, and free samples.	• Evaluate the effect of programs to enforce access laws on minors' use of tobacco. • Assess and compare the cost of different policies (e.g., local vs. state). • Determine the effects that access restrictions would have on tobacco use. • Monitor methods of youth access as the market changes.

continued on next page

TABLE 1-1 *Continued*

Chapter	Key Findings	Selected Policy Recommendations	Research Needs
8. Regulation of the Labeling, Packaging, and Contents of Tobacco Products	• Current warnings on tobacco products are inadequate. • Tobacco products are currently unregulated despite their harmfulness.	• Congress should enact legislation that delegates to an appropriate agency the necessary authority to regulate the labeling, packaging, and content of tobacco products. • Congress should strengthen the federally mandated warning labels for tobacco products. • Congress should authorize the agency to impose ceilings of tar and nicotine yields and to reduce those ceilings over time.	• Research is needed to help guide regulation of tobacco products. • Develop sound methodology for ascertaining actual yields of tar and nicotine based on human consumption.
9. Coordination of Policies and Research	• Too much focus is on programs with little impact, rather than on policies to influence large populations. • Tobacco control efforts tend to be independent and duplicated, rather than coordinated strategically. • Major policy initiatives have been made at the state and local levels.	• The federal government should provide unequivocal leadership in the effort to prevent nicotine addiction and tobacco-related disease and death. • OSH should be given the responsibility for coordinating federal tobacco control initiatives. • Funding to the non-Assist states should be increased to a level commensurate with ASSIST states. • Federal agencies should fund policy research. • The base of groups concerned with tobacco control should be broadened.	• Fund research to determine the efficacy of policy interventions for preventing youths from initiating tobacco use. • Assess the cultural and regional differences and factors influencing norms of tobacco use. • Elucidate the factors important in the initiation and prevention of tobacco use by children and youths.

(ASSIST). The Centers for Disease Control and Prevention has initiated programs in the non-ASSIST states, although funding for individual states under this program (IMPACT) is very low. In addition, the Robert Wood Johnson Foundation is collaborating with the American Medical Association to mount the SmokeLess States program. The Committee urges the federal government to broaden these initiatives with technical assistance, grants, and cooperative agreements to enable all interested states, local governments, and community coalitions to undertake youth-centered tobacco control policies.

Actions Required To Sustain Progress in the Long Term

The recommendations for immediate action will have a stronger impact if they are viewed as first steps in a long-term strategy for preventing nicotine dependence in children and youths and thereby reducing the adverse health consequences of tobacco use. Such a long-term strategy should include the key components that follow.

Congress should establish a regulatory program for tobacco products with a long-term public health objective of dramatically reducing the prevalence of nicotine addiction.

Tobacco products have been consistently exempted from coverage under consumer safety, food, and drug legislation, and as a result have been largely unregulated. This lack of regulation stands in stark contrast to other products that have far less disastrous long-term health implications than the use of tobacco products. The Committee recommends that Congress enact legislation that delegates to an appropriate agency in the Public Health Service the necessary authority to regulate tobacco products for the dual purposes of discouraging consumption and reducing the morbidity and mortality associated with their use. Such authority should encompass the packaging and constituents of all tobacco products, including the possibility of prescribing ceilings on yields of tar and nicotine. The regulation of tobacco products is discussed in chapter 8.

Congress and state legislatures should eliminate all features of advertising and promotion of tobacco products that tend to encourage initiation of tobacco use among children and youths.

Children and youths believe that adults and even their peers smoke and use tobacco products far more than they actually do. Ubiquitous messages that associate tobacco use with images of youthfulness, athletic prowess, and sexuality reinforce a social norm that encourages tobacco use. Once initiated on a regular basis, tobacco use becomes further reinforced by the physiological and psychological processes of nicotine addiction. The pro-tobacco messages in advertising and promotion are particularly difficult to combat among children and youths. The Committee therefore concludes that advertising and promotion of tobacco products should be severely curtailed. A more detailed discussion of this issue, and a series of relevant recommendations, can be found in chapter 4.

> *Governments and voluntary organizations at all levels should sustain and reinforce the continued evolution of a tobacco-free norm in American society.*

Within a relatively short period of time, tobacco use has declined in prevalence and has become widely disapproved. Only a few decades ago, smoking was the social norm; now it is approaching a status of social deviance. The continued evolution of a tobacco-free norm is a potentially powerful component of a long-term strategy for reducing the prevalence of tobacco use among children and youths. This tobacco-free norm also protects children's health by reducing their exposure to environmental tobacco smoke. It is therefore important for governments and private organizations to promote and reinforce the evolving tobacco-free norm by implementing smoke-free policies in schools, workplaces, fast-food restaurants, and all other places where children and youths spend their time. A detailed discussion of the many opportunities for promoting a tobacco-free norm appear in chapter 3.

> *Agencies and foundations that sponsor tobacco-related research should implement a youth-centered research agenda including studies of the efficacy of policy interventions. These efforts must recognize cultural differences among members of the major ethnic groups and attempt to develop culturally appropriate strategies.*

The above recommendations, and many others in this report, focus on setting social parameters to reduce the likelihood that children and youths will begin to use tobacco or that they will "graduate" into a lifetime of addiction. These recommendations are based on the knowledge at hand. Research to improve prevention and cessation interventions can help improve those efforts over time. Understanding the reasons for the remarkable decline in smoking prevalence among African-American youths is a major research priority. A better understanding of the molecular and cellular correlates of nicotine addiction, and the factors that mediate the adverse health effects of tobacco use can also provide helpful clues to guide future efforts. Moreover, improving smoking cessation treatments to help the 49 million Americans who smoke will benefit the smokers and foster knowledge about nicotine addiction as well. Finally, some of the data most useful to the Committee came from studies of tobacco control policy, such as epidemiologic studies and risk-factor analyses that monitor the effects of policy change. For example, decisions about which policies are most likely to succeed were aided by assessments of the large-scale programs undertaken in Canada and California, measurements of the effects in local jurisdictions where youth access laws have been rigorously enforced, and studies describing the political influences that shape tobacco policy. The State of California and the Robert Wood Johnson Foundation have been leaders in promoting such policy research, joined recently by the National Cancer Institute. Recommendations and a discussion about research on the addictive process are presented in chapter 2, on prevention and cessation interventions in chapter 5, and on policy intervention throughout the report.

During the course of its deliberations, the Committee was mindful that many youth-centered policy recommendations will also tend to reduce tobacco use by adults. However, the Committee does not think that justified youth-centered interventions should be weakened simply because they will make tobacco use more costly or inconvenient for adults. After all, the ultimate goal of a youth-centered prevention strategy is to reduce the health toll associated with tobacco use. Indeed, the Committee came to understand that the relationship between a youth-centered prevention strategy and a broader tobacco control policy is a reciprocal one. On the one hand, reducing the onset of tobacco use by youths is an essential element of a successful strategy of long-term tobacco control. On the other hand, successful tobacco control initiatives in the society as a whole—such as the widespread adoption of tobacco-free policies establishing a normative climate unfavorable to smoking—play an important role in preventing nicotine addiction among youths. In both respects, a successful youth-centered prevention policy is the most expeditious way to reduce tobacco-related disease.

REFERENCES

1. Centers for Disease Control and Prevention. "Cigarette Smoking—Attributable Mortality and Years of Potential Life Lost—United States, 1990." *Morbidity and Mortality Weekly Report* 42:33 (27 Aug. 1993): 645-649.

2. Centers for Disease Control. *Reducing the Health Consequences of Smoking: 25 Years of Progress. A Report of the Surgeon General.* DHHS Pub. No. (CDC) 89-8411. Washington, DC: U.S. Department of Health and Human Services, 1989.

3. National Cancer Institute. *Smokeless Tobacco or Health. Monograph 2.* NIH Pub. No. 93-3461. Washington, DC: U.S. Department of Health and Human Services, Sept. 1992.

4. Winn, D. M., W. J. Blot, C. M. Shy, L. W. Pickle, et al. "Snuff Dipping and Oral Cancer Among Women in the Southern U.S." *New England Journal of Medicine* 304:13 (1981): 745-749.

5. Herdman, Roger, Maria Hewitt, and Mary Laschober. *Smoking-Related Deaths and Financial Costs: Office of Technology Assessment Estimates for 1990.* Testimony before the Senate Special Committee on Aging. Hearing on *Preventive Health: An Ounce of Prevention Saves a Pound of Cure.* 6 May 1993. 2-4.

6. Manning, Willard, Emmett B. Keeler, Joseph P. Newhouse, Elizabeth M. Sloss, and Jeffrey Wasserman. "The Taxes of Sin: Do Smokers and Drinkers Pay Their Way?" *Journal of the American Medical Association* 261:11 (17 Mar. 1989): 1604-1609. Compare with: Hodgson, Thomas A. "Cigarette Smoking and Lifetime Medical Expenditures." *The Milbank Quarterly* 70:1 (1992): 110-113.

7. *Herdman.*

8. Hodgson.

9. Centers for Disease Control and Prevention. *Preventing Tobacco Use Among Young People: A Report of the Surgeon General.* Washington, DC: U.S. Department of Health and Human Services, 1994. 65.

10. Centers for Disease Control and Prevention. "Cigarette Smoking Among Adults— United States, 1991." *Morbidity and Mortality Weekly Report* 42:12 (2 Apr. 1993): 230-233.

11. Centers for Disease Control and Prevention. "Use of Smokeless Tobacco Among Adults— United States, 1991." *Morbidity and Mortality Weekly Report* 42:14 (16 Apr. 1993): 263-266.

12. U.S. Department of Health and Human Services. Public Health Service. *Healthy People 2000. National Health Promotion and Disease Prevention Objectives.* USDHHS Pub. No. (PHS) 91-50212, 1990. 140, 147.

13. Pierce, John P., Michael C. Fiore, Thomas E. Novotny, Evridiki J. Hatziandreu, and Ronald M. Davis. "Trends in Cigarette Smoking in the United States." *Journal of the American Medical Association* 261:1 (6 Jan. 1989): 61-65.

14. Johnston, Lloyd, P. O'Malley, and J. Bachman. "Monitoring the Future Study." Press release. The University of Michigan, Ann Arbor. January 31, 1994.

15. Cummings, K. Michael, Terry Pechacek, and Donald Shopland. "The Illegal Sale of Cigarettes to U.S. Minors: Estimates by State." *American Journal of Public Health* 84:2 (1994): 300-302.

16. Johnston et al., 1994.

17. DiFranza, Joseph R., and Joe B. Tye. "Who Profits from Tobacco Sales to Children?" *Journal of the American Medical Association* 263:20 (1990): 2784-2787.

18. Johnston et al., 1994.

19. Marcus, Alfred C., Lori A. Crane, Donald R. Shopland, and William R. Lynn. "Use of Smokeless Tobacco in the United States: Recent Estimates from the Current Population Survey." In *Smokeless Tobacco Use in the United States: National Cancer Institute Monographs 8* (1989): 17-23.

20. Johnston et al., 1994.

21. Johnston, Lloyd D., Patrick M. O'Malley, and Jerald G. Bachman. Data supplied by the Office on Smoking and Health, Centers for Disease Control and Prevention, Atlanta.

22. Federal Trade Commission. *Report to Congress for 1991 Pursuant to the Federal Cigarette Labeling and Advertising Act.* Washington, DC: Federal Trade Commission, 1994: 5. The percentage has been adjusted for inflation.

23. M. Joycelyn Elders, "Preface," Centers for Disease Control and Prevention, *Preventing Tobacco Use,* iii.

24. Gallup Organization, Inc. *The Public's Attitudes Toward Cigarette Advertising and Cigarette Tax Increase.* Conducted for Coalition on Smoking or Health. Princeton, NJ: Gallup Organization, Inc., Apr. 1993. 3, 10, 17.

25. Marttila & Kiley, Inc. *Highlights From an American Cancer Society Survey of U.S. Voter Attitudes Toward Cigarette Smoking.* Boston: Marttila and Kiley, Inc., Sept. 1993. 26.

26. *Ibid.* 28.

27. SmithKline Beecham. *Gallup Report: A National Survey of Americans Who Smoke.* New York, 1993.

28. National Cancer Institute. *Major Local Tobacco Control Ordinances in the United States. Monograph 3.* NIH Pub. No. 93-3532. Washington DC: U.S. Department of Health and Human Services, May 1993.

29. Rabin, Robert, and Stephen D. Sugarman. *Smoking Policy: Law, Politics, and Culture.* New York: Oxford University Press, 1993; and Goodin, Robert E. *No Smoking: The Ethical Issues.* Chicago: University of Chicago Press, 1989.

30. Feinberg, Joel. *Harm to Self. Volume 3.* New York: Oxford University Press, 1986. 128-134; and Viscusi, W. Kip. *Smoking: Making the Risky Decision.* New York: Oxford University Press, 1992.

31. See for example: Schelling, Thomas C. "Addictive Drugs: The Cigarette Experience." *Science* 255 (Jan. 1992): 430-433; and Robert Goodin, *ibid.*

32. Escobedo, L. G. "Sports Participation, Age at Smoking Initiation, and the Risk of Smoking Among U.S. High School Students." *Journal of the American Medical Association* 269:11 (1993): 1391-95.

33. Office of Technology Assessment. "Consent and Confidentiality in Adolescent Health Care Decisionmaking." *Adolescent Health: Vol. 3. Crosscutting Issues in the Delivery of Health and Related Services.* Chapter 17. Pub. No. OTA-H-467. Washington, DC: U.S. Congress, 1991. III.141-III.150; and Quadrel, Marilyn J., Baruch Fischhoff, and Wendy Davis. "Adolescent (In)vulnerability." *American Psychologist* 48:2 (1993):102-116.

34. Viscusi.

35. Benthin, Alida, Paul Slovic, and Herbert Severson. "A Psychometric Study of Adolescent Risk Perception." *Journal of Adolescence* 16 (1993): 153-168; and Eiser, J. Richard. "Smoking, Seat-Belt Use and Perception of Health Risks." *Addictive Behaviors* 8:1 (1983): 75-78.

36. Levanthal, Howard, Kathleen Glynn, and Raymond Fleming. "Is the Smoking Decision an 'Informed Choice'? Effect of Smoking Risk Factors on Smoking Beliefs." *Journal of the American Medical Association* 257:24 (26 June 1987): 3373-3376.

37. Centers for Disease Control and Prevention. *Preventing Tobacco Use,* 80.

38. 32. Slovic, Paul. *What Does It Mean to Know a Risk? Adolescents' Perceptions of Short-Term and Long-Term Consequences of Smoking.* Report No. 94-4. Eugene, OR: Decision Research, June 1994.

39. Allen, Karen, A. Moss, G. A. Giovino, D. R. Shopland, and J. P. Pierce. "Teenage Tobacco Use Data. Estimates from the Teenage Attitudes and Practices Survey, United States, 1989." *Advance Data* No. 224 (1993): 9.

40. Centers for Disease Control and Prevention. *Preventing Tobacco Use,* 84.

41. Johnston et al., 1994.

42. Centers for Disease Control and Prevention. *Preventing Tobacco Use,* 76.

43. Allen et al., 9.

44. Centers for Disease Control and Prevention. *Preventing Tobacco Use,* 78.

45. Centers for Disease Control and Prevention. Division of Adolescent and School Health. Youth Risk Behavior Survey, unpublished data, 1994.

46. Centers for Disease Control, *MMWR* 42:33.

47. USDHHS, 143.

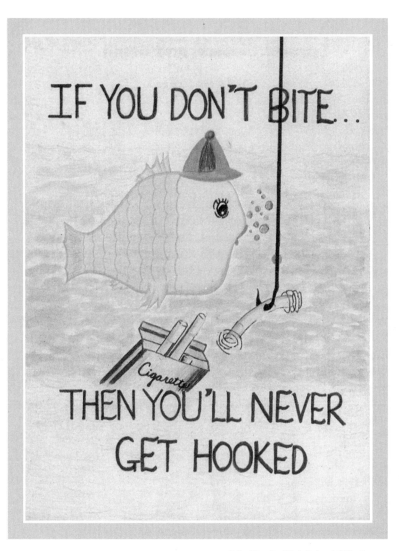

Lily Lin, Jr. High School 158, Queens

CONTENTS

2 | THE NATURE OF NICOTINE ADDICTION*

Cigarettes and other forms of tobacco are addicting. Most smokers use tobacco regularly because they are addicted to nicotine. Furthermore, most smokers find it difficult to quit using tobacco because they are addicted to nicotine. Nicotine addiction develops in the first few years of cigarette smoking, that is, for most people during adolescence or early adulthood. Most smokers begin smoking during childhood or adolescence: 89% of daily smokers tried their first cigarette by or at age 18, and 71% of persons who have ever smoked daily began smoking daily by age 18 (table 2-1). The earlier in life a child tries a cigarette the more likely he or she is to become a regular smoker (that is, to smoke monthly or more frequently) or a daily smoker. For example, 67% of children who initiate smoking in the sixth grade become regular adult smokers, and 46% of teenagers who initiate smoking in the eleventh grade become regular adult smokers.[1] Furthermore, the earlier a youth begins smoking, the more cigarettes he or she will smoke as an adult.[2] Prevention of tobacco addiction and the related health consequences, therefore, requires early intervention for children and adolescents. To understand why youths use tobacco and why prevention measures are necessary and preferable to cessation measures to deter tobacco use by youths, it is useful to understand nicotine dependency. This chapter reviews (1) the general aspects of nicotine dependency, derived from research primarily in adults, and (2) the evidence of nicotine dependency and the factors that promote initiation and progression of tobacco use by youths.

---

*The terms "drug addiction" and "drug dependency" are used interchangeably in this report, as was done in the 1988 report of the surgeon general on nicotine addiction, which considered the terms to be "scientifically equivalent."

29

TABLE 2-1 Cumulative percentages of recalled age at which persons aged 30-39 first tried a cigarette or began smoking daily

Age (years)	All persons (n = 6,388)	Persons who had ever tried a cigarette	Persons who had ever smoked daily	
	First tried a cigarette	First tried a cigarette	First tried a cigarette	Began smoking daily
<12	14.1	18.0	15.6	1.9
<14	29.7	38.0	36.7	8.0
<16	48.2	61.9	62.2	24.9
<18	63.7	81.6	81.9	53.0
≤18	68.8	88.2	89.0	71.2
<20	71.0	91.0	91.3	77.0

Source: National Household Surveys on Drug Abuse, United States, 1991. Cited in Centers for Disease Control and Prevention. *Preventing Tobacco Use Among Young People. A Report of the Surgeon General.* Washington, DC: U.S. Government Printing Office, 1994. 65.

GENERAL ASPECTS OF NICOTINE ADDICTION

The Daily Nicotine Addiction Cycle

Given the pharmacologic properties of nicotine, a daily cycle of addiction can be described as follows. The first cigarette of the day produces substantial pharmacologic effects (pleasure, arousal, enhanced performance), but simultaneously the brain's chemistry changes and tolerance begins to develop. With subsequent cigarettes, nicotine accumulates in the body and is associated with the development of a greater level of tolerance. Withdrawal symptoms become more pronounced between successive cigarettes. The tolerance that develops over the day may be partially overcome by the transiently high brain levels of nicotine that occur immediately after the smoking of individual cigarettes, but the primary pleasurable effects of individual cigarettes tend to lessen throughout the day. As the day progresses, people tend to smoke more to relieve the symptoms of abstinence. Overnight abstinence allows considerable resensitization to the actions of nicotine, and the cycle begins again the next day.

What Is Addiction?

The World Health Organization (WHO) describes drug dependence as "a behavioral pattern in which the use of a given psychoactive drug is given a sharply higher priority over other behaviors that once had a significantly higher value."[3] In other words, the drug comes to control behavior to an extent considered detrimental to the individual or to society.

Historically, drug addiction meant that tolerance developed to the effects of a drug during repetitive use, and that after cessation of such use withdrawal symptoms emerged (termed physical dependence). The prototypical addictive drug was heroin, and drug addiction has had a connotation of social deviance or criminal behavior in the United States. This historical view of addiction was revised by the 1964 Expert Committee of the World Health Organization. As discussed in detail in the 1988 surgeon general's report, such a definition is narrow and does not address addictions such as cocaine or binge alcoholism. A definition based on concepts of drug dependence developed by expert committees of WHO and in publications of the National Institute on Drug Abuse (NIDA) and the American Psychiatric Association includes compulsive drug-seeking behavior, effect of the drug on the brain, and usually a need for the drug to maintain homeostasis. Specific criteria for a drug that produces dependence or addiction have been presented by the U.S. surgeon general (table 2-2), and specific criteria for diagnosing drug dependence or addiction in individuals have been presented by the American Psychiatric Association (table 2-3).

Pharmacologic Aspects of Nicotine

The pharmacologic effects of nicotine are essential to sustaining cigarette smoking.[4] Viewed another way, tobacco is used by people to deliver nicotine to

TABLE 2-2 Criteria for drug dependence

Primary criteria
  Highly controlled or compulsive use
  Psychoactive effects
  Drug-reinforced behavior

Additional criteria
  Addictive behavior often involves the following:
    Stereotypic patterns of use
    Use despite harmful effects
    Relapse following abstinence
    Recurrent drug cravings
  Dependence-producing drugs often manifest the following:
    Tolerance
    Physical dependence
    Pleasant (euphoric) effects

Source: Adapted from Centers for Disease Control. *The Health Consequences of Smoking: Nicotine Addiction. A Report of the Surgeon General.* DHHS Pub. No. (CDC) 88-8406. Washington, DC: U.S. Department of Health and Human Services, 1988. 7.

TABLE 2-3 Criteria for substance dependence

A maladaptive pattern of substance use, leading to clinically significant impairment or distress, as manifested by three (or more) of the following, occurring at any time in the same 12-month period:

1. Tolerance, as defined by either of the following:
    a. A need for markedly increased amounts of the substance to achieve intoxication or desired effect.
    b. Markedly diminished effect with continued use of the same amount of the substance.

2. Withdrawal, as manifested by either of the following:
    a. The characteristic withdrawal syndrome for the substance (refer to Criteria A and B of the criteria sets for withdrawal from the specific substance).
    b. The same (or a closely related) substance is taken to relieve or avoid withdrawal symptoms.

3. The substance is often taken in larger amounts or over a longer period than was intended.

4. There is a persistent desire or unsuccessful efforts to cut down or control substance use.

5. A great deal of time is spent in activities necessary to obtain the substance (e.g., visiting multiple doctors or driving long distances), use the substance (e.g., chain-smoking), or recover from its effects.

6. Important social, occupational, or recreational activities are given up or reduced because of substance abuse.

7. The substance use is continued despite knowledge of having a persistent or recurrent physical or psychological problem that is likely to have been caused or exacerbated by the substance (e.g., current cocaine use despite recognition of cocaine-induced depression, or continued drinking despite recognition that an ulcer was made worse by alcohol consumption)

Source: American Psychiatric Association. *Diagnostic and Statistical Manual of Mental Disorders: DSM-IV.* 4th ed. Washington, DC: American Psychiatric Association, 1994. 181.

the body. The primary physiologic effects of nicotine (reviewed in detail in the 1988 surgeon general's report) are listed below.

- Electroencephalographic desynchronization
- Increased circulating levels of catecholamines, vasopressin, growth hormone, adrenocorticotropic hormone, cortisol, prolactin, and beta-endorphin
- Increased metabolic rate
- Lipolysis, increased free fatty acids
- Heart rate acceleration

- Cutaneous and coronary vasoconstriction
- Increased cardiac output
- Increased blood pressure
- Skeletal muscle relaxation

Smokers give various explanations for their smoking. Many report that smoking produces arousal, particularly with the first few cigarettes of the day, and relaxation, particularly in stressful situations. Many smokers report that smoking helps them concentrate and lifts their mood. Nicotine has been shown to increase vigilance in the performance of repetitive tasks and to enhance selective attention. Smokers commonly report pleasure and reduced anger, tension, depression, and stress after smoking a cigarette. The extent to which the enhanced performance and mood after smoking are due to the relief of symptoms of abstinence or to an intrinsic enhancement effect on the brain is unclear. A few studies do show improvement in the performance of nonsmoking subjects after dosing with nicotine, suggesting at least some direct enhancement.

Some of the gratifying effects of nicotine are due to the relief of the symptoms of nicotine withdrawal. When nicotine use is abruptly stopped, withdrawal symptoms emerge. The typical symptoms are listed below.

- Restlessness
- Eating more than usual
- Anxiety/tension
- Impatience
- Irritability/anger
- Difficulty concentrating
- Excessive hunger
- Depression
- Disorientation
- Loss of energy/fatigue
- Dizziness
- Stomach or bowel problems
- Headaches
- Sweating
- Insomnia
- Heart palpitations
- Tremors
- Craving cigarettes[5]

Most withdrawal symptoms reach maximal intensity 24 to 48 hours after cessation of tobacco use and gradually diminish in intensity over several weeks. Some symptoms, such as eating more than usual, weight gain, and craving cigarettes (particularly in stressful situations) may persist for months or even years after cessation.

Actions of Nicotine on the Brain

The nicotine molecule is shaped like acetylcholine. Acetylcholine is a neu-rotransmitter, that is, a chemical naturally found in the body that is involved in transmitting information from one neuron to another. Receptors (specialized proteins that selectively bind drugs and initiate drug effects in the body) for acetylcholine are called cholinergic receptors. Nicotine acts on certain cholin-ergic receptors in the brain and other organs of the body. The receptors would normally be acted on by the body's own acetylcholine. By activating cholin-ergic receptors, nicotine enhances the release of other neurotransmitters and hor-mones including acetylcholine, norepinephrine, dopamine, vasopressin, seroto-nin, and beta-endorphin. The physiologic effects of nicotine include behavioral arousal and sympathetic neural activation. Release of specific neurotransmitters has been speculatively linked to particular reinforcing effects of nicotine (figure 2-1).[6] For example, enhanced release of dopamine, norepinephrine, and seroto-

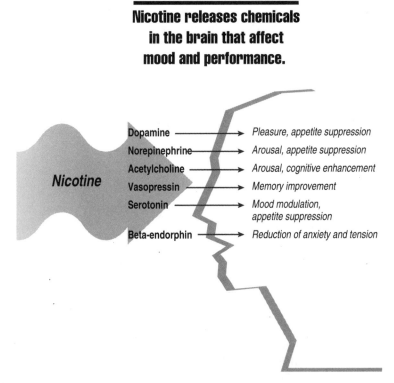

Nicotine releases chemicals in the brain that affect mood and performance.

Nicotine

Dopamine — Pleasure, appetite suppression
Norepinephrine — Arousal, appetite suppression
Acetylcholine — Arousal, cognitive enhancement
Vasopressin — Memory improvement
Serotonin — Mood modulation, appetite suppression
Beta-endorphin — Reduction of anxiety and tension

FIGURE 2-1   Source: Adapted from Pomerleau, O. F., and C. S. Pomerleau. "Neuro-regulators and the Reinforcement of Smoking: Towards a Biobehavioral Explanation." *Neuroscience Behavioral Review* 8 (1984): 503-513.

nin may be associated with pleasure as well as appetite suppression, the latter of which may contribute to lower body weight. Release of acetylcholine may be associated with improved performance on behavioral tasks and improvement of memory. Release of beta-endorphin may be associated with reduction of anxiety and tension.

Tolerance and Withdrawal

With prolonged or repetitive exposure to nicotine, the brain cells adapt in such a way as to compensate for the actions of nicotine, that is, to return brain functioning to normal. This process is called neuroadaptation. Neuroadaptation is associated with an increasing number of nicotinic receptors in the brain. Neuroadaptation results in the development of tolerance, that is, a given level of nicotine comes to have less of an effect on the body, and higher levels of nicotine are needed to produce the effects that lower doses formerly produced. Substantial tolerance develops to the behavioral arousal and cardiovascular effects of nicotine when a person smokes multiple cigarettes or uses multiple doses of smokeless tobacco, even within the course of a single day. Regular tobacco users regain sensitivity to the effects of nicotine, at least in part, after overnight abstinence from tobacco.

When the brain has adapted so as to function normally in the presence of nicotine, it also becomes dependent on the presence of nicotine for normal functioning. When nicotine is not available (such as when a smoker stops smoking), the brain function becomes disturbed, resulting in a number of withdrawal symptoms, as mentioned above.

Absorption of Nicotine from Tobacco

Nicotine from tobacco smoke is rapidly absorbed into the systemic circulation after inhalation, then is quickly carried to various body organs including the brain. Nicotine levels in the blood rise quickly after smoking, with arterial blood levels exceeding venous levels in the first few minutes (figure 2-2). Because nicotine is a weak base and is ionized at acid pH, there is little absorption of nicotine through the membranes of the mouth from the acidic smoke of blond (light-colored) tobacco. However, the smoke of pipes, cigars, and dark tobacco is more alkaline, so nicotine is absorbed through the mouth from these products. When oral snuff or chewing tobacco is used, nicotine is also absorbed through the mouth. Nicotine from oral snuff or chewing tobacco is absorbed more slowly than from cigarette smoke; peak plasma concentrations of nicotine in venous blood are similar.

Nicotine concentrations* in venous
blood during and after the use of cigarettes,
oral snuff, chewing tobacco,
and nicotine gum.

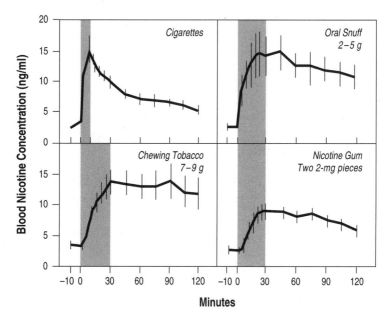

FIGURE 2-2   *Average values for 10 subjects. Shaded bars show the period of tobacco (or nicotine) use. Vertical bars indicate ranges. Source: Adapted from Benowitz, Neal L., H. Porchet, L. Sheiner, and P. Jacob III. "Nicotine Absorption and Cardiovascular Effects with Smokeless Tobacco Use: Comparison to Cigarettes and Nicotine Gum." *Clinical Pharmacology and Therapeutics* (1988): 23-28.

Distribution and Elimination of Nicotine from the Body

A cigarette delivers nicotine to the brain within 10 to 19 seconds from the start of a puff. The rapid passage of nicotine from the lungs to the arterial circulation to the brain provides for rapid behavioral reinforcement for smoking and for the possibility for the smoker to control levels of nicotine in the brain and to modulate pharmacologic effects. Nicotine is also distributed extensively to other body tissues. Slow release from tissues explains in part the elimination half-life of 2 to 3 hours.

Nicotine is eliminated primarily by liver metabolism. The rate of metabolism is quite variable from person to person, so the same level of nicotine intake may be associated with different concentrations of nicotine in the blood of different people. The main metabolite of nicotine, cotinine, has a long half-life (on average 17 hours) and has been widely used by researchers as a biochemical marker of nicotine exposure.

Intake and Accumulation of Nicotine During Cigarette Smoking

On the average, smoking a cigarette results in the absorption into the blood stream of about 1 mg of nicotine, but the range is from 0.5 to 3.0 mg. The elimination half-life of nicotine is 2 to 3 hours. This means that the level of nicotine in the blood decreases by one-half every 2 or 3 hours. It also means that after a single use of tobacco nicotine remains in the body for 8 to 12 hours. With repeated smoking, nicotine levels accumulate over 6 to 8 hours, plateauing through the remainder of the day, then gradually falling overnight. Thus, regular cigarette smoking results in continued exposure of the brain and body to nicotine.

Addiction and the Light or Occasional Smoker

Among adults the light or occasional smoker, that is, one who regularly smokes 5 or fewer cigarettes per day or who does not smoke every day, is in general less addicted than are daily smokers of more than 5 cigarettes per day.[7] Smoking appears to be reinforced for light smokers by the direct pharmacologic effects of nicotine, as described above, as well as by behavioral aspects of tobacco use, as described below. The use of tobacco in response to withdrawal symptoms is less of a factor in such tobacco users. Among adults, light or occasional smokers are relatively uncommon (less than 10% of adult smokers);[8] they have higher success in smoking cessation than do heavier smokers, although not all light smokers are able to quit. In contrast, many more children than adults are light or occasional smokers; however, light smoking by children is often not a stable pattern but, rather, represents a stage in escalation to becoming daily smokers.

Nicotine Compensation

The "Low-Yield" Cigarette

Some tobacco advertisements indicate that particular brands of cigarettes deliver less nicotine and tar than their competitors' brands, implying a health benefit to low-yield cigarettes. Some people switch to low-yield cigarettes in an attempt to reduce the health consequences of smoking, but that is an unlikely result. A daily smoker tends to regulate his or her nicotine intake to a specific level in order to achieve desired effects and to minimize withdrawal symptoms.

This nicotine regulation influences how smokers smoke cigarettes with various nicotine yields and how they respond to cutting down on the number of cigarettes they smoke per day. When smoking lower-yield cigarettes, smokers puff more frequently or more intensely than when smoking higher-yield cigarettes, presumably to obtain their usual specific level of nicotine from each cigarette. In switching from high-yield to low-yield cigarettes, smokers consume more nicotine from the low-yield cigarette than predicted by smoking machine tests. Conversely, smokers consume less nicotine than predicted from high-yield cigarettes.

The intake of nicotine, with blood cotinine or nicotine concentrations used as markers of nicotine intake, has been studied in large groups of people smoking their chosen brands of cigarettes.[9] In such studies, nicotine intake correlates only weakly with the advertised yield. The slope of the regression line between advertised nicotine yields and blood nicotine or cotinine levels is shallow, suggesting only small differences of intake from cigarettes of widely different nicotine yields. Because of this compensatory smoking, having smokers switch to low-yield cigarettes reduces the risk of smoking to a much lesser degree, if at all, than suggested by the decreases in yield.

Smoking Fewer Cigarettes

The regulation of nicotine intake by daily smokers is also apparent when the number of cigarettes available to a smoker is restricted. In one study of heavy smokers, when the number of cigarettes was reduced from unlimited (average 37 per day) to 5 cigarettes per day, the average intake of nicotine per cigarette tripled.[10] As a result, reducing the number of cigarettes to 15 per day had very little effect, and reducing to 5 cigarettes per day reduced the daily exposure to tobacco toxins only by 50%. This observation explains why many smokers who are instructed to quit report cutting down to about 10 cigarettes per day, but cannot reduce their consumption to fewer than 10. At 10 cigarettes per day smokers still can absorb adequate nicotine to maintain nicotine addiction.

Behavioral Aspects of Addiction

The behavior of smoking is maintained both by the direct pharmacologic effects of nicotine (including relief of withdrawal) and by learned responses. Anticipatory responses develop as a consequence of repetitive use of tobacco during which various kinds of gratifications from smoking occur in the presence of specific cues from the environment. For example, when a smoker encounters stressors or situational reminders of smoking, these stimuli revivify the pleasurable or other reinforcing aspects of smoking, which then generate the urge to smoke. Such recurrent anticipatory responses may persist 6 months or longer after physical dependence has been overcome, accounting for the relapses that occur beyond the first week or two after cessation of tobacco use. Such anticipatory responses probably also develop to some degree in occasional smokers.

There are various conceptualizations of the nature of the anticipatory response system. One is the conditioning model, in which learned associations between the effects of cigarette smoking and specific cues in the environment motivate smoking. Another model is self-regulation, in which high-risk situations activate cognitive processes in a form of pleasurable expectations and a reduced sense of personal control, which then increases the likelihood of smoking.[11] Examples of common anticipatory reactions include smoking after a meal, with a cup of coffee or an alcoholic beverage, during a break from work, while talking on the phone, or while with friends who smoke.

Of note, aspects of the drug-taking behavior itself often become pleasurable in addition to the pleasure afforded by the pharmacologic effects of nicotine. For example, manipulation of smoking materials or the taste, smell, or feel of tobacco smoke in the throat can become associated with the reinforcing effects of smoking and can become pleasurable in themselves. When a smoker becomes abstinent, he or she must learn not only to forego the pharmacologic pleasures afforded by the drug, but also the pleasure of engaging in those aspects of drug-taking behavior that have become pleasurable through anticipatory mechanisms.

Behavioral factors other than anticipatory mechanisms may also influence personal susceptibility to drug addiction. For example, some smokers, particularly Caucasian women, smoke as a means of maintaining lower body weight.[12] Certain characteristics of individuals appear to promote initiation of smoking and the development of nicotine addiction, as reviewed in more detail in a later section.

Addiction to Smokeless Tobacco

"Smokeless tobacco" (SLT) refers to oral and nasal snuff and chewing tobacco. Smokeless tobacco, commonly used by youths, particularly in rural areas, may be highly addicting.[13] Considerable nicotine is absorbed from smokeless tobacco. A classification scheme for levels of SLT use or addiction is problematic. The nicotine content of smokeless products is not known to the public and the nicotine content of the tobacco provides only a rough estimate of actual nicotine intake. Recent laboratory analysis of popular brands of moist snuff revealed large differences in nicotine content, from 5.7 to 30.7 mg/g.[14] Two studies found evidence for higher addiction levels and greater oral pathology among Copenhagen® users.[15] The systemic dose of nicotine derived from smokeless tobacco can be estimated by measuring blood nicotine levels after SLT use. The systemic dose of nicotine from snuff is 3.6 mg, and for chewing tobacco it is 4.5 mg; an average dose from smoking a cigarette is 1 mg.[16] No standard self-report measures exist for smokeless tobacco consumption, such as those for smoking. One way to estimate addiction level is to use the number of tins or pouches of SLT product consumed per week, the product used (high, medium, or low nicotine content), and the amount of time (minutes) the tobacco is in the mouth. In surveys, though not standardized, questions typically ask if the individual used one or more dips or chews in the past 7 days, used one or more dips or chews in the past 24 hours (or day), and uses dip or chew daily. In intervention studies, typical measures of the pattern and amount of SLT use have included the number of dips per day, the number of minutes the dip or chew is kept in the mouth, the number of days a tin or pouch lasts, and the number of tins or pouches used per week. All four measures of SLT intercorrelate significantly with saliva cotinine assays.[17] Most users report using a tin or pouch every day or two, but adolescent boys report that a tin of snuff lasts 5 days and that they use an average of five dips a day.[18]

Most cessation studies define a "regular user" as someone who has used SLT daily for the past year. Schroeder and colleagues suggest categorizing the SLT user as a light, moderate, or heavy user according to the amount of nicotine consumed per week from chewing tobacco or snuff products.[19] Other measures of the pattern of SLT use and addiction have been adapted from the smoking cessation literature. The Fagerström Tolerance Questionnaire[20] has been adapted and used with a scale applicable to SLT users by simply converting cigarette-based items to SLT-use items, for example, "I chew or dip first thing in the morning or within 30 minutes of waking up in the morning."[21] The scale has been validated by its correlation with saliva cotinine. Some items of this scale have been positively correlated with self-reported severity of nicotine withdrawal.[22]

Blood nicotine concentrations throughout the day are similar in regular smokers and people who also use smokeless tobacco.[23] Plasma cotinine levels among regular users of smokeless tobacco are in many cases similar to those of cigarette smokers.[24] Abstinence from smokeless tobacco use results in signs and symptoms of nicotine deprivation that are similar to those seen in smokers after they stop smoking.[25] These symptoms are reversed by administration of tobacco or nicotine gum. Swedish oral snuff users report difficulty in quitting and many consider themselves to be addicted, reporting as much difficulty in giving up smokeless tobacco use as is reported by cigarette smokers trying to quit smoking.[26] Finally, there is evidence that when deprived of snuff, regular snuff users will smoke cigarettes to satisfy their need for nicotine.[27] The regular use of snuff or chewing tobacco by a child therefore increases the likelihood that subsequently the person will take up regular cigarette smoking.[28]

Comparison of Nicotine Addiction with Other Drug Addictions

It is obvious that all drugs of dependence share psychoactivity, produce pleasure, and are shown to reinforce drug-taking behavior. (For a detailed review of the comparison of nicotine and other drug addictions, see the 1988 surgeon general's report.) The nature of nicotine's psychoactivity, which is generally subtle and is consistent with high levels of cognitive performance, is considerably different from that of heroin or cocaine, which produce intense euphoria and may be disruptive to performance. The subtle psychoactive effect of nicotine is experienced hundreds of times (puffs) per day, and exerts a powerful effect on behavior over time. Although the psychoactive effect of nicotine is less dramatic than that of other drugs, the strength of the addiction is as powerful or more powerful. The consequences of its addictiveness are clearly more dramatic, making tobacco use the number one health problem in the United States.

Compulsive use can be observed with all addictive drugs, but the compulsiveness is manifested in different patterns. Some drugs, such as cocaine and heroin, are used by some addicted persons only intermittently, that is, every few days or even at longer intervals, but the compulsion to use the drug does repeat. Cigarette smokers, on the other hand, rarely go more than a day without nicotine. At work or in other public places where smoking is proscribed, smokers may need to take numerous breaks throughout the day to smoke. No single physical dependence model describes the way in which drug use is continually compelled, but these compulsive behaviors are strongly controlled by the addictive actions of the drugs.

> *"Addiction is needing to smoke first thing in the morning, not just when you are bored or hanging out with your friends."*
>
> —adolescent in focus group

Use despite harmful effects confirms the difficulty that many persons have in quitting drug use. This is clearly evident to clinicians who treat alcoholics with chronic liver disease, heroin addicts with infective endocarditis, and cigarette smokers. For example, only 50% of smokers who suffer acute myocardial infarction quit smoking, despite a physician's admonition to do so.[29] It has been argued that for many activities that entail risk, such as sex, sunbathing, and skiing, the individual assumes a risk and makes a free choice, and that the same is true of cigarette smoking. However, life-long smoking results in the premature death of one in three smokers and the disability of a great number of smokers from chronic lung disease, indicating a substantially different level of risk.

Relapse rates after abstinence appear to be similar for tobacco, heroin, and alcohol; about 60% of quitters relapse within 3 months and 75% within 6 months.[30] These relapse rates have been observed in clients discharged from treatment programs. It has been argued that the relapse rate for tobacco among spontaneous quitters might be lower than these rates. Recent data indicate that relapse rates for smokers who have undergone minimal intervention treatment in a physician's office and who have successfully abstained for 24 hours are 25% at 2 days, 50% at 1 week, and 75% at 2 months,[31] whereas two-thirds of smokers who quit on their own relapse within 2 days.[32]

Recurrent drug cravings have been described for each of the addicting drugs, although there has been considerable debate about the use of the term "craving." A better term might be "strong desire" to use a drug. When desires for different drugs were compared among polydrug abusers, most of whom smoked cigarettes, the reported intensity of desire for cigarettes when they are not available was as high as or higher than for heroin, alcohol, or cocaine when the latter were not available.[33]

Tolerance to the various drugs of abuse has been well documented, although the time course varies. Different time courses of tolerance might influence the pattern of drug use. For example, tolerance to many effects of nicotine develops quickly, within the day, and there is resensitization of many responses overnight. Intermittent high levels of nicotine in the brain from individual puffs might also overcome tolerance to some extent so that effects can be experienced from individual cigarettes. Presumably because of the daily cycle of tolerance and resensitization, daily doses of nicotine tend to stabilize, and, after a period of dose escalation in the first few years, many smokers smoke the same number of cigarettes each day. In contrast, tolerance lasts longer in an alcoholic who drinks all day and whose brain is more or less continually exposed to alcohol throughout the day. Tolerance likewise occurs during cocaine binges when progressively larger doses are used in an attempt to maintain a cocaine high; however, between binges, sensitivity to cocaine may be regained. One implication of the development of tolerance is that regular smokers are able to consume far greater amounts of tobacco smoke and associated toxins than if they had not become tolerant.

Physical dependence has been well characterized for smokers as well as for other drug abusers. It has been argued that a marked stereotypic syndrome occurs in a person after stopping use of heroin or alcohol, whereas the withdrawal symptoms after stopping smoking vary widely in nature and magnitude and, in one study, were not sufficiently present in 22% of quitters to constitute a diagnosis of withdrawal.[34] Although it is true that smoking does not result in seizures or delirium tremens, withdrawal from smoking can be extremely disruptive to personal life. Nicotine withdrawal may be viewed as closer to that of withdrawal from other stimulants such as cocaine: the withdrawal syndrome is not life-threatening but it profoundly affects behavior and remains a strong impetus to recurrent drug use. Conversely, some persons dependent on heroin or alcohol stop their drug use abruptly without marked withdrawal symptoms.

Agonist drug "replacement" to modify withdrawal symptoms or to facilitate cessation has been used with narcotic abuse (methadone and L-acetylmethadol) and alcoholism (benzodiazepines) as well as with tobacco addiction (nicotine gum, transdermal nicotine, and nicotine nasal spray). In all cases the agonist relieves withdrawal symptoms. Methadone and nicotine can be used over several months, with gradual tapering, to facilitate cessation. Methadone is also used in the long term to maintain abstinence. While such use is not recommended for nicotine replacement, 6% to 38% of nicotine gum users do continue to use the gum for a year or more after stopping smoking, apparently as a sort of maintenance treatment.[35]

NICOTINE DEPENDENCY IN YOUTHS

Tobacco use begins with experimentation, often in early adolescence or in the preteen years. The immediate impetus to experiment is social, prompted by friends, or family members, or role models who smoke. Other factors involved in initiation and progression of smoking are discussed in detail in a later section. Estimates of the percentage of youths who experiment with smoking vary from 47% to 90%. Most who experiment smoke only a few cigarettes. Those who smoke three or more cigarettes have a high likelihood of becoming regular smokers.[36] Once a smoker becomes a regular smoker, the number of cigarettes smoked per day tends to escalate over several years.[37] Even when youths are smoking only a few cigarettes per day, they inhale tobacco smoke effectively and take in as much nicotine per cigarette as do adults, as shown in studies measuring salivary cotinine per cigarette smoked per day.

Epidemiology and Natural History of Cigarette Smoking

Data from the Youth Risk Behavior Survey for smoking initiation by high school youths in the United States are presented in table 2-4 (1990) and in table 2-5 (1991) for smoking within the past 30 days. Figure 2-3 shows that in 1990, by age 13, 56% of youths had tried smoking and 9% were regular smokers (that is, they smoked on 5-15 days or more in the past 30 days). The percentage of youths trying cigarettes increases with each year of age, so that by age 17, 77% of youths had tried smoking and 25% were regular smokers. This trend has been reported for current smokers (that is, who smoked within the last 30 days) in other recent surveys (table 2-5).

Data on the amount of cigarettes consumed by youths of various ages are provided in table 2-6. Younger children are less likely to be daily smokers; if they are, they smoke fewer cigarettes per day. Thus, at ages 12-13, 16.5 % of adolescent smokers are daily smokers, compared to 47.5% of teen smokers between 16-18 years old. At ages 12-13, 11% of smokers smoke 10 or more cigarettes per day, compared to 27.2% of smokers 16-18 years old.

The development of nicotine addiction has been characterized as a series of five stages:

1. Preparatory
2. Initial trying
3. Experimentation
4. Regular use
5. Nicotine addiction[38]

TABLE 2-4   Percentage of boys and girls
who initiate smoking at specific ages

Age (years)	Percentage of age group	
	Girls	Boys
<9	3.6	6.7
9–10	6.4	8.0
11–12	14.9	16.7
13–14	24.9	24.1
15–16	19.5	19.4
≥17	4.4	5.0

Note: Sample sizes for the various age groups were the
same (n = 11,241) because new smokers who emerged
from among those who had never smoked for successive
age groups were added incrementally to numerators of
older age groups.

Source: Data from the Youth Risk Behavior Survey, 1990.
In Escobedo, Luis G., Stephen Marcus, Deborah
Holtzman, and Gary Giovino. "Sports Participation, Age
at Smoking Initiation, and the Risk of Smoking among
U.S. High School Students." *Journal of the American
Medical Association* 17:11 (1993): 1391-1395.

The "preparatory" stage includes formation of knowledge, beliefs, and expectations about smoking. "Initial trying" refers to trials with the first 2 or 3
cigarettes (events that are discussed in more detail later in this section). "Experimentation" refers to repeated, irregular use over an extended period of time;
such smoking may be situation-specific (for example, smoking at parties).
"Regular smoking" by youths may mean smoking every weekend or in certain
parts of each day (such as after school with friends). "Nicotine addiction" refers
to regular smoking, usually every day, with an internally regulated need for
nicotine. Thus, for individual youths, there is a progression of smoking over
time from initiation to experimentation with light smoking to regular and heavy
smoking. Unlike adults, in whom intermittent or light smoking may be a stable
and relatively nonaddictive pattern of smoking, children who are light smokers
are often in a phase of escalation, with a typical interval from initiation to addiction of 2-3 years. The interval between initiation and addiction is based on a
comparison of the cumulative prevalence curves for trying a first cigarette and
smoking daily (table 2-1) and the interval between initiation of smoking and the
rise of salivary cotinine concentrations to adult levels (figure 2-4).

The natural history of the smoking experience for an individual provides
insight into the pharmacology of the addiction process. The first cigarette
smoked is often perceived as aversive, producing coughing, dizziness, and/or

nausea. With repeated smoking, tolerance develops to the noxious effects of cigarette smoking, and smokers tend to report positive effects of smoking. As the daily intake of nicotine increases, the development of physical dependence, that is, experiencing withdrawal symptoms between cigarettes or when cigarettes are not available, becomes established. Thus, there appears to be a progression over time from smoking initially for social reasons to smoking for pharmacologic reasons. The latter includes both smoking for positive effects of nicotine and smoking to avoid withdrawal symptoms, as discussed above in the section on general aspects of nicotine dependence.

Evidence for Nicotine Dependence in Youths

Many youths describe themselves as being dependent on tobacco, and there is evidence that nicotine dependence does become established in youthful smok-

TABLE 2-5   Percentage of youths who currently smoke cigarettes (who smoked within the last 30 days)

	Teenage Attitudes and Practices Survey 1989[a]	National Household Surveys on Drug Abuse 1991[b]	Monitoring the Future Project 1992[c]	Youth Risk Behavior Survey 1991[d]
Age (years)				
12-14	5.9	3.9		
15-16	17.5	14.0		
17-18	27.5	25.5		
Grade				
8th			15.5	
9th				23.2
10th			21.5	25.2
11th				31.6
12th			27.8	30.6

[a]Ages 12-18 years. Based on responses to the questions, "Have you ever smoked a cigarette?" and "Think about the last 30 days. On how many of these days did you smoke?"

[b]Ages 12-18 years. Based on responses to the question, "When was the most recent time you smoked a cigarette?"

[c]With the exception of data for eighth and tenth grade students reported below, all other data points for the Monitoring the Future Project survey reflect estimates for high school seniors. Based on responses to the question, "How frequently have you smoked cigarettes during the last 30 days?"

[d]Grades 9-12. Based on responses to the question, "During the past 30 days, on how many days did you smoke cigarettes?"

Source: Centers for Disease Control and Prevention. *Preventing Tobacco Use Among Young People. A Report of the Surgeon General.* Washington, DC: U.S. Department of Health and Human Services, 1994. 61.

Prevalence of smoking by students.

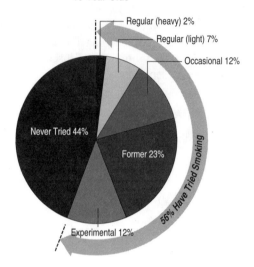

13-Year-Olds

Regular (heavy) 2%
Regular (light) 7%
Occasional 12%
Never Tried 44%
Former 23%
56% Have Tried Smoking
Experimental 12%

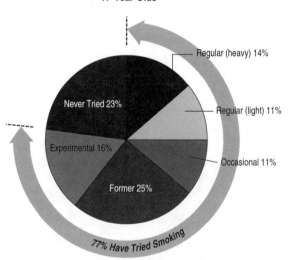

17-Year-Olds

Regular (heavy) 14%
Never Tried 23%
Regular (light) 11%
Experimental 16%
Occasional 11%
Former 25%
77% Have Tried Smoking

FIGURE 2-3 Source: Data from 1990 Youth Risk Behavior Survey, presented in Escobedo, Luis G., Stephen E. Marcus, Deborah Holtzman, and Gary Giovino. "Sports Participation, Age at Smoking Initiation, and the Risk of Smoking Among U.S. High School Students." *Journal of the American Medical Association* 17(11) (1993) 1391-1395.

TABLE 2-6 Percentage of current smokers by the number of days smoked in the past month and the average number of cigarettes smoked daily

	Number of days smoked in past month[a]				Number of cigarettes smoked daily[b]			
	<5	5–9	10–29	Every day	<5	5–9	10–19	≥20
Overall	24.1	8.7	26.4	40.8	37.9	20.4	25.7	16.0
Gender								
Boys	23.9	8.5	26.6	41.0	33.9	19.3	27.6	19.2
Girls	24.3	8.9	26.2	40.6	42.7	21.6	23.5	12.1
Age (years)								
12-13	51.9	8.3[c]	23.3	16.5[c]	64.3	24.6[c]	11.0[c]	0.0
14-15	28.4	9.8	34.5	27.3	55.5	17.2	23.0	4.3
16-18	20.0	8.4	24.1	47.5	31.6	21.1	27.2	20.1
Race								
White	23.4	8.4	26.2	42.0	36.6	20.1	26.5	16.8
African American	37.0	15.0[c]	26.5	21.6	60.3	20.5[c]	16.3[c]	2.9[c]
Hispanic origin								
Hispanic	30.7	11.2[c]	31.9	26.3	59.2	22.5	11.6[c]	6.6[c]
Non-Hispanic	23.5	8.5	26.0	42.0	36.3	20.2	26.9	16.7

[a]Excludes unknown number of days smoked.
[b]Excludes unknown number of cigarettes smoked daily and none smoked in the past week.
[c]Estimate does not meet standards of reliability or precision (<30% relative standard error).

Source: Teenage Attitudes and Practices Survey, United States, 1989. Moss, A. J., K. F. Allen, G. A. Giovino, and S. L. Mill. "Recent Trends in Adolescent Smoking, Smoking-Uptake Correlates, and Expectations About the Future." *Advance Data* 221 (1992). Cited in Centers for Disease Control and Prevention. *Preventing Tobacco Use Among Young People. A Report of the Surgeon General.* Washington, DC: U.S. Department of Health and Human Services, 1994. 118.

ers. The evidence reveals that (1) youths consume substantial levels of nicotine, (2) youths report subjective effects and subjective reasons for smoking, (3) youths experience withdrawal symptoms when they are not able to smoke, and (4) youths have difficulty in quitting tobacco use.

That youths *consume substantial amounts* of nicotine was shown in a 3-year study of 197 London schoolgirls who entered the study between the ages of 11 and 14. Saliva cotinine concentrations in girls who were smokers throughout the 3 years were higher at each year's evaluation. Average salivary cotinine levels were 103, 158, and 208 g/ml.[39] The level of 208 ng/ml is similar to that of many adult daily smokers. The ratio of salivary cotinine per cigarette per day, an index of the amount of nicotine taken in per cigarette, was similar for girls with various levels of cigarette consumption, and similar to that for adults. Thus, there seems to be the same intake of nicotine per cigarette among adolescent girls as among adults. Also of note in the study was that smokers who smoked at the time of all three surveys, as well as smokers who were occasional smokers or nonsmokers at the time of the first survey but who subsequently became daily smokers, showed escalation of cigarette consumption (figure 2-4) and saliva cotinine levels each year.

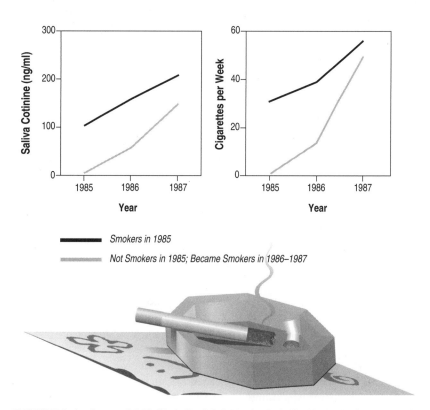

Cotinine concentrations and cigarette consumption by adolescent girls.

Smokers in 1985

Not Smokers in 1985; Became Smokers in 1986–1987

FIGURE 2-4   Source: McNeill, A. D., M. J. Jarvis, J. A. Stapleton, R. J. West, and A. Bryant. "Nicotine Intake in Young Smokers: Longitudinal Study of Saliva Cotinine Concentrations." *American Journal of Public Health* 79 (1989): 172-175.

Adolescent girls report subjective effects of smoking.

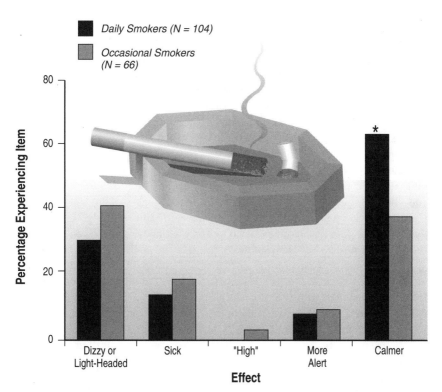

■ Daily Smokers (N = 104)

▨ Occasional Smokers (N = 66)

FIGURE 2-5 *Difference is statistically significant. Source: McNeill, Ann D., Martin Jarvis, and Robert West. "Subjective Effects of Cigarette Smoking in Adolescents." *Psychopharmacology* 92 (1987): 115-117.

That youths *experience pharmacologic effects* of nicotine from tobacco smoke was reported in an earlier study by the same researchers.[40] A smoking questionnaire asked a group of 170 British schoolgirls ages 11-17 about the five subjective effects of smoking specified in figure 2-5. Feeling high or feeling more alert, which are stimulant-like effects, were described by only a few respondents. Feeling calmer was the most common effect described, and was more likely to be reported by daily smokers than by occasional smokers. There was also a significant correlation between salivary cotinine concentrations and the response of feeling calmer. Feeling calmer may be a beneficial effect that is particularly desirable to youths with high levels of anxiety or depression (as will be discussed later). Alternatively, feeling calmer could represent the reversal of nicotine withdrawal symptoms. In any case, there is clear evidence that youthful smokers do smoke for the pharmacologic effects of tobacco, presumably the effects of nicotine.

That youths *experience withdrawal symptoms* when they try to give up smoking has been demonstrated as well. McNeill and colleagues queried 191 schoolgirls 11-17 years old who were current cigarette smokers about how they felt when they tried to stop smoking.[41] Of the group of smokers, 71% of the daily smokers and 72% of the occasional smokers had made at least one attempt to quit and had failed. Of these subjects, the average cigarette consumption by the daily smokers (69 girls) was 6.8 cigarettes per day, with an average salivary cotinine of 182 ng/ml. The average salivary cotinine concentration in the occasional smokers (47 girls) was 22 ng/ml; 74% of the daily smokers and 47% of the occasional smokers experienced one or more of the six symptoms of nicotine withdrawal graphed in figure 2-6. The withdrawal score correlated significantly with salivary cotinine concentration and with weekly cigarette consumption. This study demonstrates that adolescent smokers experience withdrawal symptoms when they try to quit and that many youths have difficulty quitting. It should be noted that the data on nicotine consumption, pharmacologic effects, and withdrawal symptoms are based on studies of schoolgirls; no data are as yet available on boys. However, based on the difficulty of quitting smoking that is experienced by both boys and girls (described below), it is likely that dependence develops to a similar degree in boys as it does in girls. This issue of the natural history of the development of addiction to nicotine in youths requires further research.

Other studies further reveal that many youths want to quit but have difficulty doing so. Townsend and colleagues reported that 60% of adolescent smokers evaluated in a general medical practice made an agreement with the practice doctor or nurse to give up smoking.[42] Stone and Kristeller surveyed tenth grade students in suburban Massachusetts; 14% of the students were daily smokers and, of these, 28% reported that they continued to smoke because they were addicted.[43] The Monitoring the Future Project, which looked at high school seniors in the United States, asked about interest in quitting smoking and prior attempts at quitting (table 2-7). Of smokers (1985-1989) who had smoked at all in the past 30 days, 42.5% reported a desire to stop smoking. Of this group, and of the subgroup who smoked daily, 28% and 39%, respectively, stated that they had tried to stop in the past and could not.[44]

Another perspective on the difficulty of quitting is youths' expectations regarding their future smoking behavior. Seniors in high school were asked, "Do you think you will be smoking cigarettes 5 years from now?" Among the respondents who were occasional smokers (less than one cigarette per day) 85%

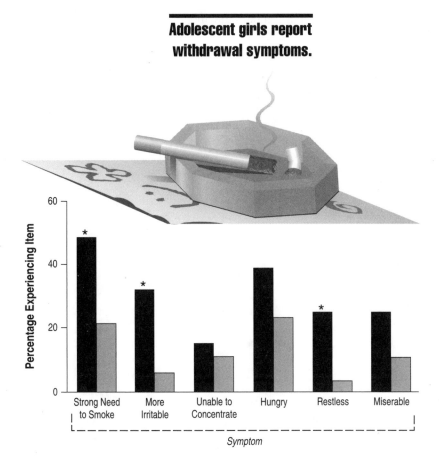

Adolescent girls report withdrawal symptoms.

FIGURE 2-6   *Difference is statistically significant. Source: McNeill, Ann D., Robert J. West, Martin Jarvis, et al. "Cigarette Withdrawal Symptoms in Adolescent Smokers." *Psychopharmacology* 90 (1986): 533-536.

stated that they probably or definitely would not be smoking in 5 years, as did 32% of those who smoked one pack per day or more (table 2-8). However, at follow-up 5-6 years later, of those who smoked occasionally only 58% had quit and 28% had actually increased their cigarette consumption. Of those who had smoked one pack or more per day, only 13% had quit and 70% still smoked one pack or more per day. Smokers of 1-5 or about 10 cigarettes per day at the time of the initial questionnaire also were less likely to quit than they had predicted, and on average escalated their smoking over the subsequent 5 years (table 2-9).[45]

TABLE 2-7   High school seniors' attempts to quit smoking

Monitoring the Future Study survey question	1976-1979	Percentage of respondents answering "Yes"	
		1980-1984	1985-1989
"Do you want to stop smoking now?"			
Among those who smoked at all during the last 30 days	46.1	47.1	42.5
Among those who smoked ≥1 cigarette/day during the last 30 days	46.1	47.6	43.9
"Have you ever tried to stop smoking and found that you could not?"			
Among those who smoked at all during the last 30 days	31.5	31.4	27.8
Among those who smoked ≥1 cigarette/day during the last 30 days	38.5	41.6	39.4

Source: Centers for Disease Control and Prevention. *Preventing Tobacco Use Among Young People. A Report of the Surgeon General.* Washington, DC: U.S. Government Printing Office, 1994. 78.

Thus, consistent with the concept of addiction, smokers' expectations of future smoking behavior shows little relationship to their actual behavior; that is, youths think that they will be able to quit but underestimate the power of their addiction. Even those who smoke only a few cigarettes per day during high school have a high risk of becoming heavy smokers as adults.

These data are evidence that nicotine addiction develops during adolescence, and that most adolescents who are daily cigarette smokers (as well as some who are occasional smokers) are addicted to nicotine. Once adolescents are addicted, cessation is difficult, as it is for adults; thus, interventions are needed at early stages to prevent an established pattern of addiction. The likelihood of successful quitting among adolescents is greater the sooner the adolescent tries to quit after initiating tobacco use, and the fewer cigarettes he or she has smoked.[46]

Risk Factors for Smoking Initiation

Understanding why children begin to smoke is important in planning and developing effective prevention strategies. The numerous major factors that influence or predict initiation and escalation of tobacco use were recently reviewed extensively in the 1994 surgeon general's report, and are listed in table 2-10. In general, the psychosocial risk factors can be described as a continuum

TABLE 2-8 High school seniors predict whether or not they will be smoking in 5 years (percentage)

Senior year smoking status (use in past 30 days)	Definitely will	Probably will	Probably will not	Definitely will not	Number
None	0.4	1.3	21.0	77.3	1,926
<1 cigarette/day	0.5	14.7	56.5	28.3	248
1–5 cigarettes/day	1.8	37.6	44.1	16.5	211
About 1/2 pack/day	0.6	57.7	30.3	11.3	197
≥1 pack/day	5.1	62.9	26.7	5.2	228
Total	0.9	14.2	27.0	58.0	2,810

Source: Monitoring the Future Project, United States, 1976-1986 senior classes. Institute for Social Research, University of Michigan (unpublished data).

TABLE 2-9 Direction of change in smoking between senior year of high school and 5-6 years later

Senior year smoking status (use in past 30 days)	Smoking status 5-6 years later (%)				Number
	Quit	Less use	Same level	More use	
None			85.6	14.4	9,238
<1 cigarette/day	57.8		14.4	27.8	1,268
1-5 cigarettes/day	29.6	8.8	17.2	44.4	1,058
About 1/2 pack/day	18.8	13.6	21.7	46.0	1,000
≥1 pack/day	13.2	17.2	40.2	29.0	869

Source: Monitoring the Future Project, United States, 1976-1986 senior classes. Institute for Social Research, University of Michigan (unpublished data).

of proximal to distal factors. Proximal factors directly affect an individual's choice to use tobacco, whereas distal factors do so indirectly. For example, being offered a cigarette at a party is a proximal factor, but prior exposure to advertising showing young adults smoking at a party would be a distal factor influencing the decision to use tobacco. Although proximal factors may seem more influential because of their immediacy, distal factors:

> . . . acquire potency if they are pervasive and provide consistent, repetitive messages across multiple channels. Distal factors are also powerful because, over time, they affect proximal factors as these influences become interpreted and internalized, particularly among adolescents as they try to shape a mature self-identity.[47]

The degree to which any of these risk factors influences smoking behavior varies for each risk factor and among research studies. The reader who wishes a de-

TABLE 2-10 Psychosocial risk factors in the initiation of tobacco use among adolescents

Risk factors	Smoking	Smokeless tobacco
Sociodemographic factors		
Low socioeconomic status	X	
Developmental stage	X	X
Male gender		X
Environmental factors		
Accessibility	X	X
Advertising	X	X
Parental use		
Sibling use	X	
Peer use	X	X
Normative expectations	X	X
Social support	X	
Behavioral factors		
Academic achievement	X	X
Other problem behaviors	X	X
Constructive behaviors	X	
Behavioral skills	X	
Intentions	X	X
Experimentation	X	X
Personal factors		
Knowledge of consequences		X
Functional meanings	X	X
Subjective expected utility	X	
Self-esteem/self-image	X	X
Self-efficacy	X	
Personality factors	X	
Psychological well-being	X	

Source: Centers for Disease Control and Prevention. *Preventing Tobacco Use Among Young People. A Report of the Surgeon General.* Washington, DC: U.S. Government Printing Office, 1994. 123.

tailed discussion of the risk factors should refer to the surgeon general's report. This section provides only an overview of those issues most pertinent to the policy questions addressed in this report.

Initiation of cigarette smoking is influenced by several kinds of factors: environmental, behavioral, personal, and sociodemographic.[48] Among the *environmental* factors that influence initiation of smoking is having friends who smoke, having a best friend who smokes, and/or having many friends who smoke strongly influences initiation. Parental smoking is more important in establishing smoking as a normative behavior, and is associated with more positive and fewer negative perceptions of the health consequences of smoking. Advertising and exposure to smoking in other mass media (for example, television, movies, and sports events) reinforces the idea that smoking is an adult, sophisticated, attractive, and sexy behavior, and downplays the adverse health consequences of smoking (see chapter 4 on advertising).

Behavioral analysis indicates that cigarette smoking is often an early manifestation of problem behavior. School children manifest such problem behaviors as poor school performance, low aspiration for future success, school absences, and the intention to drop out of school or actually dropping out. Other problem behaviors linked to cigarette smoking include alcohol and other drug use and other risk-taking or rebellious behaviors.

A number of *personal* characteristics of adolescents have been linked to cigarette smoking: (1) low self-esteem, poor self-image, low perception of self-efficacy, and susceptibility to peer pressure; (2) sensation-seeking, rebelliousness, sense of invulnerability; (3) low knowledge level of the adverse effects of cigarette smoking; (4) depression and/or anxiety; and (5) pharmacologic response. Considerable recent research has shown a high prevalence of depression among current smokers. Smokers are more likely than nonsmokers to have a history of major depression, even preceding initiation of smoking,[49] and smokers with a history of depression have been found to have lower smoking cessation rates than smokers without depression.

Various *pharmacologic* responses to smoking (presumably to nicotine) from the first cigarette may also predict the likelihood of progression to regular smoking. Hirschman and colleagues found that a report of dizziness after smoking the first cigarette predicted a high rate of progression to the next cigarette, whereas reports of adverse effects, such as coughing, were not associated with progression.[50] While the mechanism of such a link between dizziness and smoking progression is not apparent, a pharmacologic link between cigarette smoking and depression is reasonable. Nicotine is known to release dopamine, norepinephrine, and serotonin in the brain in animals. Antidepressant drugs have similar effects. Thus, it is possible that pharmacologic responses to nicotine promote tobacco use in people who are depressed.

Evidence from studies of twins suggests a moderate *genetic* influence both on initiation and on maintenance of cigarette smoking.[51] Possible mechanisms include genetically determined differences in the pharmacologic response to nicotine, differences in personality, and the presence or absence of an affective or other psychiatric disorder, particularly depression. There is a high concordance of cigarette smoking and alcoholism, and studies in twins suggest that these addictions share, to some extent, a common genetic determinant.[52] Some proportion of the genetic predisposition to tobacco addiction thus appears to be specific, but some appears to be linked to alcoholism or to other drug addictions.

The factors that influence *initiation* may be predominantly of one type, and those that influence the *progression* of cigarette smoking of another type. Hirschman and colleagues studied 386 urban public school children, grades 2-10, to determine how many had ever tried smoking, and then how many had progressed to a second and third cigarette. The main risk factors for the 47% of children who had tried at least one cigarette were grade level in school (that is, the higher the grade level and the older the child, the higher the likelihood of trying a cigarette), having a best friend who was a smoker, and risk-taking behavior (reported on a questionnaire). Progression to a second cigarette (32% of those who smoked one cigarette) was predicted by life stress (predicted rapid progression), friends who smoked (predicted slow progression), lack of negative attitudes toward smoking, and an experience of dizziness when smoking the first cigarette. Progression to a third cigarette (in 77% of those who had smoked two cigarettes) was predicted by best friend being a smoker, feelings of helplessness, and rapid progression to the second cigarette.[53] These analyses support the idea that initiation of cigarette smoking is primarily a consequence of environmental factors, whereas progression appears to be more influenced by personal and pharmacologic factors.

Sociodemographic factors that predispose youths to cigarette smoking include low socioeconomic status, low level of parental education, and the individual's developmental state of adolescence. With respect to the latter, the transition years from elementary to high school, grades 7-10, (ages 11-16) appear to be a particularly high-risk time for initiation (table 2-4).

Ethnic Differences in Nicotine Dependency

Differences in tobacco use by youths are specific to and consistent within ethnic groups. The rates for daily smoking for twelfth graders in 1991 were highest among non-Hispanic whites (21%), next among Hispanics (12%), and lowest among African Americans (5%); the rates in 1991 for smoking one or more cigarettes in the preceding 30 days were 32% for non-Hispanic whites, 25% for Hispanics, and 9% for African Americans.[54] A striking trend of decline in smoking has occurred among African-American high school seniors: from 26.8% in 1976 to 4.4% in 1993 for smoking daily during the preceding 30 days[55] (figure 2-7). Differences in the *smoking habits* of various ethnic groups are notable and may influence the addictive process. Compared to whites, African Americans show a consistent preference for menthol brands, higher tar levels, and higher nicotine levels; and they smoke fewer cigarettes per day. These factors influence inhalation patterns and health risks. For instance, because menthol cigarettes "provide a sensation of cooling when smoked," they may "promote deeper and more prolonged inhalation."[56] Although current initiation rates are lowest for African Americans, there is evidence that adult African Americans are more highly addicted to tobacco than are whites. The cotinine levels of adult African Americans are higher than those of whites, even though

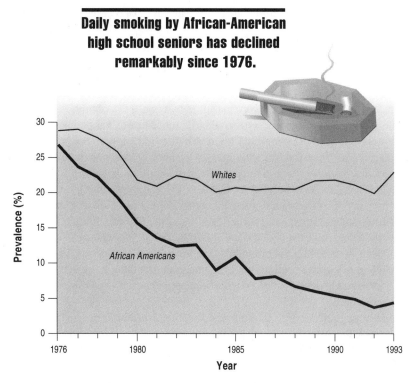

**Daily smoking by African-American
high school seniors has declined
remarkably since 1976.**

FIGURE 2-7   Source: Monitoring the Future Project, University of Michigan, 1976-1993.

they smoke fewer cigarettes;[57] this suggests that African Americans consume higher levels of nicotine from each cigarette than do whites. A greater dose of nicotine per cigarette may be explained in part by the smoking of menthol cigarettes, as discussed previously. In addition, this observation is consistent with the generally lower income level of African Americans compared to whites, and an economic pressure to extract more nicotine per cigarette. Cessation rates for African-American adults are lower than for whites, which seems to indicate a higher level of addiction for African Americans.[58] The explanation for the apparent inconsistency between lower current initiation rates but higher levels of addiction in adult African Americans is not clear. Possibly this difference reflects a cohort effect, and in the future fewer adult African Americans will be addicted. Alternatively, it may reflect initiation of cigarette smoking later in life among African Americans compared to whites. Further research is needed to clarify these issues. The use of smokeless tobacco is highest among whites and Native Americans, with relatively low levels among African Americans and

Hispanics.[59] The reasons for ethnic differences in tobacco use among youths are unclear.

Use of Smokeless Tobacco by Children and Youths

Initiation of smokeless tobacco use begins in the preteen and early teen years. In 1991 smokeless tobacco was used by about 11% of high school seniors (table 2-11). The prevalence of smokeless tobacco use varies considerably in different regions of the country, with lowest rates generally in the Northeast, and lower rates in cities than in rural areas. Of note, the prevalence of smokeless tobacco use is greater than that of cigarette smoking by youths in several states, including Alabama, Idaho, South Dakota, Colorado, Wyoming, and Montana. The prevalence of moist snuff tobacco use by youths has risen dramatically, with a 10-fold increase for 16- to 19-year-olds between 1970 and 1985.[60] There was a brief reduction in 1986-87, but sales of smokeless tobacco products are now increasing, with a 70% overall increase in moist snuff sales from 1982 to 1992.[61] Smokeless tobacco is used primarily by males in all ethnic groups except American Indians and Alaskan natives, where the prevalence of use is similar for males and females.

As discussed earlier, nicotine and cotinine concentrations in the blood of adults who use smokeless tobacco are comparable to those measured in smokers. No such data are available for children. Addiction of youths to smokeless tobacco is documented by reports that many users of smokeless tobacco have tried to quit but have been unsuccessful. According to the 1986-1989 Teenage Attitudes and Practices Survey, 21% of current smokeless tobacco users (12- to 18-year-olds) had tried to quit four or more times unsuccessfully, which is consistent with a high level of addiction.[62]

Factors influencing the initiation of smokeless tobacco are in general similar to those that are associated with initiation of cigarette smoking.[63] One difference of note, however, is that smokeless tobacco use has been associated with participation on sponsored athletic teams (for example, baseball, wrestling, football, rodeo), whereas smokers are less likely to participate in such teams. As noted earlier, smokeless tobacco use is a risk factor for cigarette smoking, and vice versa. The exchangeability of tobacco use supports the idea that nicotine addiction can be maintained by tobacco from any source.

NATURE OF TOBACCO PRODUCTS

Nicotine addiction is maintained by use of tobacco, the only significant source of nicotine. Certain teas and vegetables contain low levels of nicotine, but the amounts available are so low that it is impossible to consume pharmacologically active doses of nicotine from sources other than tobacco. Tobacco is smoked as cigarettes, cigars, and in pipes, but can also be used

TABLE 2-11 Percentage of youths who currently (within the past 30 days) use smokeless tobacco

Characteristic	Monitoring the Future Project 1992[a]	Youth Risk Behavior Survey 1991[b]
Overall	11.4	10.5
Gender		
Boys	20.8	19.2
Girls	2.0	1.3
Race/Hispanic origin		
White, non-Hispanic	13.5	13.0
Boys	23.9	23.6
Girls	2.5	1.4
African American, non-Hispanic	2.5	2.1
Boys	5.2	3.6
Girls	0.2	0.7
Hispanic	NA	5.5
Boys	NA	10.7
Girls	NA	0.6
Age		
12–14		
15–16		
17–18		
Grade		
8th	7.0	
9th		9.0
10th	9.6	10.1
11th		12.1
12th	11.4	10.7
Region		
Northeast	8.2	8.8
North Central	12.3	13.3
South	12.5	8.6
West	11.1	10.5

[a]1992 MTFP survey of high school seniors. Based on responses to the question, "How frequently have you taken smokeless tobacco during the past 30 days?" With the exception of data for eighth and tenth grade students, all other data points for the Monitoring the Future Project survey reflect estimates for high school seniors.

[b]Grades 9-12. Based on responses to the question, "During the past 30 days, did you you use chewing tobacco, such as Redman, Levi Garett, or Beechnut, or snuff, such as Skoal, Skoal Bandits, or Copenhagen?"

Source: Centers for Disease Control and Prevention. *Preventing Tobacco Use Among Young People. A Report of the Surgeon General.* Washington, DC: U.S. Department of Health and Human Services, 1994. 98.

without smoking by applying smokeless tobacco directly to mucous membranes. Several types of smokeless tobacco are available—oral snuff, nasal snuff, and chewing tobacco.

Production of Tobacco Products

Tobacco products in the United States are made by blending different types of tobacco leaf, to which sugar and other flavorings are added. Lighter tobaccos, which are found in most American cigarettes, produce acidic smoke when burned. Darker tobaccos, such as are used in cigar and pipe tobacco, produce alkaline smoke. As discussed elsewhere, the pH of the smoke determines the extent to which nicotine will be absorbed through the mouth.

In addition to different types of shredded tobacco leaf, tobacco sheet or reconstituted tobacco is also blended into many cigarettes. Tobacco sheet uses scraps and stems of tobacco as well as various additives, which are combined into a homogeneous mixture that can then be incorporated into tobacco. The manufacturing of tobacco sheet allows for production of a relatively uniform composition of tobacco, since additives can be used to achieve the end product.[64]

Reports have been made of evidence that tobacco manufacturers manipulate the nicotine content of cigarettes.[65] One way in which manufacturers control the nicotine content of tobacco is by extracting the nicotine from the tobacco, then adding it back in controlled amounts as tobacco extract. Tobacco companies also hold patents for spraying nicotine solutions onto cigarette tobacco, although it is unclear if this practice is actually used in the manufacturing of cigarettes. Tobacco manufacturers state that the reason nicotine is extracted and then reapplied to tobacco is that nicotine in the natural tobacco leaf exists in very uneven concentrations. By extracting and re-adding nicotine, it is possible to provide a more consistent tobacco product, which delivers a consistent amount of nicotine. It has also been suggested that the amount of nicotine in tobacco is controlled so as to ensure a level adequate to maintain nicotine addiction. In support of this idea was an internal memorandum, discovered in recent ligitation, from a Phillip Morris Tobacco Company scientist: "The cigarette should be conceived not as a product but as a package. The product is nicotine . . . smoke is beyond question the most optimized vehicle of nicotine and the cigarette is the most optimized dispenser of smoke."[66] That the pharmacologic actions of nicotine are important determinants of why people smoke is supported by research both by the tobacco industry and by non-industry researchers.[67]

In the United States, four primary types of smokeless tobacco are manufactured: loose leaf, plug, twist or roll, and oral snuff.[68] Loose leaf chewing tobacco consists of tobacco leaf that has been heavily treated with licorice and sugars. Plug tobacco is produced from leaves that are immersed in a mixture of licorice and sugar and then pressed into a plug. Twist tobacco is made from leaves that are flavored and twisted to resemble a rope. Oral snuff is available in dry and moist preparations. Dry snuff is powdered tobacco that contains flavor and aroma additives. Moist snuff consists of fine particles of tobacco that contain considerable moisture; many varieties are prepared with flavorings such as wintergreen or mint. The oral use of snuff, called "snuff dipping," involves placing a pinch of the tobacco between the cheek or lips and the gum, or beneath the tongue.

Starter products and distribution of free samples might introduce users to a graduation process of moving from low-nicotine to higher-nicotine snuff products. For example, products low in nicotine and low in pH (which reduces buccal absorption) and products sold in a teabag-like unit dose, would make it easier for first-time users to adapt to snuff products. The use of such low-nicotine-delivery products could be the beginning of a graduated process toward nicotine addiction.

Modifying Cigarette Yields

Tobacco smoke contains more than 4,000 chemicals, many of which are known toxins. Some of the better-known toxins include carbon monoxide, hydrogen cyanide, nitrogen oxides, ammonia, benzene, formaldehyde, nitrosoamines, vinyl chloride, polycyclic hydrocarbons, polonium-210, arsenic, and lead.

Tobacco smoke is an aerosol of droplets containing water, nicotine, and other alkaloids, and tar. Tar is what is left in the particulates after water and alkaloids are removed. Particulates are suspended in a gaseous mixture, which contains carbon monoxide, nitrogen oxides, and other gases.

To estimate the amount of various constituents that smokers are exposed to, cigarettes are routinely tested with a standardized smoking machine test. This test has been referred to as the Federal Trade Commission (FTC) method. The FTC performed and published test results in commercial cigarettes from 1967 until 1985; since that time the tobacco industry has conducted these tests. The FTC test procedure consists of placing a cigarette into a holder and igniting it; then 35-ml puffs are taken via a syringe over 2 seconds, once every minute until the cigarette is burned to a specific butt length. The smoke that is collected is passed through a filter to collect the particulate material (tar and nicotine). The gases that pass through the filter are collected for determination of carbon monoxide and other constituents. Thus, values for yields of tar, nicotine, and carbon monoxide for each cigarette are reported from this type of testing procedure.

Lowering the yields of tar and other toxic constituents of cigarettes smoke makes intuitive sense as a way to reduce the health risks of cigarette smoking. Tobacco companies widely promote cigarettes that are lower in yield, implying a health benefit compared to smoking higher-yield cigarettes. However, the low-yield cigarette concept is in many ways deceptive. To understand why this is so, it is useful to examine how low-yield cigarettes are engineered.

There are several ways in which cigarettes can be engineered to be low-yield by smoking machine tests. The most obvious way is filtration, in which case a filter is placed at the end of the cigarette. This filter can remove a significant amount of tar. In the United States, 95% of cigarettes are filtered. Another way to reduce yields is to reduce the content of nicotine or other toxic substances in tobacco per se. This appears not to be the case with commercial cigarettes. When the nicotine concentration of tobacco in cigarettes of differing yields was measured, it was found that, on average, cigarette tobacco had a nicotine concentration of about 1.6%.[69] There was a significant inverse correlation between concentration of nicotine in tobacco and yield, suggesting that low-yield cigarettes are made with tobacco that contains more, rather than less, nicotine than higher-yield cigarettes. In any case, it is clear that low-yield cigarettes are not low-yield because the contents of nicotine or tar are lower in the tobacco per se. Low-yield cigarettes are engineered to be low-yield based on the standardized smoking machine protocol. This can be done by shortening the cigarette length, increasing the burn rate of the paper, or increasing the length of the filter overwrap so that the machine is able to take fewer puffs before the cigarette is burned to its specified length. Placing less tobacco in each cigarette by using expanded tobacco and/or smaller diameters of cigarettes can also reduce yield. Diluting the mainstream smoke through the use of porous paper or ventilation holes in the filter tipping paper can substantially reduce yields. In the latter case, when the cigarette is inhaled from the tip, considerable room air is drawn in to dilute the tobacco smoke.

Unfortunately, the addicted smoker does not smoke like an FTC smoking machine. Smokers take deeper and more frequent puffs than the machine on average, and can easily alter their smoking behavior as desired. Smokers learn, without realizing what they are doing, that placing their lips or fingers over the cigarette tip improves the draw characteristics of the cigarette. They are actually blocking the ventilation holes so that they are inhaling more tobacco smoke and less room air. Many studies in which the actual intake of nicotine, carbon monoxide, or other constituents of tobacco smoke have been measured in smokers, have shown a very weak relationship, if any, to nominal nicotine yield. Thus, once a smoker becomes addicted to nicotine, he or she can easily adapt smoking behavior to obtain the desired dose of nicotine from any cigarette. Of note, the ultra-low-yield cigarettes (that is, tar less than 1 mg, nicotine less than 0.1 mg) do seem to make it more difficult for smokers to obtain levels of nicotine that they can from high-yield cigarettes.[70] The observation that sales of these ultra-low-yield cigarettes are relatively low suggests that there may be a threshold for nicotine delivery, below which nicotine addiction is not easily maintained. As typically smoked, low-yield cigarettes are not less harmful than higher-yield cigarettes. Because smokers take in much more tar and other toxins than estimated by machine yields, the risk of smoking-caused disease is not significantly reduced by using low-yield cigarettes.

In summary, people smoke cigarettes largely to obtain the nicotine they desire. They do not smoke in a standardized way as do smoking machines, and therefore machines are poor predictors of actual human exposure. Human exposures can be estimated by direct measures of levels of tobacco smoke constituents in biological fluids of smokers. Such markers include nicotine, its metabolite, cotinine, carbon monoxide, adducts of various reactive chemicals to hemoglobin or DNA, and mutagenic activity of the urine.

CONCLUSIONS AND RESEARCH RECOMMENDATIONS

Having reviewed the research literature on nicotine addiction and tobacco use, the committee finds the following conclusions to be warranted:

1. Long-term tobacco use is maintained by addiction to nicotine.

2. Use of any form of tobacco can result in addiction, and smokeless tobacco is becoming an increasingly prevalent behavior among youths. Smokeless tobacco is not a healthful alternative to cigarettes.

3. Once addicted, a person finds it difficult to quit using tobacco.

4. Children and youths begin tobacco use. Youths rapidly become addicted to nicotine; the addiction maintains their tobacco use in adulthood.

5. When youths begin using tobacco, they overestimate the proportion of tobacco use in society, underestimate the addictive nature of tobacco and the risk that they will become addicted over a long term, and underestimate the danger that they will incur tobacco-related disease. Thus, children and youths become addicted to nicotine before they are able to appreciate fully the consequences of their behavior.

6. There is considerable individual variation in susceptibility to nicotine addiction. Environmental, behavioral, personal, socioeconomic, and ethnic factors influence susceptibility to initiation and addiction.

7. The recognition that youths become addicted to nicotine should be incorporated into the design, evaluation, and dissemination of treatment programs for youths to stop tobacco use; as proven strategies emerge, they should be made easily accessible to youths.

8. Among adults the prevalence of cigarette smoking has declined from 1966 to the present. The prevalence of smoking by youths declined through 1980, but subsequently has been stable, except for African-American youths, for whom there has been a sharp decline. The prevalence of smokeless tobacco use by boys has increased steadily for the past 15 years and represents a significant growing addiction to tobacco.

9. Available evidence indicates that cigarette manufacturers control the level of nicotine in cigarettes and the nicotine delivery of their products in deliberate ways. However, "low-yield" cigarettes are not low in nicotine content and do

not in general deliver less nicotine or tar to smokers than do higher-yield cigarettes.

10. Prevention of nicotine addiction among youths is an essential part of any policy for reducing tobacco use in society as a whole. Approaches to prevention can be targeted toward the various factors that initiate and maintain tobacco addiction, as will be discussed in subsequent chapters.

The Committee makes the following recommendations for research on nicotine addiction:

1. Research should be conducted to determine individual susceptibility to nicotine addiction. Particular areas that need research are genetic factors, affective states, and ethnic influences. Such information could facilitate the identification of high-risk children and could lead to more effective prevention strategies.

2. For all forms of tobacco products, research should be conducted on the characteristics of nicotine addiction in the early stages, that is, in the first few years during which the transition between experimental and addictive nicotine use occurs. Such information could contribute to more effective intervention before youth become highly addicted adult tobacco users.

3. Research should be conducted on the relationship between the characteristics of tobacco products and addiction. For example, as a basis in developing regulatory guidelines, it would be useful to know the minimal level of nicotine delivery from a tobacco product at which addiction will develop and/ or be sustained.

REFERENCES

1. Chassin, L., C. C. Presson, S. J. Sherman, and D. A. Edwards. "The Natural History of Cigarette Smoking: Predicting Young-Adult Smoking Outcomes from Adolescent Smoking Patterns." *Health Psychology* 9:6 (1990): 701-716.

2. Tailoi, E., and E. L. Wynder. "Effect of the Age at Which Smoking Begins on Frequency of Smoking in Adulthood." *New England Journal of Medicine* 325:13 (1991): 968-969.

3. Edwards, G., A. Arif, and R. Hadgson. "Nomenclature and Classification of Drug- and Alcohol-Related Problems: A Shortened Version of a WHO Memorandum." *British Journal of Addiction* 77:1 (1982): 3-20.

4. Centers for Disease Control. *The Health Consequences of Smoking: Nicotine Addiction. A Report of the Surgeon General.* USDHHS (CDC) Pub. No. 88-8406. Washington, DC: U.S. Government Printing Office, 1988. 6-17; and Benowitz, Neal L. "Pharmacology of Smokeless Tobacco Use: Nicotine Addiction and Nicotine-Related Health Consequences." In *Smokeless Tobacco or Health. An International Perspective. Smoking and Tobacco Control Monograph 2.* NIH Pub. No. 92-3461. Washington, DC: National Cancer Institute, 1992. 219-228.

5. Gritz, Ellen H., C. R. Carr, and A. C. Marcus. "The Tobacco Withdrawal Syndrome in Unaided Quitters." *British Journal of Addiction* 86:1 (1991): 57-69.

6. Pomerleau, O. F., and C. S. Pomerleau. "Neuroregulators and the Reinforcement of Smoking: Towards a Biobehavioral Explanation." *Neuroscience Biobehavioral Reviews* 8:4 (1984): 503-513.

7. Shiffman, S. "Tobacco 'Chippers'—Individual Differences in Tobacco Dependence." *Psychopharmacology* 97:4 (1989): 539-547.

8. Centers for Disease Control. *Reducing the Health Consequence of Smoking: 25 Years of Progress. A Report of the Surgeon General.* USDHHS Pub. No. (CDC) 89-8411. Washington, DC: General Accounting Office, 1989.

9. Benowitz, Neal L., Sharon M. Hall, Ronald I. Herning, P. Jacob, III, R. T. Jones, and A-L. Osman. "Smokers of Low-Yield Cigarettes Do Not Consume Less Nicotine." *New England Journal of Medicine* 309 (21 July 1983): 139-142; Coultas, D. B., C. A. Stidley, and J. M. Samet. "Cigarette Yields of Tar and Nicotine and Markers of Exposure to Tobacco Smoke." *American Review of Respiratory Disease* 148:2 (1993): 435-440.

10. Benowitz, N. L., Jacob P., L. T. Kozlowski, and L. Yu. "Influence of Smoking Fewer Cigarettes on Exposure to Tar, Nicotine, and Carbon Monoxide." *New England Journal of Medicine* 315:21 (1986): 1310-1313.

11. Marlatt, G. A., and J. R. Gordon. *Relapse Prevention: Maintenance Strategies in the Treatment of Addictive Behaviors.* New York: Guilford Press, 1985.

12. Camp, Diane E., Robert C. Klesges, and George Relyea. "The Relationship Between Body Weight Concerns and Adolescent Smoking." *Health Psychology* 12:1 (1993): 24-32.

13. Boyd, Gayle M., and Elbert D. Glover. "Smokeless Tobacco Use by Youth in the U.S." *Journal of School Health* 59 (1989): 189-194; and Connolly, G. N., D. M. Winn, S. S. Hecht, J. E. Henningfield, B. Walker, Jr., and D. Hoffman. "The Reemergence of Smokeless Tobacco." *New England Journal of Medicine* 314:16 (1986): 1020-1027.

14. Adams, J. D., P. Owens-Tucciarone, and D. Hoffman. "Tobacco-Specific *N*-Nitrosamines in Dry Snuff." *Food and Chemical Toxicology* 25:3 (1987): 245-256.

15. Ernster, Virginia L., D. G. Grady, J. C. Greene, M. Walsh, P. Robertson, T. E. Daniels, N. Benowitz, D. Siegel, B. Gerbert, and W. W. Hauck. "Smokeless Tobacco Use and Health Effects Among Baseball Players." *Journal of the American Medical Association* 264:2 (1990): 218-224; and Connolly, Gregory N., C. T. Orleans, and M. Kogan. "Use of Smokeless Tobacco in Major-League Baseball." *New England Journal of Medicine* 318:19 (1988): 1281-1285.

16. Benowitz, Neal L., H. Porchet, L. Sheiner, and P. Jacob III. "Nicotine Absorption and Cardiovascular Effects with Smokeless Tobacco Use: Comparison to Cigarettes and Nicotine Gum." *Clinical Pharmocology and Therapeutics* 44:1 (1988): 23-28; and Benowitz, Neal L., and P. Jacob. "Daily Intake of Nicotine During Cigarette Smoking." *Clinical Pharmacology and Therapeutics* 35 (1984): 499-504.

17. Severson, Herbert H., Elizabeth G. Eakin, Edward Lichtenstein, and Victor J. Stevens. "The Inside Scoop on the Stuff Called Snuff: An Interview Study of 94 Adult Male Smokeless Tobacco Users." *Journal of Substance Abuse* 2 (1990): 77-85.

18. Ary, Dennis V., Edward Lichtenstein, and Hubert H. Severson. "Smokeless Tobacco Use Among Male Adolescents: Patterns, Correlates, Predictors, and the Use of Other Drugs." *Preventive Medicine* 16 (1987): 385-401.

19. Schroeder, Kathleen L., M. S. Chen, Jr., G. R. Iaderosa, E. D. Glover, and E. W. Edmundson. "Proposed Definition of a Smokeless Tobacco User Based on 'Potential' Nicotine Consumption." *Addictive Behaviors* 13 (1988): 395-400.

20. Fagerström, Karl-Olov. "Measuring Degree of Physical Dependence to Tobacco Smoking with Reference to Individualization of Treatment." *Addictive Behavior* 3 (1978): 235-241.

21. Boyle, Raymond, and H. Severson. *Measuring Dependence in Spit Tobacco Users.* Presentation to American Association of Public Health Dentistry. San Francisco, 4 Nov. 1993.

22. Boyle and Severson.

23. Benowitz, Neal L., P. Jacob, III, and L. Yu. "Daily Use of Smokeless Tobacco: Systemic Effects." *Annals of Internal Medicine* 111:12 (1989): 112-116.

24. Holm, H., M. J. Jarvis, M. A. Russell, and C. Feyerabend. "Nicotine Intake and Dependence in Swedish Snuff Takers." *Psychopharmacology* 108:4 (1992): 507-511.

25. Hatsukami, Dorothy K., S. W. Gust, and R. M. Keenan. "Physiologic and Subjective Changes from Smokeless Tobacco Withdrawal." *Clinical Pharmacology and Therapeutics* 41:1 (1987): 103-107.

26. Holm et al.

27. Benowitz, N. L. "Pharmacology of Smokeless Tobacco Use," 1992.

28. Ary et al., and Dent, C., S. Sussman, A. Johnson, W. Hansen, and B. R. Flay. "Adolescent Smokeless Tobacco Incidence: Relations with Other Drugs and Psychosocial Variables." *Preventive Medicine* 16 (1987): 422-431.

29. Havik, Odd E., and J. G. Maeland. "Changes in Smoking Behavior After a Myocardial Infarction." *Health Psychology* 7:5 (1988): 403-420.

30. Hunt, William A., L. W. Barnett, and L. G. Branch. "Relapse Rates in Addiction Programs." *Journal of Clinical Psychology* 27:4 (1971): 455-456.

31. Kottke, Thomas E., M. L. Brekke, L. I. Solberg, and J. R. Hughes. "A Randomized Trial to Increase Smoking Intervention by Physicians. Doctors Helping Smokers, Round 1." *Journal of the American Medical Association* 261:14 (1989): 2101-2106.

32. Hughes, John R., S. B. Gulliver, J. W. Fenwick, et al. "Smoking Cessation Among Self-Quitters." *Health Psychology* 11:5 (1992): 331-334.

33. Kozlowski, Lynn T., A. Wilkinson, W. Skinner, C. Kent, T. Franklin, M. Pope. "Comparing Tobacco Cigarette Dependence with Other Drug Dependencies: Greater or Equal 'Difficulty Quitting' and 'Urges to Use,' but Less 'Pleasure' from Cigarettes." *Journal of the American Medical Association* 261:6 (1989): 896-901.

34. Hughes, John R., and Dorothy Hatsukami. "Signs and Symptoms of Tobacco Withdrawal." *Archives of General Psychiatry* 43 (March 1986): 289.

35. Hughes, John R. "Dependence Potential and Abuse Liability of Nicotine Replacement Therapies." In O. F. Pomerleau and C. S. Pomerleau, eds. *Progress in Clinical and Biological Research: Nicotine Replacement: A Critical Evaluation.* New York: Alan R. Liss, 1988. 261-277; and Hajek, Peter, P. Jackson, M. Belcher. "Long-Term Use of Nicotine Chewing Gum: Occurrence, Determinants, and Effect on Weight Gain," *Journal of the American Medical Association* 260:11 (1988): 1593-1596.

36. Russell, M. A. H. "The Nicotine Addiction Trap: A 40-Year Sentence for Four Cigarettes." *British Journal of Addiction* 85:2 (1990): 293-300.

37. McNeill, Ann D., M. J. Jarvis, J. A. Stapleton, R. J. West, and A. Bryant. "Nicotine Intake in Young Smokers: Longitudinal Study of Saliva Cotinine Concentrations." *American Journal of Public Health* 79:2 (1989): 172-175.

38. Flay, Brian R., Judith Ockene, and Ira B. Tager. "Smoking: Epidemiology, Cessation, and Prevention." *CHEST* 102:3 (1992): 277S-301S.

39. McNeill et al., 1989.

40. McNeill, Ann D., Martin Jarvis, and Robert West. "Subjective Effects of Cigarette Smoking in Adolescents." *Psychopharmacology* 92:1 (1987): 115-117.

41. McNeill, Ann D., Robert J. West, Martin Jarvis, Paul Jackson, and Andrew Bryant. "Cigarette Withdrawal Symptoms in Adolescent Smokers." *Psychopharmacology* 90 (1986): 533-536.

42. Townsend, J., H. Wilkes, A. Haines, and M. Jarvis. "Adolescent Smokers Seen in General Practice: Health, Lifestyle, Physical Measurements, and Response to Antismoking Advice." *British Medical Journal* 303 (1991): 947-950.

43. Stone, S. L., and J. L. Kristeller. "Attitudes of Adolescents Toward Smoking Cessation." *American Journal of Preventive Medicine* 8:4 (1992): 221-225.

44. Centers for Disease Control and Prevention. *Preventing Tobacco Use Among Young People. A Report of the Surgeon General.* Washington, DC: U.S. Department of Health and Human Services, 1994. 78.

45. *Ibid.*, 84.

46. Ershler, J., H. Leventhal, Fleming R., and K. Glynn. "The Quitting Experience for Smokers

in Sixth Through Twelfth Grades." *Addictive Behaviors* 14:4 (1989): 365-378; and Ary, Dennis V., and A. Biglan. "Longitudinal Changes in Adolescent Cigarette Smoking Behavior: Onset and Cessation." *Journal of Behavioral Medicine* 11:4 (1988): 361-382.

47. Centers for Disease Control and Prevention. *Preventing Tobacco Use,* 123.

48. Perry, Cheryl L., and G. L. Silvis. "Smoking Prevention: Behavioral Prescriptions for the Pediatrician." *Pediatrics* 79:5 (1987): 790-799; van Teijlingen, Edwin, and J. A. Friend. "Children and Smoking: The Problem and the Way Forward." *Thorax* 47:7 (1992): 485-488; and Centers for Disease Control and Prevention, *Preventing Tobacco Use,* 123-146.

49. Glassman, A. H., J. E. Helzer, L. S. Covey, L. B. Cottler, F. Stetner, J. E. Tipp, and J. Johnson. "Smoking, Smoking Cessation, and Major Depression." *Journal of the American Medical Association* 254:12 (1990): 1546-1549; Anda, R. F., D. F. Williamson, L. G. Escobedo, E. E. Mast, G. A. Giovino, and P. L. Remington. "Depresssion and the Dynamics of Smoking: A National Perspective." *Journal of the American Medical Association* 264:12 (1990): 1541-1545; and Breslau, Naomi, Marlyne Kilbey, and Patricia Andreski. "Nicotine Dependence, Major Depression, and Anxiety in Young Adults." *Archives of General Psychiatry* 48 (1991): 1069-1074.

50. Hirschman, Robert S., H. Leventhal, and K. Glynn. "The Development of Smoking Behavior: Conceptualization and Supportive Cross-Sectional Survey Data." *Journal of Applied Social Psychology* 14:3 (1984): 184-206.

51. Carmelli, D., G. E. Swann, D. Robinette, and R. Fabsitz. "Genetic Influence on Smoking—A Study of Male Twins." *New England Journal of Medicine* 327:12 (1992): 829-833.

52. Swan, G. E., D. Carmelli, R. H. Rosenman, R. R. Fabsitz, and J. C. Christian. "Smoking and Alcohol Consumption in Adult Male Twins: Genetic Heritability and Shared Environmental Influences." *Journal of Substance Abuse* 2:1 (1990): 39-50.

53. Hirschman et al.

54. Johnston, Lloyd D., P. M. O'Malley, and Jerald G. Bachman. *Smoking, Drinking, and Illicit Drug Use Among American Secondary School Students, College Students, and Young Adults, 1975-1991. Volume I, Secondary School Students.* NIH Pub. No. 93-3480 Washington, DC: National Institute on Drug Abuse, 1992. 64.

55. Johnston, Lloyd D., P. M. O'Malley, and Jerald G. Bachman. *Monitoring the Future Project.* Institute for Social Research. University of Michigan, 1994. Unpublished data.

56. Robinson, Robert G., Michael Pertschuk, and Charyn Sutton. "Smoking and African Americans." In Samuels, Robert G., Michael Pertschuk, and Charyn Sutton. eds. *Improving the Health of the Poor: Strategies for Prevention.* Menlo Park, CA: Henry J. Kaiser Family Foundation, May 1992. 131.

57. Wagenknecht, L. E., G. R. Cutter, N. J. Haley, S. Sidney, T. A. Manolio, G. H. Hughes, and D. R. Jacobs. "Racial Differences in Serum Cotinine Levels among Smokers in the Coronary Artery Risk Development in (Young) Adults Study." *American Journal of Public Health* 80:9 (1990): 1053-1056.

58. Centers for Disease Control. "Smoking Cessation During Previous Year Among Adults—United States, 1990 and 1991." *Morbidity and Mortality Weekly Report* 42:26 (1993): 504-507.

59. Schinke, S. P., R. F. Schilling, II, L. D. Gilchrist, M. R. Ashby, and E. Kitajima. "Native Youth and Smokeless Tobacco: Prevalence Rates, Gender Differences, and Descriptive Characteristics." *NCI Monographs* 8 (1989): 39-42; and Centers for Disease Control and Prevention, *Preventing Tobacco Use,* 97.

60. Marcus, Alfred C., L. A. Crane, D. R. Shopland, and W. R. Lynn. "Use of Smokeless Tobacco in the United States: Recent Estimates from the Current Population Survey." *Smokeless Tobacco Use in the United States. NCI Monographs* 8 (1989): 17-23.

61. Sullivan, Louis W. "Keynote Address." In *Smokeless Tobacco or Health: An International Perspective.* Smoking and Tobacco Control Monograph 2. NIH Pub. No. 92-3461. National Cancer Institute, 1992. iv.

62. Centers for Disease Control and Prevention. *Preventing Tobacco Use.* 101.

63. Jones, Rhys B., and D. Paul Moberg. "Correlates of Smokeless Tobacco Use in a Male Adolescent Population." *American Journal of Public Health* 78:1 (1988): 61-63.

64. Slade, John. "Nicotine Delivery Devices." In C. Orleans and J. Slade, eds. *Nicotine Addiction: Principles and Management.* New York: Oxford University Press, 1993. 6.

65. American Broadcasting Corporation. *Day One.* February 28, 1994; and Slade, *ibid.*

66. *Cipollone v. Ligget Group, Inc.* 112 S. Ct. 2608 (1992).

67. Robinson, J. H., W. S. Pritchard, and R. A. Davis. "Psychopharmacological Effects of Smoking a Cigarette with Typical Tar and Carbon Monoxide Yields But Minimal Nicotine." *Psychopharmacology* 108:4 (1992): 166-172; Robinson, J. H., and W. S. Pritchard. "The Role of Nicotine in Tobacco Use." *Psychopharmacology* 108:4 (1992): 397-407; and Centers for Disease Control. *The Health Consequences,* 1988.

68. Brunnemann, Klaus D., and Dietrich Hoffman. "Chemical Composition of Smokeless Tobacco Products." In *Smokeless Tobacco or Health: An International Perspective.* NIH Pub. No. 92-3461. Washington, DC: National Cancer Institute, 1992. 96.

69. Benowitz et al., 1983.

70. Benowitz, Neal L., P. Jacob, III, L. Yu, R. Talcott, S. Hall, and R. T. Jones. "Reduced Tar, Nicotine, and Carbon Monoxide Exposure While Smoking Ultralow—but Not Low-Yield Cigarettes." *Journal of the American Medical Association* 256:2 (1986): 241-246.

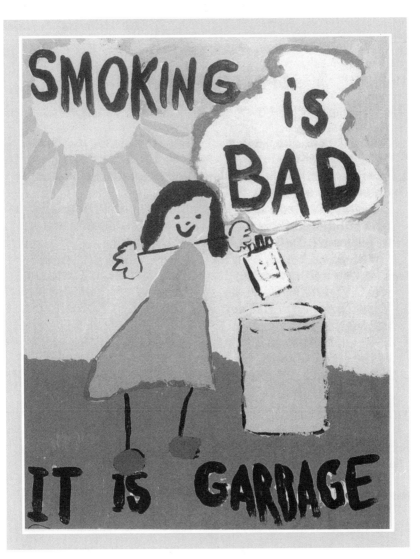

Erin Fels, P.S. 52, Brooklyn

CONTENTS

3 | SOCIAL NORMS AND THE ACCEPTABILITY OF TOBACCO USE

Tobacco use is a learned and socially mediated behavior. Experimenting with tobacco is attractive to children and youths because of associations they learn to make between tobacco use and the kind of social identity they wish to establish. Repeated and ubiquitous messages reinforcing the positive attributes of tobacco use give youths the impression that tobacco use is pervasive, normative in many social contexts, and socially acceptable among people they aspire to be like. Youths are led to believe that tobacco consumption is a social norm among attractive, vital, successful people who seek to express their individuality, who enjoy life, and who are socially secure. Several factors are involved in maintaining this impression among youths and in fostering tobacco use as a social norm at a time when public health messages are calling attention to the serious health risks associated with tobacco consumption. These factors will be highlighted in this chapter, and attention will also be called to a growing, largely local, movement calling for the exercise of greater social responsibility in the reduction of environmental cues that reinforce tobacco use in public spaces frequented by children and youths. At issue is an ecology of representations, ideas, images, cues, and the like, that foster tobacco use as normative behavior.

THE FUNCTION OF SOCIAL NORMS

The term "norms" has a broad range of meaning, with very specific connotations applied in the social sciences. In general, however, and for the purposes of discussion in this report, social norms are at once descriptive, that is, normative in a statistical sense denoting majority approval, and prescriptive, that is, guidelines for acceptable behavior associated with sociocultural values. Norms are maintained both by social reinforcements and social sanctions. A social learning analysis of tobacco use takes into account the different types of social reinforcement that coincide with the development of tobacco use from experimentation to initiation to maintenance of regular use. Experimentation typically occurs under conditions of peer reinforcement; usually the initial inhalation of smoke is aversive but eventually the youth develops a tolerance to it. In other words, the adolescent "learns" in a peer context that tobacco use is an acceptable or desirable behavior, despite initial negative physiological reactions. Continued use produces pharmacologic reinforcement to sustain the behavior independent of social reinforcement. The behavior then occurs in different situations, where new learning takes place. The young smoker discriminates between situations in which smoking is socially acceptable or unacceptable. At the same time, various environmental or situational cues, such as an ashtray, or an empty cigarette pack, or a party, not only can suggest acceptability but can also stimulate physiological responses that reinforce the addiction to nicotine.[1] Hence, whereas the addictive power of nicotine drives a person to use tobacco regularly and to maintain that regular use, it is the power of these perceived social norms that persuades children and youths to experiment with and initiate use of tobacco.

The development of these perceived norms among children and youths is influenced by pervasive images and messages of everyday life. These messages come from numerous sources: friends, peers, family, school, the workplace, church, films, magazines, radio and television, billboards, electronic media, advertisements, sports events, arts performances, and so on. These messages typically have a prescriptive influence on social norms; in other words, in addition to characterizing what members of society do, they suggest to people what they *should* do. As standards set by a society or social group, norms define the boundaries of behavior; they dictate etiquette, protocol, and a sense of what is normal, natural, expected, and acceptable in given contexts. Because the norms of society are in large part prescribed through public sources, they are subject to the influence of interest groups that seek to legitimize an agenda and to engineer behavior.

Social groups are influenced by, but do not passively accept, prescribed norms. They mark their identity by selectively adopting and appropriating behaviors and images that take on meaning in opposition to behaviors and images adopted by other groups. Markers of group identity and conventions of group membership are not fixed, but rather change over time. Images associated with tobacco use are not stable, if not reinforced.

For adolescents, norms are particularly complex, for two reasons. First, adolescence is a transitional period "shaped by prior development in childhood and the future requirements of adulthood, as well as by current expectations and opportunities."[2] Second, adolescence itself is a complex developmental period, marked by physiological, emotional, and psychological changes. Adolescents are establishing their sense of self and redefining themselves socially in the contexts of family, peers, school, the workplace, and the local community.[3] Parents and peers contribute in different ways to the development of adolescents' values. Adolescents tend to hold values similar to those of their parents regarding education, religion, and work, but are more similar to their peers in aspects of adolescent culture, such as music and appearance.[4] Peers find security, identity, and a sense of wellness by constructing peer groups and group norms dictating valued behaviors.[5] These behaviors have more potency if they are also perceived as normative for adults, yet not acceptable for children.[6] If an adolescent perceives a specific behavior, such as drinking alcohol or using tobacco, to be normative in the peer group, he or she might adopt the behavior in order to belong to the group or to feel relaxed when with the group.

In developing peer norms, adolescents look to the greater social environment for concepts of adult identity, particularly in the behavior of leaders, heroes, and film stars, and in the media. Messages, especially repeated messages, that associate behaviors with maturity, peer approval, and independence tend to be the most influential. An overabundance of such messages in relation to a given behavior can result in a youth's misperception of how pervasive the behavior actually is. Misperception of the pervasiveness of tobacco use can be a powerful influence on behavior.

What are the current norms regarding tobacco use? How do social norms influence, or make children and youths susceptible to adopting, tobacco use? How can actions by parents, social groups, and communities set and reinforce social norms and thereby prevent the initiation of tobacco use by children and youths?

THE EMERGING TOBACCO-FREE NORM

The Decline of Tobacco Use

A useful scientific descriptor of the pervasiveness of behaviors is statistical trend data, which describe patterns of behavior with information obtained in an objective manner through surveys. A review of trend data on tobacco use reveals that currently the norm for three-quarters of the population in the United States is *non-use* of tobacco. The survey data describe the overall decrease in smoking prevalence in the general population from 40% in 1965 to 26% from 1990 to 1992.[7] In the military, prevalence of any smoking decreased from 51% in 1980 to 35% in 1992; the prevalence of heavy smoking (one or more packs per day) decreased from 34% in 1980 to 18% in 1992.[8] Among high school seniors, the prevalence of daily smoking was 29% in 1976, 21% in 1980, 17% in 1992, and 19% in 1993.[9]

Youths and adults alike want to quit using tobacco. A 1993 national Gallup poll reported that 76% of adult smokers have tried to quit smoking. Despite past failures, 73% believe that they will be nonsmokers within 5 years, and 30% were trying to quit at the time of the survey.[10] Similarly, in a 1994 *USA Today*/CNN Gallup poll, 70% of smokers expressed interest in quitting; 48% had tried to do so but failed. About the same percentage (76%) of adolescent girls (smokers and ex-smokers) in the Teen Lifestyle Study had attempted to quit.[11] Two large national surveys of teens also reveal that youths want to and try to quit. The 1989 TAPS (Teenage Attitudes and Practices Survey) data show that 74% of 12-through 18-year-old smokers had seriously thought about quitting; 64% had tried at some time to stop smoking and 49% had tried during the preceding 6 months (figure 3-1).[12] The Monitoring the Future Project data show that nearly half of smokers who were seniors in high school between 1976 and 1989 wanted to quit, and about 40% had tried unsuccessfully to do so.[13]

As discussed above, social norms vary among groups, and the trend data describe a variety of tobacco use patterns in different groups identified by gender, ethnicity, and socioeconomic status. Knowing what the trends are for specific groups is important in determining what the social norms are perceived to be, and what factors may reinforce tobacco use, so that counter-strategies can be developed and implemented. For example, important racial/ethnic differences in cigarette smoking have become apparent among high school seniors during the

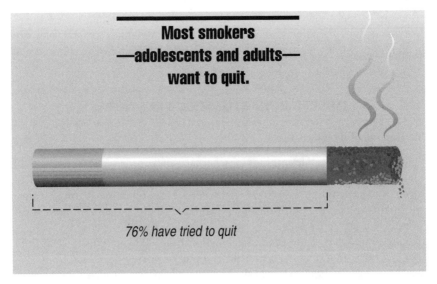

FIGURE 3-1   Sources: Nichter, Mark, Mimi Nichter, C. Ritenbaugh, and N. Buckovic. *The Teen Lifestyle Project: Preliminary Report.* Tucson: University of Arizona. 1994 (unpublished); and SmithKline Beecham. *Gallup Report: A National Survey of Americans Who Smoke.* New York, 1993.

life of the Monitoring the Future Project. In the late 1970s three student ethnic groups—non-Hispanic whites, African Americans, and Hispanics—had fairly similar smoking rates; all three mirrored the general decline in adult smoking from 1977 to 1981. Since 1981, however, a considerable divergence has emerged: smoking rates have declined very little for non-Hispanic white and Hispanic youths, but the rates for African-American youths have continued to decline steadily. As a result, in 1992, the smoking rates for African-American students were about one-fifth to one-third of those for white students; specifically, for African-American high school seniors, the prevalence of daily cigarette smoking reported is 4%, whereas for non-Hispanic whites it is 21%.[14] Currently, there is no explanation for this difference. Data from the Monitoring the Future Project also reveal a striking difference between levels of education and amount of cigarettes smoked daily. For example, smoking half a pack or more a day is nearly three times as prevalent among the noncollege-bound youths (19% versus 7%) and these differences persist after high school.[15]

What little information is available on the smoking habits of American-Indian groups shows large regional and tribal variations. For instance, one study found tobacco use to be very high among girls, and daily cigarette smoking higher among girls than among boys, after the seventh grade. Daily cigarette smoking rose from 8.9% for girls and 8.1% for boys in junior high to 17.8% and 15.0%, respectively, for high school students. Elsewhere rates of about 20% were reported for regular smoking among American-Indian youths, and the rates seem to be increasing.[16]

It is clear that the use of smokeless tobacco by young American Indians and Alaskan Natives, boys and girls, is higher than by any other ethnic group. In studies of communities, weekly use of smokeless tobacco by boys was 43% and by girls 34%.[17] Furthermore, a study found rates of occasional use of smokeless tobacco by American Indians to be astonishingly high among the *very* young: 74% of girls and 90% of boys who reported weekly use of smokeless tobacco began using it before the age of 10.[18] Other studies have documented that American-Indian children may initiate smokeless tobacco use before kindergarten.[19]

What are the reasons behind this diversity in tobacco use among the various age, gender, and ethnic groups? Why are some members of the population more susceptible to becoming addicted to this health risk? No clear answers have emerged. Several studies have shown that perceptions of vulnerability vary with ethnicity and that African-American and Hispanic adolescents feel more susceptible than their white peers to a variety of health outcomes, including cancer, AIDS, and pregnancy.[20] One study found that differences in perceived vulnerability are a function of knowledge.[21] Youths acquire knowledge through many cultural social systems, systems that also can convey erroneous impressions of the trends in tobacco use, as described in the section below.

The military services historically have reinforced a pro-tobacco norm, and had a smoking prevalence about 10% higher than that in the general population. Cigarettes have traditionally been cheaper in commissaries and post exchanges than in retail outlets, and cigarettes were distributed free to the troops during wartime. A high prevalence of tobacco use continued after World War II, and in 1980 was 51% for military men. (This finding was followed by a Department of Defense (DoD) memorandum requesting that an intensive antismoking campaign be carried out at all levels of DoD.)[22] Studies by the Naval Health Research Center found that young men between the ages of 18 and 24 entering the Navy in 1986 smoked at the same rate (28%) as civilians of that age group, but that one year later the same group of naval recruits had a smoking rate of 41%.[23] The reasons given for the smoking initiation were "curiosity" and "friends smoking." The researchers conclude that social factors may have a fairly strong influence on smoking behavior of new Navy personnel, especially given that the Navy encourages cohesiveness and uniformity. Fortunately, in the past few years, the prescribed norm for the military has been a tobacco-free environment, and research studies have shown that prevention interventions can be successful in reducing the percentage of recruits who take up smoking.

The Social Unacceptability of Tobacco Use

The social unacceptability of tobacco use throughout society in the United States is anchored in changing attitudes toward health and personal responsibility:

> The contemporary place of the cigarette in American life is a distant shout from its accepted position in the 1950s. Despite the opposition of the tobacco industry, the public health campaigns of the past three decades have brought about a remarkable change in attitudes and meanings toward smoking. The health movement has produced a cultural shift in the meaning of health and patterns of living that would have seemed impossible 30 years ago.[24]

The emergent tobacco-free norm reflects two distinct links between personal responsibility and health. First and least controversial is the idea that it is socially, and perhaps morally, irresponsible to expose nonsmokers to the risks of disease associated with environmental tobacco smoke (ETS). In the wake of the 1993 report of the Environmental Protection Agency confirming the harmful effects of ETS, public support for laws and policies guaranteeing smoke-free environments is now nearly universal among nonsmokers, and even very high among smokers. In a recent Gallup poll of smokers, 42% of smokers said that nonsmokers' rights in public places should supersede smokers' rights.[25] In a national poll of U.S. voters, 72% of voters believe that second-hand smoke can give nonsmokers cancer and other serious diseases, and 64% favored banning smoking in all public places, such as restaurants, stores, and government buildings.[26] The apparently high level of compliance with public smoking restrictions reflects a widespread acceptance of both the norm favoring smoke-free environments and of its legitimacy. Indeed a norm of civility—obligating a smoker to request permission of nonsmokers to light up and enabling companions and social hosts to deny permission—has taken root throughout society.[27]

The second concept about health and personal responsibility underlying the emerging tobacco-free norms is that exposing one's own health to the risk of diseases, including tobacco-related diseases, is itself socially unacceptable. This attitude reflects a marked shift from the traditional libertarian intuition that tobacco use (or other personal risk-taking) is "no one else's business." It now seems that tobacco use, just as other health-related behaviors, is seen as "everyone's business" because the costs of tobacco-related disease are borne by the whole society.[28] In general, the public seems to have accepted the idea that unhealthy personal choices are of public concern. This attitude is associated with widespread acceptance of the legitimacy of public policies aimed at discouraging people from using tobacco, particularly through taxes that require tobacco users to absorb the social costs of their unhealthy choices.

Thus, the emerging tobacco-free norm has two underlying values. First, no one should be exposed to tobacco smoke, because it puts everyone exposed to it at risk; therefore the environment should be smoke-free. People who smoke should do so only in environments that protect others from exposure, for example, in areas with separate ventilation systems. Second, because the aggregate effects of tobacco-related health consequences affect everyone, society as a whole has an interest in discouraging tobacco use and in supporting the efforts of people who are trying to stop using tobacco. This means instilling and supporting the idea that to stop using tobacco is "the right thing to do."

TOBACCO USE AS PERCEIVED BY CHILDREN AND YOUTHS

Increasingly, through a variety of channels, the message is being conveyed that tobacco is not used by the majority of people and that it is not socially acceptable. The public health values underlying this tobacco-free norm are steadily growing stronger and are being articulated more emphatically. Nevertheless, youths do not perceive the norm to be tobacco-free; rather, they commonly overestimate the percentage of their peers and adults who use tobacco.

The Perception of Tobacco Use

In an interview study of 895 urban children and youths, the respondents greatly overestimated the prevalence of adult and peer smoking. The mean estimate for adult smoking was 66% at a time when 30% of adults were cigarette smokers. Estimates of peer smoking were about double the real figure by students in high school and higher by students in grade school.[29] Other studies show similar results. Findings from the 3-year (1990-1992) Teen Lifestyle Project reveal that, although only 5% of adolescent girls in a Tucson sample smoked regularly and another 20% smoked only occasionally or only at parties, 31% of their peers thought that 51-75% of girls at their school smoked and another 10% thought that 75-90% smoked. The estimates about percentages of boys who smoke were similar, as they were for adult men and women. For example, 28% thought that 51-75% of women were smokers and 15% thought that 75-90% were smokers.[30] A study of over 200 adolescents in Michigan found that youths' perceptions of the prevalence of smoking were "highly inaccurate": 79% of the youths thought that over half of all adults smoke and 68% thought that over half of all teens smoke.[31]

Adolescents who smoke overestimate smoking prevalence by a greater margin than do nonsmokers. A study of 5,351 sixth to twelfth graders from a midwestern and a southwestern community found that adolescents who smoked estimated significantly higher numbers of smokers than did adolescents who did not smoke (table 3-1). For example, middle school students who smoke estimated that 48.9% of boys smoke, whereas nonsmokers estimated that 27.2% of boys smoke, a difference of 21.7%. Smokers estimated that 66.8% of men smoke, whereas nonsmokers estimated 56.5%.[32] Similarly, a study of 5,610 students from the Los Angeles area found that students in the eighth and ninth grades greatly overestimate the number of adolescents and adults who smoke regularly. Adolescent smokers who were regular smokers made the greatest

TABLE 3-1 Estimates by youths of the percentage of boys, girls, men, and women who smoke

| | Middle school students | | | | High school students | | | |
	Boys	Girls	Men	Women	Boys	Girls	Men	Women
Midwest Sample								
Nonsmokers	27.2	21.3	56.5	50.9	38.3	34.5	50.8	47.6
Smokers	48.9	41.8	66.8	58.1	50.6	44.7	60.1	54.2
Smoker-nonsmoker difference	21.7^c	20.5^c	10.3^c	7.2^c	12.3^c	10.2^c	9.3^c	6.6^c
Southwest Sample								
Nonsmokers	34.4	26.6	60.6	55.2	44.7	43.0	59.6	56.1
Smokers	49.0	47.1	68.7	64.3	48.6	48.0	63.5	57.5
Smokers-nonsmoker difference	14.6^c	20.5^c	8.1^a	9.1^b	3.9	5.0^a	3.9	1.4

^{a}p < .05; ^{b}p < .01; ^{c}p < .001.

Source: Sherman, Steven J., Clark C. Presson, Laurie Chassin, Eric Corty, and Richard Olshavsky. "The False Consensus Effect in Estimates of Smoking Prevalence: Underlying Mechanisms." *Personality and Social Psychology Bulletin* 9:2 (1983): 201.

overestimates. Whereas in fact 9% and 12% of eighth and ninth graders, respectively, were regular smokers, students who were regular smokers estimated that 55% smoke regularly. Whereas 33% of adults were smokers at that time (1981 Los Angeles data), the students who were regular smokers estimated the figure to be 66-70% (figure 3-2). Interestingly, nonsmokers *under*estimated the percentage of adolescents who have ever tried smoking, whereas regular smokers

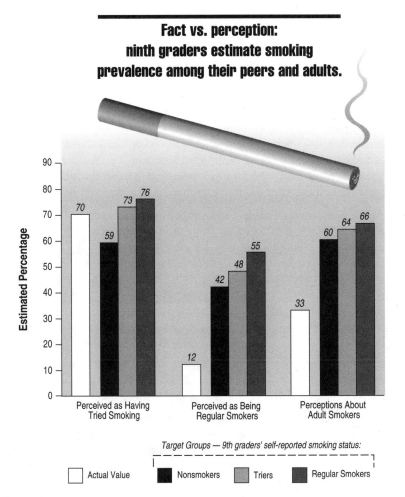

FIGURE 3-2 Fact: 12% of 9th graders are regular smokers. Perception: 9th graders who are regular smokers estimate that 55% of their peers are also regular smokers. Source: Adapted from Sussman, S., C. W. Dent, J. Mestel-Rauch, et al. "Adolescent Nonsmokers, Triers, and Regular Smokers' Estimates of Cigarette Smoking Prevalence: When Do Overestimations Occur and by Whom?" *Journal of Applied Psychology* 18(7) (1988): 542-543.

overestimated the percentage by 6-9%. In addition, the study found that inflated estimates, relative to the adolescent's stage of smoking development, were significantly associated with future onset of smoking. The researchers concluded that "the provision of accurate norms regarding regular smoking by adolescents and adults might be extremely beneficial to prevention efforts."[33] In fact, overestimating smoking prevalence is one of the strongest predictors of smoking initiation.[34]

Spreading a False Impression: The Ubiquitous Pro-Tobacco Message

The misperception of youths that the large majority of peers and adults use tobacco may well derive from the near-constant exposure youths experience to pro-tobacco messages and images, which make tobacco use seem common. (See chapter 4 on advertising for a full discussion.) Pro-tobacco messages are ubiquitous in the American environment. Children walking home from schools see billboards in their neighborhoods promoting tobacco products (figure 3-3). Children themselves become walking billboards by wearing t-shirts, caps, and other clothing items that display tobacco logos. Children watch film and sports stars smoke and chew tobacco products. They read magazines with ads that either

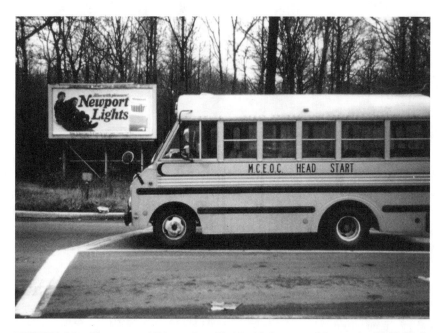

FIGURE 3-3 The young children who will ride this bus to and from school will likely be exposed to a number of tobacco advertisements along the way. Source: Courtesy of John Slade.

directly or indirectly promote tobacco products. They eat in restaurants that permit tobacco use. They frequent and linger in shopping malls where tobacco use is permitted. Many even attend schools where smoking is permitted on the grounds and where teachers smoke even if the students are prohibited from smoking. Youths attend cultural events, such as music concerts, and sporting events, such as rodeos and car racing, either sponsored by the tobacco industry or where billboards, scoreboards, or contestants display tobacco logos. Furthermore, tobacco products are displayed in many stores frequented by youths and are easily purchased by youths. As a result, children learn early and erroneously that tobacco use is widespread and acceptable, especially as an adult behavior.

The primary concept conveyed by the multitude of pro-tobacco messages is that there are benefits to using tobacco. The repetition of these messages reinforces the perception of benefits, and that perception influences youths, making them susceptible to tobacco use. The importance of the perceived benefits of smoking as a predictor of susceptibility to smoking was examined in a study of teen smoking in California. That study defined "susceptibility" as "the absence of a determined decision not to smoke in the future."[35] In surveys conducted in 1990 and 1992, adolescents were asked if they believed that smoking helps people when they are *bored*, helps them *relax*, helps people feel more *comfortable at parties* and in other social situations, and helps them keep their *weight down*. The findings were as follows:

1. In each year, over 40% of adolescents felt that smoking helped people socialize; over 30% felt that it helped people relax. The benefit least endorsed by teenagers related to weight control, with percentages at about 16%.

2. In each year, only one-third of adolescents did not perceive that smoking provided any of these benefits.

3. One-quarter of adolescents reported one benefit of smoking, 30% reported two or three benefits, and 12% reported four or five benefits.

4. Adolescents who were 12-13 years old were just as likely to perceive benefits of smoking as those who were 16-17 years old. This result suggests that the belief that smoking has utility is established before the adolescent years.[36]

The belief that there are benefits to smoking was a major predictor of both susceptibility and smoking in the last month in the 1990 and 1992 surveys. The univariate statistics from the 1992 survey indicate that, of those who did not perceive any of these benefits, 24% were susceptible to smoking; of those who perceived one benefit, 38% were susceptible to smoking; of those who perceived two benefits, 41% were susceptible; and of those who perceived three or more benefits, 57% were susceptible. In cross-sectional analyses of the 1992 survey data, the proportion of susceptible youth who experimented with cigarettes rose dramatically with age (14% of 12-year-olds versus 90% of 19-year-olds) compared to experimentation among those not susceptible (5% of 12-year-olds versus about 25% of 19-year-olds). The investigators conclude that, "these data suggest that the susceptibility measure includes adolescents who may smoke in the future but have not yet tried a cigarette."[37]

The five most commonly presented "benefits" (discussed in more detail in chapter 4 on advertising) are presented as image messages in advertising:

1. Tobacco use is a rite of passage to adulthood.
2. Successful, attractive people use tobacco.
3. Tobacco use is normal.
4. Tobacco use is safe and healthful.
5. Tobacco use is relaxing in social situations.

In the Teen Lifestyle Study, about half of those adolescents who smoked said that they started smoking because they had stress in their lives and they thought that smoking would be relaxing. Over half of them smoke when they are with friends.[38] In another study, to determine the power of image messages in reinforcing tobacco use, Pierce and colleagues related trends in smoking initiation to the sales of leading cigarette brands targeted to women in advertisements from 1944 through the mid-1980s. The analysis revealed gender-specific relationships with the tobacco advertising campaigns that targeted women and were launched in 1967.[39] (See chapter 4 for details.)

A common practice of the tobacco industry, which has the effect of infusing society with pro-tobacco messages, is to sponsor or cosponsor cultural events. This sponsorship not only provides an opportunity for direct marketing to specific market segments but also creates a dependency on the industry for continuation of such events. For example, Philip Morris Inc. has sponsored performances of the Alvin Ailey Dance Theatre and a photographic exhibit of the late Dr. Martin Luther King, Jr. R.J. Reynolds Tobacco Co. and United States Tobacco sponsor Hispanic street fairs and festivals, such as Cinco de Mayo celebrations. Brown and Williamson Tobacco Corp. presents "Kool Achiever" awards to persons who want to improve the "quality of life in inner-city communities" and has enlisted the National Urban League, the NAACP, and the National Newspaper Publishers Association in the nominating process. Contributions to African-American groups by Philip Morris and R.J. Reynolds in 1987 totalled $4.3 million.[40]

The ubiquity of the pro-tobacco message is an important influence on youths' desire to experiment with and to continue using tobacco products. The pro-tobacco environment leads youths to misperceive tobacco use as the public norm and to interfere with youths' perception of the serious, mortal consequences of tobacco use. The appropriate preventive public health approach, therefore, and the most effective approach given the large numbers of individuals involved and the variations in their group characteristics, is to change the environment or social context so that it fosters and reinforces the majority's value of a tobacco-free norm. We must also correct misperceptions of the pervasiveness of tobacco use. As mentioned in chapter 4 on advertising, one important approach for competing against the pro-tobacco messages is an aggressive, ongoing counter-tobacco advertising campaign that promotes and reinforces the tobacco-free norm and presents its benefits.

OPPORTUNITIES FOR PROMOTING A TOBACCO-FREE NORM

Establishing a tobacco-free norm clearly and strongly in the lives of children and youths requires measures to counter all sources of pro-tobacco messages to which youths are exposed. The environmental conditions that reinforce tobacco use must be either eliminated or rendered ineffectual. Efforts to make the tobacco-free norm highly visible and ubiquitous must be persistent and continuous.

Messages countering pro-tobacco messages and images must be as pervasive and frequent and as imaginative as the pro-tobacco messages themselves. Counter-tobacco advertising through media-based approaches has included anti-smoking messages in newspapers and on television and radio broadcasts. Typically these take the form of brief announcements but also occasionally are developed as special programs and curricula. Mass-media messages were included in early smoking prevention efforts of the federal government and voluntary health organizations. The effectiveness of counter-smoking advertising was demonstrated from 1967 to 1970, soon after the release of the landmark surgeon general's report on smoking but during a time when the tobacco industry still aired pro-smoking advertisements. Antismoking messages were widely aired on television and radio as a result of the FTC's Fairness Doctrine. A study of nearly 7,000 adolescents found that the teenage smoking rate was 3 percentage points smaller during the period of the Fairness Doctrine than during the preceding 16-month period. The Fairness Doctrine had its greatest impact during its first year, in something of a "shock" effect.[41] These study findings "suggest that a nationwide, well-funded antismoking campaign could effectively counter the effects of cigarette advertising in its currently permitted media forms."[42]

Counter-tobacco messages should especially address the "benefits" commonly presented in pro-tobacco advertisements, and reverse the perception that tobacco use is normal, attractive, safe, and healthful. The most effective use of mass-media interventions has been in conjunction with other materials and programming, such as school-based programs.[43] Messages in the media should be coordinated to enhance and support other efforts to promote a tobacco-free norm at home and in schools, workplaces, public buildings, shopping malls, restaurants, sports arenas, and entertainment facilities. Youths should be involved in the development of the design and evaluation of health messages and programs. (See chapters 4, 5, and 7 for potential applications of the concept of including youths in developing research questions and message concepts.)

Families

The degree of parental influence on tobacco use by youths is not clear; in fact, research studies have reported contradictory effects and different effects for different ethnic groups. For example, in southern California, a longitudinal study of 11- through 14-year-olds found parental smoking to be predictive of a child's smoking for non-Hispanic whites but not for Hispanics, African Americans, or Asians.[44] Similarly, a longitudinal study of 8- through 17-year-olds in the southern United States found parental behavior to be predictive of children's smoking initiation for whites but not for African Americans.[45] The 1994 surgeon general's report presents the results of 27 prospective studies on the onset of smoking. In 15 of the studies investigating parental smoking as a factor in initiation, 7 studies showed that parental smoking was predictive; 2 studies suggested that it was predictive only for girls. Six of the studies did not show parental smoking as a predictive factor in onset.[46]

Parental attitudes and reactions to tobacco use may be a stronger influence on adolescent smoking than the actual smoking status of parents. Parental disapproval toward smoking was shown to indirectly predict low levels of use in a study that investigated parental actions toward smoking among 10- to 12-year-olds.[47] Comparison of parental strictness toward smoking among different age groups indicates that 14- to 16-year-olds are less likely to begin smoking if they perceive that parents disapprove.[48] In a survey of teens in Fond du Lac, Wisconsin, parental disapproval was an important reason that teens did not smoke—for 45% of eighth graders, 33% of tenth graders, and 27% of twelfth graders. For teens in Manitowoc, Wisconsin, the percentages were even higher—62% of eighth graders, 60% of tenth graders, and 48% of twelfth graders. In both places, parental influence was greatest for the younger adolescents.[49]

A study in Norway demonstrated that when parents set clear standards disapproving of tobacco use, adolescents responded to those standards by subsequently being less likely to take up smoking, regardless of parental smoking status.[50] Similarly, a study of 10,000 adolescents in the United Kingdom found that parental opposition to smoking was a more important direct predictor of the adolescents' intention to smoke than was parental smoking behavior.[51] Thus, one opportunity for establishing a tobacco-free norm is for parents to establish and consistently reinforce a standard of no tobacco use for their children. Even parents who smoke can be effective in doing this if the standard is accompanied by an explanation of the regrettable addictiveness of nicotine, which is controlling their own tobacco use. It is the *lack* of a parent's general concern for his or her child that seems to increase the risk of tobacco use,[52] whereas general parental support appears to decrease risk. Parents, like children, are influenced by their environment. In a Gallup poll for adult smokers, 50% reported that "pressure from family and friends" was a major reason for wanting to quit and 70% were concerned (53% saw this as a major concern) that their children might start smoking because they see them doing it.[53]

Peer Context

Although the influence of peers is a common factor in determining the circumstances of tobacco experimentation—that is, when and how the tobacco will be tried—it is important to remember that children and youths who choose to use tobacco have already been influenced by the norms of the larger society and, in particular, by continuous exposure to pro-tobacco messages. Experimentation is preceded by a preparatory stage during which a child or adolescent forms attitudes and beliefs about the benefits of smoking. The child or adolescent who chooses to smoke probably sees smoking as functional: as a way to appear mature, as a way to display either independence or bonding, as a way to cope with stress, and as a way to be relaxed in a social situation by having something to do.[54] Thus, whereas the ritual of experimentation commonly is peer-influenced, the predisposition to use tobacco is generated and reinforced by multiple environmental factors. The peer environment often serves as a convenient context in which to mimic a seemingly adult behavior.

Even within this broader frame of reference, the role of peer influence may be less robust than is commonly assumed. In the Teen Lifestyle Study, although the adolescents' perception of peer and adult smoking prevalence was highly exaggerated, the perception was not based on their best friends' behavior or their parents' behavior: 62% said that their best girlfriend never smokes and only 10.7% said that their best friend smokes regularly; 56% reported that their parents are nonsmokers. Thus, the girls' erroneous perception that the majority of people smoke must be deriving from sources other than immediate friends and families.[55] Data from the Monitoring the Future Study show that peer *disapproval* of cigarette smoking is rather high: in 1993 71% of high school seniors and 80% of eighth graders said that they disapprove of people who smoke a pack of cigarettes a day; 74% of tenth graders and 77% of eighth graders disapprove of using smokeless tobacco regularly.[56]

Studies of adolescent decision-making do not provide clear-cut evidence of the role of peer influence on risk-taking. In a review of the empirical evidence on risk-taking and decision-making in adolescence, Furby and Beyth-Marom reported mixed results about peer influence on risky behaviors:

> In sum, adolescents may care very much what their peers think of them, but that apparently does not necessarily mean that their decisions about engaging in risky behaviors are heavily influenced by peers. In most studies, perception of influence has been measured, but actual influence on behavior has not been assessed. Furthermore, the emphasis has usually been on whose advice adolescents *follow*. However, they might not necessarily *seek* that advice.[57]

Interestingly, adolescents report that they are more influenced by *prosocial* or *neutral pressures* from peers than by pressures toward misconduct.[58] The positive influence of peers may be reflected in surveys of teens in Fond du Lac and Manitowoc, Wisconsin. The percentages of nonsmokers who gave as a reason for *not* smoking the fact that their friends do not smoke averaged 29% in Manitowoc and in Fond du Lac, 23% for eighth and tenth graders, and 13% for twelfth graders.[59] Thus, the peer context can become an opportunity for prevention and reinforcement of a tobacco-free norm if youths are taught refusal skills (as discussed in chapter 5 on prevention), especially when peer leaders play an active role in the teaching. Youths with such skills who are either indecisive or who feel pressured to respond to the experimental context would not only be able to resist in an acceptable manner but would also be communicating thereby that tobacco use is not the norm. In the study of Michigan youths mentioned above, 54% of current smokers suggested having "a friend to quit with" as a potentially successful approach to smoking cessation.[60]

Furby and Beyth-Marom suggest that altering various aspects of the social-structural environment in which adolescents find themselves may be equally, or even more, effective in improving the quality of their choices than attempts to influence individual decison-making processes.[61] An example of the power of peer rejection of smoking as a norm and of the capability of teens to influence their social-structural environment occurred in 1990 in Bozeman, Montana. A stringent tobacco-free policy was adopted in Bozeman via a referendum voted on by students and staff, at the request of student representatives to the Board of Trustees. The district's 1,900 students in grades 7-12 and 300 staff members and the trustees agreed in advance to abide by the results of the referendum. The tobacco-free schools policy was ratified by a vote of 79% of students and 77% of staff. The staff and students implemented the policy themselves. A second referendum, this time regarding sales of tobacco products to youths under age 18, was authorized by the 1991 Montana legislature. Approximately 60% of 50,000 students voting in grades 7-12 voted "Yes—I do favor requesting that stores refuse to sell cigarettes and tobacco to persons under 18 years of age."[62]

The School Environment

Outside of the home, the principal consistent environment of children and adolescents is the school. The school environment, as a social organization, prescribes social norms, whether stated directly in school policies, implied in the expectations and behavior of teachers, or promoted by peer groups. The school therefore offers an important opportunity for promoting the tobacco-free norm, for countering pro-tobacco messages, and for creating a health-promoting environment in general. As discussed in chapter 5, schools are the natural setting for educating children and youths about the consequences of tobacco use and for teaching them refusal and other social skills. In addition, schools should establish no-smoking policies that apply to students and all school personnel alike. Tobacco-free policies have been endorsed by educational organizations such as the National School Boards Association and the American Association for Health, Physical Education, and Recreation. Among the Healthy People 2000

Objectives for the Nation, Objective 3.10 specifically addresses tobacco-free environments in the school: "Establish tobacco-free environments and include tobacco use prevention in the curricula of all elementary, middle, and secondary schools, preferably as part of quality school health education."[63] School policies can and do have an impact on tobacco use behavior. In California, the written smoking policies of 23 schools (over 4,000 adolescents) were evaluated on whether they banned smoking on school grounds, banned smoking near school, and included an education program on smoking prevention. The schools that had significantly lower smoking rates had policies in all of these areas and emphasized prevention and cessation.[64] In 1992, 28 states had state-level mandates to offer tobacco-use education in the schools, and 31 had statewide restrictions on tobacco use in schools.[65]

The state of Colorado provides an example of how a serious commitment by interested organizations can take action to establish a tobacco-free school environment. A 1988 survey by the Colorado Department of Health revealed that only eight Colorado school districts (5% of the total) had comprehensive tobacco-free policies. The Colorado School Health Council, a state constituent of the American School Health Association, in response to their concern, developed the Colorado Tobacco-Free Schools and Communities Project. With the support of over 25 collaborating agencies statewide, Colorado has moved from 8 to 81 tobacco-free school districts in a little over 4 years. The Colorado program defines "tobacco-free" as "no use of any tobacco products in school buildings, on school grounds or at school-sponsored activities by students, staff, and visitors."[66] In Minnesota, the tobacco-free school environment is already statewide.

Activity to require tobacco-free school policies is also occurring at the federal level. On March 23, 1994, the House and Senate included a provision in an education bill that would ban smoking in all public schools that receive federal money, including Head Start Centers, day care centers, and most community health centers. The Lautenberg amendment is part of the Goals 2000: Educate America Act, which sets national education goals. Although federal and state requirements are effective means of instituting tobacco-free policies in schools, another important means should also be considered: involving students in establishing the policies, as was done in the Bozeman referendum described above.

The Community Environment

The daily life of adolescents extends broadly into the local community, as they progressively take on greater autonomy and require less adult supervision. Yet, certain restrictions continue to apply to them (for example, restrictions on smoking and drinking), and these restricted behaviors become symbols for adult status.[67] Therefore, as adolescents venture more and more into the community, their perceptions that certain norms seem to apply only to them and not to adults may promote health-compromising behaviors. On the other hand, public restrictions that apply to all persons in an environment can enhance the adolescent's perception of himself or herself as emerging toward an adult role in society.

Restrictions on tobacco use in public places are statements of the preferences of the larger community. Restrictions on smoking in public places state and reinforce the norm that tobacco use is not acceptable, and create a social climate where not using tobacco is considered normal.[68] Social policy thereby communicates the message that tobacco use causes health problems for everyone exposed to it, even to environmental tobacco smoke. The restrictions also reduce the number of opportunities to use tobacco; thus, tobacco use is not only a behavior disapproved by society but also an inconvenient behavior. These messages counter the pro-tobacco message and diminish the perception that psychosocial benefits are associated with tobacco use.

Currently there is broad public support for restricting tobacco use in public places. In the American Cancer Society's Survey of American Voters, 64% of all voters polled said that they favor banning smoking in all public places, such as restaurants, stores, and government buildings.[69] Results from a 1994 *USA Today*/CNN Gallup poll of adults nationwide reveal that support for a ban on smoking in public places has doubled in the last 7 years, with a majority favoring restrictions in restaurants, offices, and hotels.[70] A large percentage of smokers (42%) polled in a 1973 Gallup survey felt that nonsmokers' rights in public places should supersede smokers' rights.[71] The more these public attitudes are expressed in actual tobacco control ordinances—and enforced—the more children and youths will encounter a tobacco-free environment and will perceive that tobacco use is not normative. In the Fond du Lac and Manitowoc surveys mentioned earlier, about 20% of the teens in the former and 29% in latter said that they do not smoke because it bothers others.[72]

The community environments in which youths spend much of their time, and which are therefore the environments that provide their context for tobacco use, are workplaces, shopping malls, fast-food restaurants, sports facilities, and community and youth organization meeting places.

The Workplace

The workplace is an important social context for adolescents for two reasons. First, more than half of high school students hold part-time jobs; they work in a wide variety of places, such as restaurants, offices, and stores. Second, as part of their developmental task of social redefinition, adolescents are preparing for responsible roles in society as adults, and even more specifically, in school they are learning skills that prepare them for work. Thus, while still in high school, adolescents are exposed to the norms of the work environment and they experience what will be expected of them in the future in the workplace.

Increasingly, workplaces have adopted no-smoking policies, particularly since the publication of the Environmental Protection Agency's report on environmental tobacco smoke. Usually, these policies are initiated by management, but recently, in March 1994, employees took the initiative to make their workplace smoke free. The last United Auto Workers local to settle with General Motors voted, as part of its contract, to prohibit smoking at its plant.[73] In adopting tobacco-free policies, employees and employers are not only literally protecting employees from the elements in smoke that are harmful to one's health, but they are also clearly stating and promoting the public health norm that an individual should not impose health risks on other individuals. The worksite objective in the Healthy People 2000 proposal is "to increase to at least 75% the proportion of worksites with a formal smoking policy that prohibits or severely restricts smoking at the workplace."[74] The objective is not unrealistic if current momentum can be maintained.

On March 25, 1994, the Department of Labor proposed a virtual ban on smoking in the workplace as part of a comprehensive plan to increase the air quality in workplaces. The proposed ban would be instituted through the Occupational Safety and Health Administration (OSHA) and would cover approximately 6 million workplaces. The OSHA regulation would apply to private-sector employers everywhere and to public-sector employers in the 25 states and territories that have their own OSHA programs.[75] Meanwhile, Washington will likely be the first state to have a statewide ban on smoking in workplaces. On March 16, 1994, Washington State Labor Director Mark Brown signed into law a directive to ban smoking in the workplace, effective September 1, 1994.[76]

The Department of Defense (DoD) is the largest employer in the United States, with nearly 3 million employees. DoD implemented a far-reaching smoke-free workplace policy in April 1994, banning smoking of tobacco products in all DoD work facilities worldwide. The policy is intended to meet three objectives: (1) to provide a safe and healthy workplace for all DoD employees, (2) to contribute to the readiness of the armed forces by maintaining healthier personnel, and (3) to be a leader in creating a smoke-free workplace.[77] The leadership role of this policy will carry over to the general population to the families and friends of the military personnel, as well as to prospective recruits in the general population.

Prohibiting tobacco use in the workplace has proven to be an effective way of reinforcing society's tobacco-free norm and decreasing tobacco consumption. A study in California of the relationship between workplace smoking policies and smoking prevalence and cigarette consumption found that employees in smoke-free workplaces have a lower smoking prevalence and, among continuing smokers, lower cigarette consumption than individuals working where smoking is permitted. The researchers estimate that cigarette consumption among employees indoors is 21% below that which would occur if there were no smoking restrictions in California workplaces.[78] In a recent Gallup poll, 23% of smokers reported bans on smoking in the workplace as a major reason for wanting to quit smoking and 21% reported lack of locations in which to smoke as a major reason (multiple reasons were allowed in the survey question).[79]

As youths encounter a tobacco-free workplace norm, they will become increasingly aware that tobacco use is not an adult norm and is becoming less socially approved. They will also be cognizant of the fact that they will have to forego tobacco use in the workplace themselves. This recognition provides an important opportunity for schools and parents to help adolescents. For example, a technical institution in Minnesota implemented a smoking prevention project because women attending technical institutes often enroll in training programs for occupations with traditionally high smoking rates, at a time when no-smoking policies are increasingly being adapted in the workplace. Entitled "Smoking Doesn't Work," the program used employability as the central theme in schoolwide events and classroom activities. The intervention resulted in significant increases in knowledge and awareness of smoking and employability issues; the young women had not been highly aware of the relationship between smoking status and employability.[80] In a 1994 national poll, 20% of respondents said that they would be less likely to hire an applicant who is a smoker.[81]

Fast-Food Restaurants

Fast-food franchise restaurants estimate that as many as 25% of their customers are under the age of 18, with 10% under the age of 10. These children not only eat at the restaurants but also spend extended time there in special play areas for children, complete with jungle gyms and slides. Additionally, 40% of employees in fast-food restaurants are under age 18. In 1993, after reviewing these and other data supplied by the industry, the attorneys general of 16 states made the following observations in a preliminary report, "Fast Food, Growing Children, and Passive Smoke: A Dangerous Menu":

• The overwhelming majority of fast-food restaurants permit smoking on the premises.
• No major fast-food chain prohibits smoking altogether.
• Only 25% of customers smoke.
• Most fast-food companies would ultimately like to go smoke free.
• Most companies would prefer to wait until legislative smoking bans are in place before mandating a smoke-free policy for their customers.
• The companies would not oppose legislation to ban smoking in restaurants.
• The companies are concerned that they would lose business if they implemented a smoke-free policy before their competitors.[82]

In the report, the attorneys general requested fast-food establishments to enact smoke-free policies, recommending specific steps of a staged implementation plan.

A number of fast-food chains responded quickly to the appeal. In March 1994, Taco Bell banned smoking in all of its 3,300 company-owned restaurants, and expects its 1,000 franchise stores will also go smoke free. The company said its decision was based, in part, on a year-long customer survey which found that 70% of smokers and 84% of nonsmokers found smoking in fast-food restaurants to be offensive.[83] As of March 1994, one-third of the members of the National Council of Chain Restaurants had banned smoking, and the council endorsed a proposed federal bill that would ban smoking in restaurants.

Though fast-food companies are inclined to go smoke free, apparently a concern holding them back is that of diminished sales, a concern that is unwarranted. Although smoking customers had reported that they would not frequent the restaurants, several studies have shown that restaurants do not suffer loss of sales when they go smoke free. For example, a recent study found that the first 13 U.S. cities (10 in California, 3 in Colorado) to ban smoking in restaurants are not losing customers or sending money to neighboring communities that allow diners to smoke, countering the claim of the tobacco industry and other opponents of smoke-free ordinances that such bans have caused up to a 30% dip in restaurant business.[84]

Shopping Malls

Popular places for adolescents to congregate are shopping malls; adolescents congregate in the open areas, arcades, food court areas, and movie theaters. Malls are areas in which youths can socialize, entertain themselves, and pass time in an unsupervised setting. The circumstances are conducive to tobacco use both by the youths and adults in the malls. One of the first counties to prohibit smoking in enclosed private malls was Howard County, Maryland in 1992. Since then many malls across the country have enacted smoke-free policies. Maine, New York, and Washington include shopping centers in their legislation for clean indoor air. One of the largest malls in Virginia (home to Philip Morris) went smoke free on April 4, 1994. The manager of Potomac Mills Mall stated the following reason:

> We value all of our customers and employees, including those who choose to smoke. However, Potomac Mills must do everything possible to maintain the healthiest environment possible for our visitors and employees.[85]

Tobacco-use restrictions in malls are important not only because they reinforce the smoke- free norm in an adult environment but also because they considerably diminish the opportunity for tobacco use.

Sports Facilities

Sports, both participatory and spectator sports, are a favorite pastime of youths. Sports stars are heroes and role models for youths. The arena of sports offers three distinct opportunities to promote a tobacco-free norm. First, one's physiologic performance while participating sports is diminished by tobacco use. By recognizing that participation in sports can be a receptive learning moment for an adolescent, peers, parents, and coaches could have an important influence on a youth who is active in sports. Second, many youths imitate the behavior of sports stars, including the use of spitting tobacco and cigarettes. In 1993, professional baseball minor-league teams adopted a total ban on smoking or chewing by all players, coaches, and umpires anywhere in the ballparks. Third, two-thirds of major-league stadiums have voluntarily eliminated smoking from their seating areas; 18 stadiums have eliminated tobacco advertising. At least half of the 50 states restrict smoking in gymnasiums and arenas as part of their clean indoor air legislation.[86] A Current Population Survey survey of youths asked if they thought that smoking should be allowed in indoor sporting events; 65% replied "not at all," and 28.6% replied "to allow in some areas."[87]

Community and Youth Organizations

One of the highest rates of tobacco use is among youths who have dropped out of high school; they are of course the least likely group to be reached through school programs. It might be possible to reach some of these youths through their communities, that is, through organizations or events sponsored by community groups. Youths who remain in school may be likely to participate in organizations for youths. Thus, community groups and youth organizations provide an important means of promoting the tobacco-free norm to youths at all risk levels and of providing alternative behaviors to tobacco use through organizational activities that allow youths to have a sense of belonging and to be relaxed among their peers. Organizations can also provide opportunities for youths to become active in promoting the tobacco-free norm to their peers.

Organizations have begun to recognize their potential for preventing tobacco use by children and youths and a number of them have begun to affiliate in order to enhance their resources and effect. For example, a national alliance of organizations that serve youths or have youth memberships, the Coalition for America's Children, was founded in 1991 "to promote health, education, safety, and security for all American children" by increasing public awareness of children's issues through member organizations and by providing materials and technical assistance to member organizations. In 1993-1994, the Coalition adopted prevention of tobacco use by children as a major issue. The Institute of Medicine collaborated with the Coalition to conduct a survey of the Coalition's member organizations to determine their level of involvement in tobacco control issues and the level of interest in becoming more involved. The results indicate that while there is some interest and activity in tobacco issues, organizations that serve children are not fully aware of the seriousness of the issues. For example,

66% of the responding organizations have a formal policy on tobacco use that is enforced; an effort is made to prevent the use of tobacco by staff in 47% of the organizations and by the general public in 28%; however, only a few provide assistance for tobacco cessation. Sixty-three percent of the respondents felt that tobacco use by children was less important than other issues in which their organizations were involved; another 34% felt the issue was of about the same importance. (Note that staff size, minimal funds, and specificity of mission may be factors influencing their thinking and activities.) Nevertheless, 81% indicated that they would be very likely or somewhat likely to distribute information on tobacco issues to members, and 77% indicated that they would be very likely or somewhat likely to incorporate tobacco into their health materials. According to 68% of the respondents, public awareness in their community of the issues surrounding children's use of tobacco is less than that for other children's issues; 45% feel that there is little or no media coverage devoted to this topic.

The Join Together Project, funded by the Robert Wood Johnson Foundation, is a national resource for information and technical assistance to coalitions of community organizations that combat tobacco, alcohol, and other drug abuse. In 1993 Join Together surveyed 12,000 collaborative agencies nationwide, soliciting information on how their coalitions are organized and what they do.[88] Of the 5,475 responding agencies, 2,196 are lead agencies or sponsoring agencies of coalitions or organizations. Of this subset, 23% (779) reported having extensive programs on tobacco prevention, and some were considering expanding their activities. Most of those agencies are attempting to reach high-risk populations, such as pregnant teens, juvenile offenders, and dropouts, as well as the general youth populations. They focus on the community environment as opposed to needs of individuals, and on system-wide change rather than on specific areas. Among the policy barriers most frequently identified by the agencies was the need to break down barriers that exist between organizations and governments.

The community coalitions are broad-based collections of public and private agencies and many volunteers, and most have either equal participation by professionals, government officials, and lay people or are led mostly by lay people. Local police and schools are represented in a high percentage of the coalitions; however, participation should be broadened in two respects. Local recreation departments, where youths may spend time after school and on weekends, are active in less than one-third of all substance abuse coalitions. The mass media were reported to be active in less than one-half (41%) of the community coalitions, even though they can be influential in helping set the tone for a community's approach to substance abuse.

ADVOCACY FOR A TOBACCO-FREE NORM

Many organizations and coalitions have taken on advocacy roles, promoting a tobacco-free norm. For example, some religions have begun to unite in their efforts to prevent tobacco use by youths. The Interreligious Coalition on Smoking OR Health represents 15 religious organizations. In supporting tobacco control initiatives, the coalition holds that there is "an obligation to preserve the quality of human life" and "a moral obligation to protect the vulnerable, such as the young."[89] Similarly, the Union of American Hebrew Congregations adopted a resolution in 1987 to promote tobacco control. The resolution includes implementing tobacco education for youths and enacting smoke-free policies in public places.[90] Churches and church-affiliated activities and organizations are important norm-setting sources of influence on children and youths.

Coalitions have also been established through government-supported tobacco control initiatives. State and local coalitions support policy change on a large-scale basis by involving communities. Staffed by state and local government health officials, these coalitions are composed of a spectrum of organizations and individuals concerned with tobacco control. Examples are regional coalitions such as the Rocky Mountain Tobacco-Free Challenge, the Tobacco-Free Heartland Coalition, and the National Cancer Institute's American Stop Smoking Intervention Project (ASSIST). ASSIST, which is conducted in partnership with the American Cancer Society, provides funding to 17 states to support community-based tobacco control interventions. The $150 million project, to be implemented from 1993 to 1998, aims to reduce tobacco use through policy interventions and media advocacy mobilized by statewide and local coalitions. Youths are a priority prevention group in the ASSIST effort. The 17 states are Colorado, Indiana, Maine, Massachusetts, Michigan, Minnesota, Missouri, New Jersey, New Mexico, New York, North Carolina, Rhode Island, South Carolina, Virginia, Washington, West Virginia, and Wisconsin.

A state-initiated and state-supported program resulted from California's Proposition 99. In 1988, California voters approved Proposition 99, an excise tax on tobacco products that earmarked 20% of the revenue to support tobacco control efforts. Enabling legislation provided funding of approximately $14 million in 1990-1991 and $79 million in 1991-1992. As a major component of the tobacco control program, the state health department funds 61 local coalitions supported by local health departments, 10 regional coalitions staffed by administrative agencies, and 4 ethnic networks.[91]

Other combined local and national efforts are being implemented by voluntary health organizations and by health and health professionals' organizations. For example, tobacco control is an important issue for the American Heart Association, the American Cancer Association, and the American Lung Association. These organizations, which traditionally have focused on public education and research, are increasingly pursuing public policy initiatives to tobacco control.

Health and health professionals' organizations, at national, state, and local levels are drawing on their memberships to support policy efforts. These include organizations such as the American Medical Association, American Public Health Association, American Medical Women's Association, American Academy of Family Physicians, American Dental Association, American Association of Occupational Health Nurses, and Doctors Ought to Care (DOC). The American Medical Association (AMA) took a major step into the realm of tobacco control advocacy when it sponsored the Tobacco Use in America Conference in 1989, which brought together tobacco control advocates and members of Congress. The 100 invited conference participants formed workgroups around major tobacco control policy issue areas and developed recommendations.[92] In 1993, the AMA sponsored a second conference, again promoting collaboration among legislators and advocates and producing a series of recommendations. Special tobacco editions of the *Journal of the American Medical Association* are important sources of research and draw media attention to tobacco issues. The AMA serves as the administrative agency for the $10 million Robert Wood Johnson Foundation SmokeLess States program. This program will support statewide coalitions to reduce tobacco uptake and use and increase public awareness of the role of tobacco control policy in health care reform.

Supporting organizations are not frontline advocacy groups themselves, but support the efforts and coordinate advocacy groups. At the national level, the Advocacy Institute's Smoking Control Advocacy Resource Center (SCARC) plays a unique role by bringing together disparate parts of the tobacco control movement. Its electronic communications network, SCARCNet, provides advocates with timely, concise strategic resources and offers them the opportunity to confer about strategic questions and share advocacy successes and failures. Over 400 U.S.-based advocates representing all areas of tobacco control have joined the network, and hundreds more receive periodic mailings updating them on tobacco control strategies. Other organizations have taken frontline positions as advocates of tobacco control, for example ANR, ASH, and GASP.

Foundations and others have also increased funding for advocacy activities. The Robert Wood Johnson Foundation (RWJ) now plays the leading foundation role in supporting these efforts. RWJ funded the Tobacco Policy Research Project in 1991, which brought together committees of researchers and experts in tobacco control policy to assess research needs; the committee reports were published as a supplement to the journal *Tobacco Control*. Following this project, RWJ launched a 4-year, $5 million program to support policy-related research. Most recently, RWJ launched its SmokeLess States initiative, a 4-year, $10 million program to support up to 18 statewide coalitions. Grantees will implement comprehensive tobacco control programs including education, treatment, and policy initiatives.

All tobacco control policies, either directly or indirectly, affect youths. To that extent, the range of groups described above all address issues concerning youths. For many, however, their youth-focused activities are not primary. A few groups do focus on youths in particular, including the following. Stop Teenage Addiction to Tobacco (STAT) focuses primarily on the issue of tobacco and youth. STAT advocates directly for policy changes at the federal, state, and local levels In 1989 STAT began hosting an annual conference focused on advocacy activities around youth tobacco use; at the 1993 conference, attendees included approximately 100 youths who participated in a separate youth track. Through a 3-year, $1 million grant from the Robert Wood Johnson Foundation, STAT also funds four youth-involved local initiatives to reduce youth tobacco use prevalence. Smokefree Educational Services (SES), a relatively small-scale organization with an all-volunteer staff, has scored many policy victories in New York City. SES works with hundreds of youths on youth-focused advocacy efforts and disseminates information on its efforts and other important issues to over 13,000 advocates nationally through its newsletter. The North Bay Health Resources Center's STAMP (Stop Tobacco Access for Minors Project), funded through Proposition 99, distributes signs to stores regarding youth access in a 6-county (approximately 40-city) region of Northern California.

Across the nation, youths themselves are becoming involved and carrying the issue forward. Involving youths in working on tobacco control efforts has been a way to empower them and to increase youth awareness of tobacco issues. For example, the Gold Country, a 13-county region in California, has active youth coalitions in each county and holds an annual youth summit that provides advocacy training.   Additionally, many statewide and local coalitions such as those established for ASSIST and California have youth representatives. Youths are involved in all phases of advocacy, including documenting the problem in the community, developing strategies for addressing the problem, and presenting their ideas to the community, media, and policymakers. Youths who have been willing to speak out for their own concerns have inspired respect for their cause. For example, testimony before the city council by teens from San Jose STAT proved important in convincing the San Jose City Council to implement a vending machine ban.[93]

While youths have been central in these efforts, until recently they have only been part of organizations run and funded by adults, and their numbers are small compared to SADD and other anti-drug efforts. At the 1993 annual STAT conference, a group of 20-30 youths from across the country decided that it was time to establish an organization created and run by youths. They formed their own organization—Students Coalition Against Tobacco (SCAT)—which aims to establish nationwide chapters that will focus on peer education as well as advocacy efforts. SCAT's young chairperson has expressed the need for youth involvement as follows:

> The next step must be to create school based clubs, following the model of SADD, that will advocate for social change on the level where the problem is originating. We must empower young people to work within their domain—the school system. These teens can conduct peer educational programs and work to enhance comprehensive health educational programs. The mere presence and advertisement of such a group will bring an awareness to students of the issues. Young people know where the problems lie and upon mobilization can enact

change more rapidly than any organization acting on behalf of young people. It will be the job of these young people to target their peers for a smoke-free lifestyle before the industry . . . can get to them.[94]

In summary, there has been an initiation of community activity supporting tobacco control policies. The efforts of community organizations, coalitions, and advocacy groups have been successful in establishing hundreds of ordinances that seek to improve the public health through a tobacco-free norm. In the process, the public has become somewhat more aware of the problems of tobacco and more supportive of tobacco control efforts. Those activities are an important beginning because they demonstrate that the public will support tobacco control measures and that youths are responsive to helping set the tobacco control agenda. However, the efforts to date are not sufficient in themselves to counter the pro-tobacco messages in our culture and to correct the misperception of the level of tobacco use. Community organizations and coalitions are potentially the most effective means of accomplishing those objectives, but they need support to broaden their bases.

REINFORCING THE TOBACCO-FREE NORM: CONCLUSIONS AND RECOMMENDATIONS

We must not become complacent about the downward trend of smoking prevalence during the past two decades. To the contrary, the public should be concerned about the fact that prevalence has leveled off and that there was a slight increase in youth smoking in 1993. Renewed efforts are required to once again start the downward trend and to prevent youths from ever initiating tobacco use.

The forces influencing tobacco use originate well beyond a youth's immediate personal environment of family and peers; youths encounter pro-tobacco messages everywhere and repeatedly in the social environment. Therefore, countermeasures should be actively undertaken to promote a tobacco-free norm. The Committee recommends that:

1. Public education programs and messages should be increased and implemented on a continuous basis to (a) inform the public about the hazards of tobacco use and of environmental tobacco smoke and (b) promote a tobacco-free environment. In particular, mass media campaigns, including paid counter-tobacco advertisements, should be intensified to reverse the image appeal of pro-tobacco messages, especially those that appeal to children and youths.

2. Tobacco-free policies should be adopted and enforced in all public locations, especially in those that cater to or are frequented by children and youths, including all educational institutions, sports arenas, cultural facilities, shopping malls, fast-food restaurants, and transit systems.

3. All levels of government should adopt tobacco-free policies in public buildings. The Department of Defense should continue its aggressive efforts to adopt tobacco-free policies in all military services.

4. All workplaces should adopt tobacco-free policies.

5. All organizations involved with youths should adopt tobacco-free policies that apply to all persons attending or participating in all events sponsored by the organizations, and should actively promote a tobacco-free norm.

6. Parents should clearly and unequivocally express disapproval of tobacco use to their children, and, if smokers themselves, should quit smoking.

To advance understanding of how best to promote a tobacco-free social norm, the Committee recommends that the following research approaches be undertaken:

7. Research should be conducted to determine the factors influencing the substantial decline in tobacco use by African-American youths, with particular attention to the role of social norms.

8. Youths should be involved in the development of research questions and approaches and in designing and evaluating health messages and programs.

REFERENCES

1. U.S. Department of Health, Education, and Welfare. *Smoking and Health. A Report of the Surgeon General, 1979.* DHEW Pub. No. (PHS) 79-50066. Rockville, MD: Office on Smoking and Health. 16-5, 6.

2. Crocket, Lisa J., and Anne C. Petersen. "Adolescent Development: Health Risks and Opportunities for Health Promotion." In Millstein, Susan, Anne C. Petersen, and Elena O. Nightingale, eds. *Promoting the Health of Adolescents: New Directions for the Twenty-first Century.* New York: Oxford University Press, 1993. 13.

3. Hurrelmann, Klaus. "Adolescents as Productive Processors of Reality: Methodological Perspectives." In Hurrelmann, K., and U. Engel, eds. *The Social World of Adolescents: International Perspectives.* Berlin: Walter de Gruyter, 1989.

4. Kandel, D. B. "Processes of Peer Influences in Adolescence." In Silbereisen, R. K., K. Eyferth, and G. Rudinger, eds. *Development as Action in Context..* Berlin: Springer-Verlag, 1986. 203-227; Lerner, R., M. Karson, M. Meisels, and J. R. Knapp. "Actual and Perceived Attitudes of Late Adolescents: The Phenomenon of the Generation Gap." *Journal of Genetic Psychology* 126 (1975): 197-207.

5. Leventhal, Howard, and Patricia Keeshan. "Promoting Healthy Alternatives to Substance Abuse." In Millstein, Susan, Anne C. Petersen, and Elena O. Nightingale, eds. *Promoting the Health of Adolescents: New Directions for the Twenty-first Century.* New York: Oxford University Press, 1993. 260-284.

6. Jessor, Richard, and S. L. Jessor. *Problem Behavior and Psychosocial Development: A Longitudinal Study of Youth.* New York: Academic Press, 1977.

7. Centers for Disease Control. "Cigarette Smoking Among Adults—United States, 1992." *Morbidity and Mortality Weekly Report* 43:19 (20 May 1994): 342-346.

8. Bray, Robert M., L. A. Kroutil, J. W. Luckey, S. C. Wheeless, V. G. Iannacchione, D. W. Anderson, M. E. Marsden, and G. H. Dunteman. *Highlights: 1992 Worldwide Survey of Substance Abuse and Health Behaviors Among Military Personnel.* RTI/5154/06-17FR. Research Triangle Institute, December 1992. 45.

9. Johnston, Lloyd, P. O'Malley, and J. Bachman. "Monitoring the Future Study." Press release. The University of Michigan, Ann Arbor. January 27, 1994.

10. SmithKline Beecham. *Gallup Report: A National Survey of Americans Who Smoke.* New York, 1993.

11. Manning, Anita. "Poll Shows More Back Smoking Ban." *USA Today* (16 Mar. 1994): D1; and Nichter, Mark, Mimi Nichter, C. Ritenbaugh, and N. Vuckovic. "The Teen Lifestyle Project: Preliminary Report, 1994." University of Arizona, Dept. of Anthropology. Unpublished data.

12. Allen, Karen, A. Moss, G. A. Giovino, D. R. Shopland, and J. P. Pierce. "Teenage Tobacco Use: Data Estimates From the Teenage Attitudes and Practices Survey, United States, 1989." *Advance Data* 224 (1 Feb. 1993): 9.

13. Centers for Disease Control and Prevention. *Preventing Tobacco Use Among Young People. A Report of the Surgeon General, 1994.* S/N 017-001-004901-0. Washington, DC: U.S. Department of Health and Human Services, 1994. 78.

14. Johnston, Lloyd D., P. M. O'Malley, and J. G. Bachman. *National Survey Results on Drug Use from Monitoring the Future Study, 1975-1992; Vol. II.* NIH Pub. No. 93-3598. Washington, DC: National Institute on Drug Abuse, 1993. 15-17.

15. *Ibid.*, 15.

16. Schinke, Steven P., Robert F. Shilling, Lewayne D. Gilchrist, Marianne R. Ashby, and E. Kitajima. "Native Youth and Smokeless Tobacco: Prevalence Rates, Gender Differences, and Descriptive Characteristics." *NCI Monograph 8: Smokeless Tobacco Use in the United States.* NIH Pub. No. 89-3055. (1989): 39-42.

17. Schinke, Steven P., Robert F. Schilling, Lewayne D. Gilchrist, Marianne R. Ashby, and Eiji Kitajima. "Pacific Northwest Native American Youth and Smokeless Tobacco Use." *International Journal of Addiction* 22:9 (1987): 881-884; Bruerd, B. "Smokeless Tobacco Use Among Native American School Children." *Public Health Reports* 105:2 (1990): 196-201.

18. Schinke et al., 1989.

19. Centers for Disease Control. "Smokeless Tobacco Use in Rural Alaska." *Morbidity and Mortality Weekly Report* 36:10 (20 Mar. 1987): 140-143.

20. Eisen, M., G. L. Zellman, and A. L. McAlister. "A Health Belief Model Approach to Adolescents' Fertility Control: Some Pilot Program Findings." *Health Education Quarterly* 12:2 (1985): 185-210; Michielutte, R., and R. A. Diseker. "Children's Perception of Cancer in Comparison to Other Chronic Illnesses." *Journal of Chronic Diseases* 35:11 (1982): 843-852; and Price, James H., S. M. Desmond, M. Wallace, D. Smith, and P. M. Stewart. "Differences in Black and White Adolescents' Perceptions about Cancer." *Journal of School Health* 58:2 (1988): 66-70.

21. DiClemente, Ralph, Cherrie Boyer, and Edward Morales. "Minorities and AIDS: Knowledge, Attitudes, and Misconceptions Among Black and Latino Adolescents." *American Journal of Public Health* 78:1 (1988): 55-57.

22. Bray, Robert M., L. A. Kroutil, J. W. Luckey, S. C. Wheeless, V. G. Iannacchione, D. W. Anderson, M.E. Marsden, and G. H. Dunteman. *1992 World Survey of Substance Abuse and Health Behaviors Among Military Personnel.* RTI /5154/06-16FR Research Triangle Institute, December 1992. 6-2, 6-3.

23. Cronan, Terry A., Terry L. Conway, and Suzanne L. Kaszas. "Starting to Smoke in the Navy: When, Where, and Why?" *Social Science and Medicine* 33:12 (1991): 1349-1353.

24. Gusfield, Joseph R. "The Social Symbolism of Smoking and Health." In Rabin, Robert L., and Stephen D. Sugarman, eds. *Smoking Policy: Law, Politics, and Culture.* New York: Oxford University Press, 1993. 67.

25. SmithKline Beecham.

26. Marttila & Kiley, Inc. *Highlights From an American Cancer Society Survey of U.S. Voter Attitudes Toward Cigarette Smoking.* Boston, MA: Marttila & Kiley, Inc., 9 Sept. 1993. 25-26.

27. Kagan, Robert A., and Jerome H. Skolnick. "Banning Smoking: Compliance Without Enforcement." In Rabin, Robert L., and Stephen D. Sugarman. eds. *Smoking Policy: Law, Politics, and Culture.* New York: Oxford University Press, 1993. 83.

28. Bonnie, Richard J. "The Efficacy of Law as a Paternalistic Instrument." In Melton, Gary, ed. *Nebraska Symposium on Human Motivation, 1985.* Lincoln: University of Nebraska, 1986: 131-211.

29. Leventhal, Howard, Kathleen Glynn, and Raymond Fleming. "Is the Smoking Decision an 'Informed Choice'? Effect of Smoking Risk Factors on Smoking Beliefs." *Journal of the American Medical Association* 257:24 (1987): 3373-3376.

30. Nichter, Mark, Mimi Nichter, C. Ritenbaugh, and N. Vuckovic. *The Teen Lifestyle Project: Preliminary Report,* 1994. (Unpublished.)

31. Tuakli, Nadu, M. A. Smith, and C. Heaton. "Smoking in Adolescence: Methods for Health Education and Smoking Cessation." *Journal of Family Practice* 31:4 (1990): 369-374.

32. Sherman, Steven J., Clark C. Presson, Laurie Chassin, Eric Corty, and Richard Olshavsky. "The False Consensus Effect in Estimates of Smoking Prevalence: Underlying Mechanisms." *Personality and Social Psychology Bulletin* 9:2 (1983): 197-207.

33. Sussman, Steve, Clyde W. Dent, Jill Mestel-Rauch, C. Anderson Johnson, William B. Hansen, and Brian R. Flay. "Adolescent Nonsmokers, Triers, and Regular Smokers' Estimates of Cigarette Smoking Prevalence: When Do Overestimations Occur and by Whom?" *Journal of Applied Social Psychology* 18:7 (1988): 537-551.

34. Chassin, Laurie, Clark C. Presson, Steven J. Sherman, Eric Corty, and Richard W. Olshavsky. "Predicting the Onset of Cigarette Smoking in Adolescents: A Longitudinal Study." *Journal of Applied Social Psychology* 14:3 (1984): 224-243; Collins, Linda M., Steve Sussman, Jill Mestel Rauch, Clyde W. Dent, C. Anderson Johnson, William B. Hansen, and Brian R. Flay. "Psychosocial Predictors of Young Adolescent Cigarette Smoking: A Sixteen-Month, Three-Wave Longitudinal Study." *Journal of Applied Social Psychology* 17:6 (1987): 554-573.

35. Pierce, John P., A. Farkas, N. Evans, C. Berry, W. Choi, B. Rosbrook, M. Johnson, and D. G. Bal. *Tobacco Use in California 1992. A Focus on Preventing Uptake in Adolescents.* Sacramento, California: Department of Health Services, 1993. 43.

36. *Ibid.* See tables B-6, B-7.

37. *Ibid.,* 48.

38. Nichter et al.

39. Pierce, John P., Lora Lee, and Elizabeth Gilpin. "Smoking Initiation by Adolescent Girls, 1944 Through 1988." *Journal of the American Medical Association* 271:8 (1994): 608-611.

40. Robinson, Robert G., Michael Pertschuk, and Charyn Sutton. "Smoking and African Americans." In Samuels, Robert G., Michael Pertschuk, and Charyn Sutton, eds. *Improving the Health of the Poor: Strategies for Prevention.* Menlo Park, CA: Henry J. Kaiser Family Foundation, May 1992. 157.

41. Lewit, Eugene M., Douglas Coate, and Michael Grossman. "The Effects of Government Regulation on Teenage Smoking." *Journal of Law and Economics* 24:3 (1981): 545-573.

42. Centers for Disease Control and Prevention. *Preventing Tobacco Use,* 188.

43. Flay, Brian R. "Mass Media Linkages with School-Based Programs for Drug Abuse Prevention." *Journal of School Health* 56:9 (1986): 402-406; Leventhal, Howard, and Paul D. Cleary. "The Smoking Problem: A Review of the Research and Theory in Behavioral Risk Modification." *Psychological Bulletin* 88:2 (1980): 370-405; and Warner, K. E., and H. A. Murt. "Impact of the Antismoking Campaign on Smoking Prevalence: A Cohort Analysis." *Journal of Public Health Policy* 3:4 (1982): 374-390.

44. Sussman, Steve, Clyde W. Dent, Brian R. Flay, William B. Hansen, and C. Anderson Johnson. "Psychosocial Predictors of Cigarette Smoking Onset by White, Black, Hispanic, and Asian Adolescents in Southern California." *Morbidity and Mortality Weekly Report* 36:4 (1987): 11S-17S.

45. Hunter, Saundra, Janet B. Croft, Igor A. Vizelber, and Gerald S. Berenson. "Psychosocial

Influences on Cigarette Smoking Among Youth in a Southern Community: The Bogalusa Heart Study." *Morbidity and Mortality Weekly Report* 36:4S (1987): 17S-24S.

46. Centers of Disease Control and Prevention. *Preventing Tobacco Use*, 130.

47. Hansen, W. B., J. W. Graham, J. L. Sobel, D. R. Shelton, B. R. Flay, and C. A. Johnson. "The Consistency of Peer and Parent Influences on Tobacco, Alcohol, and Marijuana Use Among Young Adolescents." *Journal of Behavioral Medicine* 10:6 (1987): 559-579.

48. Pandina, R. J., and J. A. Schuele. "Psychosocial Correlates of Alcohol and Drug Use of Adolescent Students and Adolescents in Treatment." *Journal of Studies on Alcohol* 44:6 (1983): 950-973.

49. Cismoski, Joseph. *Addendum to Michigan Alcohol and Other Drugs School Survey*. Western Michigan University, 1994. (Unpublished data.); Cismoski, Joseph, and Marian Sheridan. *Alcohol and Tobacco Survey*. Fond du Lac Public Health Nursing Department. 1994. (Unpublished data.)

50. Aaro, Leif, Arne Hauknes, and Else Berglund. "Smoking Among Norwegian Schoolchildren 1975-1980. II. The Influence of the Social Environment." *Scandinavian Journal of Psychology* 22:4 (1981): 297-309.

51. Eiser, J. Richard, Michelle Morgan, Philip Gammage, and Elspeth Gray. "Adolescent Smoking: Attitudes, Norms and Parental Influence." *British Journal of Social Psychology* 28 (1989): 193-202.

52. Swan, A. V., R. Creeser, and M. Murray. "When and Why Children First Start to Smoke." *International Journal of Epidemiology* 19:2 (1990): 323-330.

53. SmithKline Beecham.

54. Perry, Cheryl L., David M. Murray, and Knut-Inge Klepp. "Predictors of Adolescent Smoking and Implications for Prevention." *Morbidity and Mortality Weekly Report* 36:4S (1987): 41S-46S.

55. Nichter et al.

56. Johnston et al., January 27, 1994.

57. Furby, Lita, and Ruth Beyth-Marom. "Risk-Taking in Adolescence: A Decision-Making Perspective." Carnegie Council on Adolescent Development Working Papers. Washington, DC. June 1990. 39.

58. Berndt, T. "Developmental Changes in Conformity to Peers and Parents." *Developmental Psychology* 15 (1979): 608-616; Brown, B., M. Lohr, and E. McClenahan. "Early Adolescents' Perceptions of Peer Pressure." *Journal of Early Adolescence* 6 (1986): 139-154.

59. Cismoski; and Cismoski and Sheridan.

60. Tuakli et al.

61. Furby and Beyth-Marom, 68.

62. Males, Mike. "Use of a School Referendum to Deter Teen-age Tobacco Use." *Journal of School Health* 62:2 (Aug. 1992): 229-232.

63. U.S. Department of Health and Human Services. *Healthy People 2000. National Health Promotion and Disease Prevention Objectives*. USDHHS Pub. No. (PHS) 91-50212. Washington, DC: U.S. Department of Health and Human Services, 1990. 147-148.

64. Pentz, Mary A., B. R. Brannon, V. L. Charlin, E. J. MacKinnon, D. P. Barrett, and B. R. Flay. "The Power of Policy: The Relationship of Smoking Policy to Adolescent Smoking." *American Journal of Public Health* 79:7 (1989): 857-862.

65. Association of State and Territorial Health Officials. *State Tobacco Use Prevention and Control Activities. Progress Report 1990 to 1992*. Washington, DC: ASTHO, 1994.

66. Colorado State University Cooperative Extension. *Colorado Tobacco-Free Schools and Communities: A Collaborative Community Approach*. Brochure. Fort Collins: Colorado State University, 1993.

67. Jessor, Richard "Adolescent Development and Behavioral Health." In Matarazzo, J., S. Weiss, J. Herd, N. Miller, and J. M. Weiss, eds. *Behavioral Health: A Handbook of Health Enhancement and Disease Prevention*. New York: Wiley, 1984. 69-90.

68. Rigotti, N. A. "Trends in the Adoption of Smoking Restrictions in Public Places and

Worksites." *New York State Journal of Medicine* 89:1 (1989): 19-26; Simonich, William L. *Government Antismoking Policies.* New York: Peter Lang Publishing, 1991; Wasserman, Jeffrey, Willard G. Manning, Joseph P. Newhouse, and John D. Winkler. "The Effects of Excise Taxes and Regulations on Cigarette Smoking." *Journal of Health Economics* 10:1 (1991): 43-64; and Emont, Seth L., Won S. Choi, Thomas E. Novotny, and Gary A. Giovino. "Clean Indoor Air Legislation, Taxation, and Smoking Behaviour in the United States: An Ecological Analysis." *Tobacco Control* 2:1 (1993): 13-17.

69. Marttila & Kiley.

70. Manning.

71. SmithKline Beecham.

72. Cismoski; and Cismoski and Sheridan.

73. Upton, Jodi. "Contract Snuffs Out Smoking." *Lansing State Journal* (3 Mar. 1994): A1.

74. USDHHS, 148.

75. Seelye, Katharine. "Labor Dept. Agency Proposes Ban on All Smoking in the Workplace." *New York Times* (26 Mar. 1994): A1.

76. "Smoking Ban." *USA Today* (16 Mar. 1994): A3.

77. Department of Defense. *Instruction No. 1010.15.* 7 Mar. 1994. (And attached news release, 8 Mar. 1994.)

78. Woodruff, Tracey J., Brad Rosbrook, John Pierce, Stanton Glantz. "Lower Levels of Cigarette Consumption Found in Smoke-free Workplaces in California." *Archives of Internal Medicine* 153 (28 June 1993): 1485-1493.

79. SmithKline Beecham.

80. Moore, Susan Morton, Kathy Daly, Colleen M. McBride, and Michelle S. Lodahl. "'Smoking Doesn't Work:' A Smoking Prevention Project for Women Attending a Technical Institute." *Journal of School Health* 62:2 (1992): 55-58.

81. Manning.

82. Attorneys General. *Fast Food, Growing Children and Passive Smoke: A Dangerous Menu. Findings and Preliminary Recommendations for Implementing Smoke Free Policies in Fast Food Restaurants.* 8 Nov. 1993. 6, 8, 10, 13. Available through New York Attorney General's Office.

83. "PepsiCo's Taco Bell Bans Smoking in Its Restaurants." *Wall Street Journal* (15 Mar. 1994).

84. Glantz, Stanton A., and Lisa R. A. Smith. "The Effect of Ordinances Requiring Smoke Free Restaurants on Restaurant Sales in the United States." *American Public Health Association* (27 Oct. 1993).

85. "Potomac Mills to Prohibit Smoking." *Arlington Journal* 1 Mar. 1994.

86. Coalition on Smoking OR Health. "State Legislated Actions on Tobacco Issues." Washington, DC, 1992.

87. Current Population Survey Tobacco Use Supplement 1992-1993. Courtesy of National Cancer Institute. (Unpublished data.)

88. Join Together. *1993 Report to the Nation: Community Leaders Speak Out Against Substance Abuse.* Boston, MA: Join Together, 1993.

89. Interreligious Coalition on Smoking or Health. *Religion & Tobacco Control Newsletter* (Jan. 1994).

90. Union of American Hebrew Congregations. *Resolution Adopted by the General Assembly.* Chicago. 29 Oct. 1993.

91. Tobacco Education Oversight Committee. *Toward a Tobacco-Free California: Exploring a New Frontier, 1993-1995.* Sacramento, CA. 1993.

92. Houston, Thomas P., ed. *Tobacco Use: An American Crisis. Final Conference Report and Recommendations from America's Health Community.* Washington, D.C., American Medical Association. January 9-12, 1993.

93. Butler, Judy. "The Role of Advocacy in Reducing Tobacco Addiction in Youth." Paper commissioned by the Committee on Preventing Nicotine Addiction in Children and Youths, 1993.

94. Dubner, David P. Letter to the Committee on Preventing Nicotine Addiction in Children and Youths. 19 Apr. 1994.

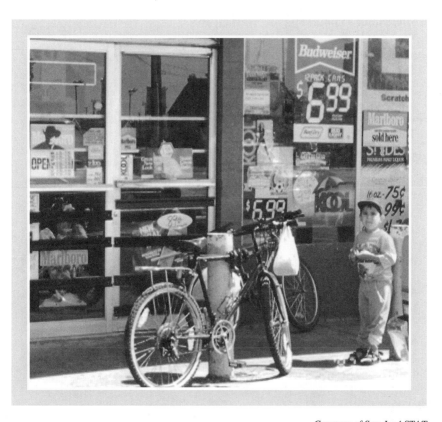

Courtesy of San José STAT

CONTENTS

4

TOBACCO ADVERTISING AND PROMOTION

INTRODUCTION: MAINTAINING THE MARKET

Every day, children and youths in the United States are exposed to a wide array of persuasive, carefully crafted commercial messages encouraging the use of tobacco products. In 1991 the tobacco industry spent $4.6 billion—more than $12.6 million a day, $8,750 a minute—on advertising and promoting* cigarette consumption, and over $100 million on advertising and promoting smokeless tobacco products.[1] During the past 15 years, the tobacco industry has nearly quadrupled** its marketing expenditures, at a time when tobacco consumption has been declining. Each day, approximately 3,500 Americans quit smoking and an additional 1,200 tobacco customers and former customers die of smoking-related illness; therefore, maintaining current levels of tobacco use and revenues requires that approximately 5,000 new smokers be recruited every day (about 2 million a year).[2] Children and youths constitute the most likely source of new smokers. The 1991 National Household Surveys on Drug Abuse data reveal that the large majority (89%) of persons ages 30-39 who ever smoked daily tried their first cigarette by age 18, and 62% by age 16; over three quarters (77%) were smoking daily before age 20.[3] At least 3 million

---

*As used in this report, "advertising" refers to expenditures for advertisements in newspapers and magazines and on billboards and transit systems; "promotions" refers to all other expenditures to promote tobacco consumption, especially point-of-sale displays, distribution of samples and specialty items, sponsorship of public entertainment, direct mail, coupons, and retail value-added products.

**All figures have been converted from nominal to real dollars with a base of 1991, the year for which the most recent data are available from the Federal Trade Commission.

American teenagers smoke regularly and 3 million people who regularly use smokeless tobacco are under age 21.[4]

Three trends have caused a growing number of public health professionals to call attention to the role of marketing (advertising and other promotional approaches) in making tobacco use attractive to children and youths and in encouraging them to use cigarettes and smokeless tobacco. First, boys and girls are beginning to use tobacco at ever younger ages. The average age at which boys and girls initiate smoking has declined over the past 4 decades by 2.4 years overall for whites, 1.3 years overall for African Americans, and 5.4 and 4.6 years for white girls and African-American girls, respectively.[5] The trend for girls to begin smoking at an earlier age began between 1955 and 1966,[6] and the likelihood of becoming a daily smoker at an earlier age increased sharply in the early to mid-1970s both for boys and girls.[7] During the same period, a second alarming trend in tobacco use has been noted: more and more, youths began using smokeless tobacco products. Half of the nation's 6 million smokeless tobacco users are under the age of 21, and several national surveys show an increase in prevalence, especially among boys.[8] A third trend, which has occurred over the past 10 years, entails a slowing down of the rate at which smoking prevalence by youths had been decreasing. Between 1977 and 1981, daily smoking among high school seniors dropped a total of about 9% (from 29% to 20%), an average of 2.25 percentage points per year. Yet during the following 11 years, 1981 to 1992 (during which time the tobacco industry more than doubled its advertising and promotion expenditures) smoking by high school seniors fell by only a total of about 3% (to 17.2%), or only 0.26 percentage points per year. Among college students, from 1980 to 1992, the decrease in daily smoking was about the same as for high school seniors, except that for 1989-1992 there was a slight upward trend in prevalence of cigarette use.[9] Notably, during this same period (1981-1991), the per capita cigarette consumption fell 28% among adults.[10]

What factors have contributed to stable smoking rates and to increased rates of smokeless tobacco use among children and youths, but have proven to be less effective in sustaining tobacco use by adults? Public health advocates suggest that youths have a heightened sensitivity to image advertising and promotion themes at a time in their lives when they are struggling to define their own identities. Adolescence is characterized by three major types of developmental challenges: (a) physical maturation, (b) cultural pressures to begin the transition to adult roles and emotional independence from parents, and (c) establishment of a coherent self-concept and values.[11] Cigarette advertisements are often evocative and play off these challenges in addition to being positioned to appeal to specific groups defined by social class and ethnic identity. Early adolescence (ages 11-14) in particular may be a time of increased susceptibility to the appeal of image advertising and promotions. The possible effects of marketing techniques on youths are considered below, following a brief review of shifting trends in the appropriation of tobacco marketing dollars.

SHIFTING TRENDS IN TOBACCO MARKETING

Tobacco advertising and promotions are clearly on the rise in the United States. In 1991, expenditures ($4.65 billion) on advertising and promotion of tobacco products were almost four times the amount ($1.22 billion) invested in 1980 (figure 4-1). From 1990 to 1991 alone, expenditures increased 13%.[12] The current annual expenditures amount to $18 for every man, woman, and child in the United States. Promotional activities take many forms and are the fastest growing mode of product marketing; they have been found to be effective in leading consumers to act once exposed to advertising.[13]

The tobacco industry's *distribution* of marketing expenditures over the past 2 decades represents a major shift in marketing trends; overall, the ratio of promotional expenditures to advertising expenditures has reversed. Whereas in

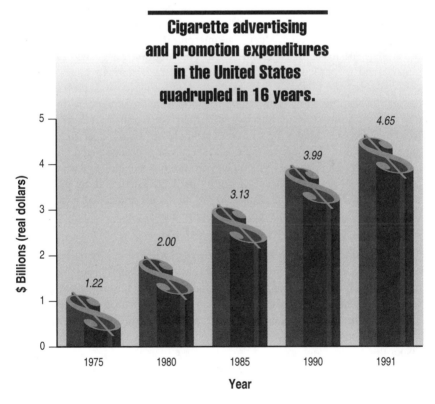

FIGURE 4-1   Source: Federal Trade Commission. *Report to Congress for 1991: Pursuant to the Federal Cigarette Labeling and Advertising Act.* Washington, D.C.: Federal Trade Commission, 1994.

1970 advertisements represented 82%* of total spending on tobacco marketing, they were down to 67% in 1980, 21% in 1990, and 17% in 1991. Although advertising expenditures per se have decreased, overall spending on marketing (advertising plus promotional activities) has increased. Of the $4.6 billion spent annually on tobacco marketing, about $700 million is spent on advertising. The remaining $4 billion is spent on a variety of promotional activities designed to: (a) place cigarettes and chewing tobacco in the hands of prospective users, (b) position cigarettes and chewing tobacco in prominent locations in shops and other points of sale where they will be psychologically appealing and physically available to customers, and (c) create good will for the tobacco industry among the public, community leaders, and politicians.

Promoting Tobacco Use to Consumers

The goal of marketing is to increase the appeal and acceptability of a product as well as to make the product available to the potential consumer. Tobacco marketing strategies (a) establish attitudinal predispositions that lead nonusers to experiment with tobacco products and interpret their experience as positive and rewarding, (b) foster the perception that consumption of tobacco products in general and in particular contexts (places, times) is normative, (c) minimize concern about the potential risks associated with tobacco use, propagating the perception that there are "safe" smoking options, and (d) reassure smokers and users of smokeless tobacco that possible risks are worth the benefits received from tobacco use. Marketing strategies promote both brand-specific and aggregate tobacco use. The impression that tobacco use is desirable and normative is conveyed through image advertising and promotions that make tobacco products highly visible in public spaces—if not by their presence, then by proxy in the forms of brand trademarks, insignia, logos, and items associated with preestablished brand images (for example, adventure scenarios). The major forms of marketing are highlighted below.

1. Retail value-added promotions and specialty items. Dramatically on the rise are retail value-added promotions such as multiple packs (buy one, get one free), cents-off coupons, and a free key chain or lighter blister-packed to a cigarette pack. Value-added promotions and coupons constituted the largest marketing expenditure (40% of total marketing expenditures) by the tobacco industry in 1991. Promotional items have special appeal to youths. Since youths have less disposable income and are more price-sensitive than adults, promotions such as discount buy-one-get-one-free schemes may be especially attractive to them. Coupons are easily accessible to youths through direct-mail promotions. (See figure 4-2 for expenditure data for this section.)

---

*The 1970 figure includes radio and television advertising. Broadcast advertising was banned after January 1, 1971.

109

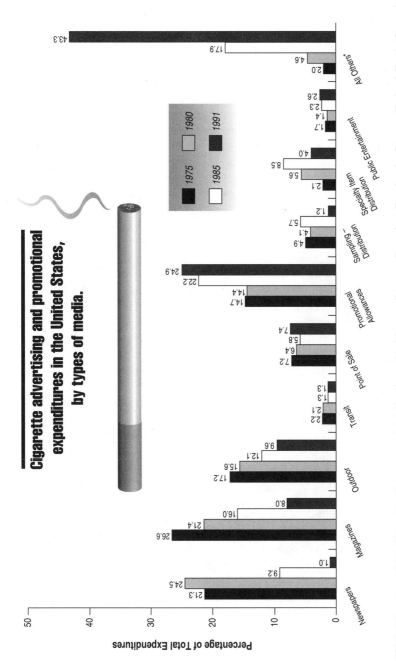

FIGURE 4-2 Note: "All Others" = Coupons and retail value-added items, direct mail, and audio-visuals. Source: Federal Trade Commission. *Report to Congress for 1991 Pursuant to the Federal Cigarette Labeling and Advertising Act.* Washington, D.C.: Federal Trade Commission, 1994.

Attractive specialty items—such as T-shirts, caps, calendars, and sporting goods—are distributed by the tobacco industry through the mail and at promotional events. These items, which sport a logo or brand name, become walking advertisements capable of penetrating areas of a child's world that might be off-limits to other forms of advertising. The ubiquity of such speciality items conveys the impression that tobacco use is the norm. Spending for specialty items accounted for 4% of expenditures in 1991. A 1992 Gallup survey found that half of all adolescent smokers and one-quarter of adolescent nonsmokers owned at least one promotional item from a tobacco company.[14] Similar data were reported in a survey of almost 8,000 ninth graders in Erie County, New York: 65% of regular smokers, 48% of occasional smokers, and 28% of nonsmokers reported owning clothing with a cigarette brand logo.[15] Although most youths seem to find logo clothing appealing, some high school students in focus groups (conducted under the auspices of the Committee) found them "tacky" and would not consider wearing them. Notably, however, these same teens save Marlboro Miles and Camel Cash coupons in order to acquire other types of goods. In a 1993 survey of 1,047 respondents ages 12-17, ownership of an average of 3.2 tobacco promotional items was reported by 10.6% of the sample. While 68.2% of current smokers reported participating in promotional campaigns, 28.4% of *non*smoking teens were also active participants. These promotional items carry no warning labels and provide free advertising.[16]

> *"My brother gets the Camel Cash. He's got stacks and stacks of them to get hats or whatever."*
>
> —adolescent in focus group

2. *Promotional allowances* constitute the second largest tobacco marketing expenditure—25% of all marketing-related expenditures. Through this form of promotion, tobacco companies pay retailers for shelf space, engage in cooperative advertising with retailers, and offer trade promotions to wholesalers, etc. Retailers are rewarded for stocking a wide variety of brands, even brands with low market demand. For example, a convenience store owner who sells 2,000 packs per week may be motivated to stock over 180 different brand packings (some having only 0.1% market share) in order to be eligible to receive incentive payments, which might be as high as $8,000 per year for a moderate-size retailer.[17]

As a result of trade incentives, cigarettes and other tobacco products are displayed prominently where adults as well as youths of all ages can see them. Self-service displays are an important source of tobacco products for minors.[18] Cigarettes are commonly displayed near checkout counters, and flavored chewing tobacco has been reported to be displayed near candy racks in convenience shops. A survey in California of stores near high schools found chewing tobacco next to candy and snacks in 42% of the stores.[19] In addition to catching the eye of a potential buyer who may not consciously be in the market for a tobacco product, the positioning of tobacco with other commodities conveys subtle associational meanings. For example, when placed near liquor, as they often are, cigarettes come to be associated with adult status as well as with products promoted to shift one's consciousness away from the stress, strains, anxieties, and boredom of routine existence, as a means of providing some temporary release and relief.

3. Point-of-sale advertising showcases particular brands of cigarettes in shops to stimulate impulse purchases. Since the 1971 ban on broadcast advertising, tobacco companies have made marketing through distribution a major function of their sales forces, which numbered more than 9,000 industry wide in the early 1980s.[20] This marketing technique places the tobacco products in convenient, visible racks, usually self-service, and in point-of-purchase displays. Point-of-sale promotions tend to involve the retailer, as well as the consumer, in a brand product. Support of brands through point-of-sale advertising helps to bolster the legitimacy of a brand in the eyes of retailers who make stocking decisions.[21] Point-of-sale materials are coordinated with national advertising campaigns to tie retailers in with the image-building for the product. In this sense, point-of-sale advertising both influences product distribution and directly induces consumption.[22] Point-of-sale advertising in retail establishments has been increasing and in 1991 represented 7.4% of advertising and promotional expenditures.

4. Magazine and newspaper advertising accounted for about 7% of marketing expenditures in 1991, when expenditures on *newspaper* ads reached an all-time low of 1.0%, a large drop since the 1980 high of 24.5%. *Magazine* ads were down to 6% of marketing dollars in 1991, from 21.4% in 1980. Nevertheless, expenditures on tobacco advertising in the print media do continue to be substantial and the decreases are not occurring at the same rate across all market segments; for example, while the number of ads per magazine issue has declined in men's and women's magazines, it has remained relatively stable in those magazines having substantial African-American and youth readerships.[23] In addition, advertisements are often combined with interactive promotional items that appeal to children and youths. For example, many magazine advertisements feature giveaway, non-cigarette utility items (calendars, lighters, T-shirts, and "action products") associated with "cash coupon" catalogue offers. Magazines often inform potential customers to be on the lookout for additional information about these offers at point-of-sale locations.

> *"They advertise a lot. Every magazine I have—there's an ad for Camels, Marlboros, Newports."*
>
> —high school girl in focus group

5. The tobacco industry was the number one spender for *outdoor advertising* in 1989;[24] of the approximately 3 million billboards in the United States, 30% were allocated to tobacco and alcohol products.[25] Advertising through the use of outdoor billboards and transit system signs accounted for 9.6% of all tobacco marketing expenditures in 1991. The industry has saturated African-American neighborhoods with cigarette billboards. Studies reveal that the intensity of cigarette billboard advertising is 2.6 times greater in African-American than in white neighborhoods in Columbia, South Carolina,[26] and 3.8 times greater in Baltimore.[27] Despite supposed industry standards to the contrary, billboards advertising tobacco products can be found next to homes, schools, churches, parks, playgrounds, health centers, stadiums, shopping centers, and along rural and city streets. More permanent than magazine advertising, and seen over and over again by youths, billboard ads expose children repeatedly to pro-tobacco messages and give the erroneous impression that smoking is pervasive and normative.

6. *Sponsorship of sporting events and public entertainment* associates tobacco with (a) all-American cultural events, such as music concerts and art exhibits, where fundamental social values are celebrated, and (b) high-risk sporting events, such as rodeos and car racing, where risks are socially approved and taken by individuals who brave the odds. The tobacco industry sponsors opera and ballet performances, and concerts of rock, rap, country and western, blues, jazz, and classical music, making tobacco products highly visible to diverse populations and strengthening the association between cigarettes, artistic expression, entertainment, glamour, and individuality.

Expenditures on the promotion of sports and sporting events are growing. The 1994 surgeon general's report has called special attention to sponsorship of sporting events associated with a company's brand name and/or logo, noting that this constitutes one of the most effective means of *covert* advertising. Even during events that are not sponsored by the tobacco industry, tobacco products are permanently displayed: tobacco billboards are the dominant form of advertisement in many major professional stadiums. Youths attend such sporting events, and watch them on television; many seek to emulate sports superstars, such as baseball players, who visibly chew and spit tobacco during these sports events, thereby actually demonstrating the use of the products on the billboards. Each 3-second exposure of a billboard in a ballpark has a marketing impact similar to a 10-second TV commercial.[28]A widely cited example of just how much product exposure is realized through covert advertising during sporting events is the 1989 Marlboro Grand Prix: when the event was televised, the Marlboro logo could be seen for 46 of the 94 total minutes of this sport event's broadcast time.[29] In the 1987 NASCAR Stock Race Circuit the Winston logo appeared for a total of 6 hours and 22 minutes—nonpaid covert advertising on the air valued at $7.5 million.[30] In 1992, 354 motorsports broadcasts were quantitatively measured for estimates of product exposure value. The programs had a total viewing audience of 915 million, 7% of whom were children and teens, and an overall tobacco product exposure value of $68 million ($41 million for Winston, $12 million for Marlboro, $7 million for Skoal, $4 million for Camel, and $4 million for others).[31]   Studies have found that youths accurately associate sporting events with tobacco brands.[32]

   7. Distribution of free samples of cigarettes in public places, for "adults only," was at its highest percentage (about 7%) of total marketing dollars in the early 1970s, and has stayed about 2% since the late 1980s. Monitoring of who is given free samples has been poor, and tobacco companies who contract-out sample distribution have taken no responsibility for cited violations in which minors have been given samples.

   8. Expenditures for *direct-mail promotions* are on the rise; $65 million was spent in 1991, an increase of 22% over 1990. All five major cigarette companies actively compile mailing lists of customers, largely from coupons, which ask for name, address, usual brand, etc; from promotion redemptions; from the return of "smoker surveys" in magazines; and from the return of more general consumer information questionnaires. The forms sometimes ask detailed questions about brand use and about demographic characteristics.   Brown & Williamson, Lorrilard, and American Brands use their lists occasionally to send out coupons. R. J. Reynolds Tobacco Company (RJR), Philip Morris Tobacco Company, and United States Tobacco Company (UST) have made more substantial use of their mailing lists. UST sends its listees a slick quarterly magazine, *Heartland*, which puts Skoal and Copenhagen in a pleasant context and contains various offers. RJR and Philip Morris mount regular mailings promoting a variety of brands, depending on the characteristics of the persons on the lists. RJR promotes Camel and discount brands, and sometimes sends out coupons good for any top-of-the-line RJR cigarette product.   Philip Morris has distinct mail programs for Marlboro, Virginia Slims, Merit, and Benson & Hedges.   Individuals on the Camel lists have received at least six mailings in the past year apart from any coupon redemptions.

   These direct-mail efforts are large undertakings. Philip Morris, in a letter to its retailers dated July 20, 1993, indicated that it had 26 million people on its mailing lists. While a large number of teenagers may be included on these mailing lists, the tobacco companies has no mechanism for purging minors from their lists. Slade and colleagues conducted a nationally representative, random-digit dial survey of 1,047 respondents aged 12 to 17 to assess participation in promotional activities.[33] They found that 7.6% of the sample had received mail from a tobacco company. Extrapolating this figure to the entire 12- to 17-year-old population, they estimate that 1.6 million teens are on tobacco industry mailing lists.

   Direct mail may be a form of promotion that tobacco companies will pursue more aggressively if restrictions on conventional advertising are adopted. The expenditure data show a continuing trend toward advertising and promotional practices that are not required to carry health warnings.

Inhibiting Opposition to Tobacco Use

The tobacco industry's spending on advertising inhibits dissemination of anti-tobacco messages. *Billboard companies* allegedly have expressed reluctance to rent space for antismoking ads because they are well paid to saturate African-American neighborhoods with smoking ads and believe that they cannot afford to lose tobacco conglomerate accounts. *Magazines* that receive sizable revenues for advertising tobacco are less likely to run articles that discuss the negative aspects of tobacco use than magazines not dependent on tobacco industry revenue.[34] When articles are run that could potentially shed a negative light on tobacco use, they are toned down through editing.[35] This practice, termed "latent censorship," gives the public a distorted view of the dangers of smoking. For example, during the first 7 years after cigarette ads were banned on television (in 1971), the only two magazines (*Reader's Digest* and *The New Yorker*) that carried accurate articles on the link between tobacco and disease refused to accept cigarette ads.[36] A study of tobacco advertising in 99 magazines between 1959 through 1969 and 1973 through 1986 noted and confirmed a tendency toward latent censorship in women's magazines regarding the health effects of smoking as a result of their large amount of advertising income: "Magazines that did not carry advertisements for cigarettes were more than 40% more likely to cover the hazards of smoking than were magazines that carried cigarette advertisements. . . . women's magazines that did not carry cigarette advertisements were 2.3 times more likely to cover the risks of smoking."

Magazines for African Americans have earned revenues from tobacco ads since at least 1950. A study of patterns of tobacco advertising in magazines from 1950 to 1965 found that African Americans were at first subject to less, then to more, advertising than whites.[37] The greatest concentration of tobacco company advertising is in African-American publications such as *Jet, Essence*, and *Ebony*, but many small, local publications and other media serving the African-American community have found it extremely difficult to find other means of financial support, and might not survive without tobacco advertisements.

A similar effect of "latent censorship" results when revenue for advertising comes from one of the numerous companies that belong to tobacco industry conglomerates (for example, Nabisco, General Foods, Kraft). In 1988, after the ad agency Saatchi and Saatchi prepared ads touting the no-smoking policy of its client Northwest Airlines, RJR/Nabisco cancelled an $80 million annual contract with that agency for advertising food products.[38] A study of advertising executives found that they do fear economic reprisals from tobacco conglomerates should they print articles unfavorable to the tobacco industry.[39]

THE TOBACCO MARKET AND
MARKET SEGMENTATION

Tobacco has been aggressively marketed to the American public through a number of different channels and interactive modalities in order to foster demand for particular brands of tobacco products, create a more permissive environment in which to engage in tobacco use, and establish tobacco use as a norm of acceptable social behavior if not a "habit" to be emulated. Ever sensitive to social and cultural differences, the tobacco industry has gone to great pains to position tobacco products through market segmentation. Tobacco products are marketed to appeal to specific market niches; to existing smokers as well as potential smokers.

Tobacco: A Mature and a Growth Market

The tobacco industry claims that its primary, if not sole, purposes for advertising and promoting tobacco products are to (a) provide information to tobacco consumers regarding product choice, (b) capture brand share from competitors, and (c) maintain product loyalty in a mature market. Identifying a market as "mature" bears close examination for what the term both reveals and conceals. Some, but not all, products are categorized by marketing experts as constituting either a "mature" or "growth" market. In mature markets, awareness of a product is nearly universal and demand is relatively stable. Most of the market segment is already using the product, rises in product use are not dramatic, and expansion results from getting consumers to use a product more often or in new ways. In growth markets, new market segments are identified, new users are a source of significant market expansion, and rises in product use are significant.[40]

The cigarette market simultaneously displays characteristics of being both a mature and a growth market. The industry calls attention to the fact that cigarette sales have been fairly consistent over the last decade; however, it is clear that per capita consumption has decreased, and that the tobacco industry loses 2 million smokers a year—those who quit and those who die (about 44 million and 9 million, respectively, since 1964).[41] Consequently, market expansion must be occurring to maintain total tobacco sales at a consistent level. Adults are not a likely population for that market expansion because few new smokers are adults. Furthermore, for three decades the trend among adults has been to quit smoking. In fact, most new smokers are youths: 77% of daily smokers are daily smokers by age 20.

Market Segmentation to Reach Youths

Considerable research on the part of the tobacco industry has resulted in the positioning of specific brands in different market segments. This entails vigilant monitoring of changing responses to brand images and consumption patterns among specific populations in a competitive market. Particular market niches are targeted for intensive advertising activities. Capturing a share of the starters market, which is predominantly under age 20, is important to tobacco companies because of the amount of brand loyalty and switching within brand families. Several studies have been specially commissioned by the tobacco industry to study the youth market,[42] although the tobacco industry has claimed that it does not target underage youth in its advertising campaigns. Youths constitute not only a market segment in their own right but also a subgroup of market segments defined in relation to gender, socioeconomic status, ethnicity, etc. Research suggests that, regardless of intent, marketing pitches aimed at young adults ages 20-25 are also appealing to youths of the same class, gender, and ethnic group. For example, the tobacco industry heavily advertises in magazines that appeal to youthful readerships, for example *Spin, Rolling Stone, Cycle World, Mademoiselle, Glamour*, and *New Woman*.[43] A consideration of the impact of advertising on children and youths therefore demands an understanding of those subpopulations targeted by the industry as market growth segments: women, the less educated, and ethnic groups. A method for identifying which market segments are specially targeted by the tobacco industry would entail trend surveillance of two elements of tobacco advertising and promotion: (1) where the ads are being placed and therefore who is likely to see the ads, and (2) to whom the context and message of the ads appeal.

An example of research that has considered the power of image messages in reinforcing tobacco use is a study by Pierce and colleagues that found an association between trends in female smoking initiation and the sales of leading cigarette brands targeted to women through image advertisements from 1944 through the mid-1980s. Age-specific rates of smoking initiation for boys and girls ages 10-20 were constructed from National Health Interview Survey data. The analysis revealed gender-specific relationships with the tobacco advertising campaigns that targeted women and were launched in 1967. Specifically, in girls under 18, smoking initiation increased abruptly around 1967 and peaked around 1973, at about the same time that sales of such brands as Virginia Slims peaked. The increase was especially marked among girls who never attended college (1.7-fold higher). The trend did not apply to women 18-20 years old, nor to men. The investigators concluded that "tobacco advertising has a temporal and specific relationship to smoking uptake in girls younger than the legal age to purchase cigarettes."[44]

THE APPEAL OF TOBACCO ADS TO
CHILDREN AND YOUTHS

The recent success of the Old Joe Camel campaign, introduced in 1987, has rekindled a longstanding debate on what role advertising plays in predisposing youths to use tobacco, and to use specific brands of tobacco products. Choices to smoke are often spontaneous and based on psychological and social processes of identification, individuation, and differentiation. The effect of advertising is complex, and measuring the relative magnitude of any one type of influence on human behavior in isolation from other influences is difficult. Nevertheless, research data suggest that adolescents are more responsive than adults to advertisements. Surveys conducted between 1976 and 1990 among seventh to twelfth graders suggest an association between an explosive growth in the use of Camel cigarettes and the Old Joe Camel campaign. A study of this age group in 1990 found that 32.8% of children who smoked reported smoking Camel cigarettes.[45] While there is some debate about the underage market for Camel cigarettes before the campaign, that market was very small.[46] Furthermore, the study found that the market share for Camels decreased abruptly with age. Camel was the brand choice of 24.5% and 21.7% of boys and girls, respectively, ages 12-17, but of only 12.7% and 5.0% of youths ages 18-24. Thus, it would seem that, whether or not youths are a targeted market segment, advertisements present images that appeal to children and youths and are seen and remembered by them. Concern has been expressed that while smoking advertisements may not have had an immediate effect on smoking uptake, they may increase susceptibility to smoking, which over time translates into behavior.[47]

> *"Camel's cartoons are for the younger kids. Joe Camel's a cool person—a model."*
>
> —adolescent in a focus group

Psychosocial Mechanisms Through Which Advertising Influences the Behavior of Children and Youths

Advertising may influence consumer behavior in two broad ways—either cognitively or affectively. A cognitive influence convinces an individual that there are benefits to be derived from purchasing (or consuming) a particular product. These benefits may be related to (a) a specific need or desire that an individual maintains, or (b) an ideal image that the individual would like to adopt and convey to others. An affective response to a product is fostered by psychological conditioning: an advertisement sets up a positive evocative response.[48] The affective appeal of an advertisement is often unconscious and automatic, apparent when individuals identify a particular advertisement as their "favorite."[49] Both advertising pitches are used to encourage potential consumers to smoke or chew tobacco as well as to buy a particular brand of cigarettes.

Psychologists have described specific mechanisms by which advertising makes tobacco use appear attractive to smokers and potential smokers. Ajzen and Fishbein's *theory of reasoned action* postulates, in brief, that intentions to perform a particular act are predicted both by a person's attitude toward the act and by normative beliefs about it, concordant with "what others think."[50] Ajzen and Fishbein argue that personal attitudinal factors are probably more important in decisions that adults make concerning smoking, whereas social normative factors are more important in the decisions of children. Other psychologists have suggested that children understand the intent of image advertising at a young age.[51] According to the theory of reasoned action, advertising can function either as a direct normative influence by shaping a child's image of what it means to be a smoker or as an indirect normative influence by increasing peer pressure associated with the emulation of role models provided by cigarette advertising. In his exhaustive 1976 review of the literature, Fishbein noted: "there can be little question that cigarette ads attempt to create a positive image of the 'smoker.'" He concluded that "our review suggests that cigarette advertising does affect cigarette consumption."[52]

Bandura's *social cognitive theory* emphasizes the central role played by modeling influences in shaping human thinking, values, and patterns of behavior.[53] Through modeling, one learns behavior and develops preferences as well as a sense of what is normative. The process of social modeling exerts its effects in several different ways.

One way in which the power of modeling is substantially increased is by showing that the modeled behavior produces desired benefits. In image advertising, smoking is portrayed as an expression of independence, individualism, and social sophistication. It engages the consumer in a fantasy and invites the consumer to participate in a promise "that the product can do something for you that you cannot do for yourself."[54] A self-image that the target audience already desires is reinforced.[55] For example, smoking is associated with a strong masculine self-conception. It is depicted as relieving stress, and as winning the admiration of wholesome, fun-loving peers. The models in cigarette ads appear healthy and happy, in stark contrast to the negative health consequences of smoking. Adolescents who evaluate positively the attributes of models used in cigarette advertising strongly overestimate the prevalence of smokers and give less thought to long-term consequences of risky behavior.[56] Associating the names and logos of tobacco products with sporting and musical events serves as yet another vehicle for framing tobacco use around images.

Another way in which social modeling exerts itself is through belief of personal efficacy. According to social cognitive theory, behavior is regulated, in large part, by belief of personal efficacy to exercise control over events and the consequences expected to flow from one's behavior. After people develop a dependence on smoking, their beliefs about personal efficacy affect every phase of their efforts to quit the habit. Such beliefs influence whether they even try to quit smoking, whether they can enlist the motivation and perseverance needed to succeed should they choose to do so, and whether they are vulnerable to relapse after they have given up the smoking habit.[57]

Adolescence is marked by cognitive developmental stages that in turn affect one's concept of self. Early adolescence has been characterized as a period of heightened self-awareness as well as preoccupation with one's self-image. Elkind and Bowen described the notion of the imaginary audience, wherein young adolescents feel that they are always on a stage with imaginary others monitoring and evaluating their appearance and activity.[58] Indeed, studies have shown that adolescents whose actual self-concepts are consistent with their perceptions of "stereotypic" smokers (derived from advertisements) are more likely to smoke.[59] Among nonsmokers, teens who admire the attributes depicted by smokers in ads are also more likely to intend to smoke in the future.[60] In order to acquire selected attributes of model smokers, adolescents may be motivated to use tobacco, even when they view smoking as negative.[61]

Social psychologists have found that the tendency to choose behaviors that are consistent with self-concept is stronger when one's self-concept is threatened.[62] Smoking experimentation commonly occurs at transition points in adolescence when there is a threat to a teen's emerging self-concept: "Teenagers are typically less secure in their identities than most groups in the population, and their age-appropriate task is in part to experiment with different adult identities. They are more subject to social pressure and more attuned to advertising than most groups in the population."[63] For example, Imperial Tobacco Limited's Project Sting tested "overtly masculine imagery, targeted at young males." Young males were seen as "going through a stage where they are seeking to express their independence and individuality under constant pressure of being accepted by their peers. . . . very young starter smokers choose Export A because it provides them with an instant badge of masculinity, appeals to their rebellious nature, and establishes their position amongst their peers."[64] Advertisers recommended that ads be designed for the company's Player's brand that showed someone "free to choose friends, music, clothes, own activities, to be alone if he wishes"; who can manage alone and "be close to nature" with "nobody to interfere, no boss/parents; someone self reliant enough to experience solitude without loneliness."[65] The theme of independence is appealing to those teens that exhibit a proclivity toward "destructive deviance" (low self-esteem, reactant nonconformity) and "constructive deviance" (high self-esteem, autonomy, independence).[66] Most research on tobacco use among teen subgroups has found the highest levels of tobacco use among "dirts" (problem prone) and "skaters" (skateboarders)[67] but one study found that 28% of "hot shots" (academic and social leaders) currently smoked (and 62% of "dirts" currently smoked).[68] What these data suggest is that a wide range of youths are attracted to tobacco advertisements that play up the theme of independence.

Themes and Images

Considerable psychographic research underlies tobacco ad designs.[69] Image advertising tends to appeal to youths.[70] Notably, each of the three brands

(Marlboro, Newport, Camel) most popular among youths maximizes a considerable amount of image-based advertising.[71] Even children ages 6-10 are able to identify the images and slogans associated with popular brands of cigarettes.[72] The symbols of the most popular cigarettes among youths, a cowboy and a camel cartoon character, are more likely to appeal to children than to adults.[73] In addition to the theme of independence noted above, five other themes are pervasive in tobacco ads: that tobacco use is a rite of passage to adulthood, that successful people use tobacco, that tobacco use is relaxing in social situations, that tobacco use is normative, and that tobacco use is safe.

1. *"Tobacco use is a rite of passage to adulthood."* Advertising associates smoking with a passage from childhood to adulthood through sets of images and messages. Smoking is portrayed as a marker of social status (adulthood) and of pleasure appreciated by popular young adults whom teens wish to emulate. Market research has found that teens are more attracted to young adult models in advertisements than to other teens.[74] "Adult themes"—adventure, rugged individualism, independence, sophistication, glamour, and sex—appeal to youths, a fact well established by research of the youth market.[75] Indeed, the popularity of the Marlboro cowboy dispels the myth that in order to appeal to young people as potential smokers, the ad must show young people.[76]

2. *"Successful, popular people use tobacco."* Advertisements effectively associate smoking with sophistication in social and sexual relations. Tobacco image advertisements are appealing to those who are young and impressionable, who would like to acquire the attributes of the models in the ads. The brands most successful with teenagers commonly employ evocative images in their advertising, whether in the form of models or cartoon characters that depict success, sophistication, and self-reliance.[77] Quality of life is an attribute often depicted in smoking ads. Tobacco industry support of cultural events further conveys the impression that smoking is socially acceptable to successful people who patronize the arts and have a high quality of life.

3. *"Tobacco use is relaxing in social situations."* Advertisements position cigarettes and other forms of tobacco as products facilitating peer acceptance. Associating cigarettes with a sense of carefree belonging is reassuring to adolescents at a time of identity construction when social relations are extremely important and teens often feel awkward in social situations. In addition to gaining social approval, ads depict cigarettes as a means of initiating social exchanges and sharing in a relaxed social environment.[78]

4. *"Tobacco use is the norm."* By associating tobacco use with commonplace activities, events, social spaces, or mind-sets, advertising reassures users that smoking and chewing are normal, pervasive, and socially acceptable. Advertising links tobacco consumption to routine social activities and transition points in the daily work-play cycle. For example, cigarettes are depicted as going with a coffee break, an after-work drink, and time off. The sheer volume

of tobacco advertising contributes to the false impression that smoking is normative in a wide variety of contexts.[79]

5. *"Tobacco use is safe and healthful."* Tobacco-related imagery saturates
the public world, leading many potential consumers to believe that its use must
be less dangerous than health messages make it out to be. In ads, tobacco use is
associated with healthy, outdoor activities, leaving the impression that tobacco
use is not only safe but the choice of healthy, vigorous people. Healthiness has
been a manifest theme in cigarette ads for at least 60 years. Images of healthy
smokers offer reassurance to would-be quitters. Such imagery undermines the
effects of public health programs to inform the public of the hazards of tobacco
use and to discourage youths from initiating smoking.

Cigarette advertising has persistently used images and language to reassure
smokers and would-be smokers that one can engage in "healthy smoking." Cigarettes have been described over the years as being "mild," " light," "fresh,"
"smooth," "clean," "pure," "soft," and "natural." The history of cigarette advertising is punctuated by a steady stream of "news" announcements about scientific discoveries and modern materials reducing the hazards and increasing the
pleasures of smoking. The public has been exposed to "miracle tip filters,"
descriptions of "20,000 filter traps," and filters made of activated charcoal,
"selectrate," "millicel," "cellulose acetate," or "micronite," described as "effective," "complete," "superior," etc.[80] The inferred, perhaps implied, benefit of
such filtration systems is reduction if not elimination of cancer-causing agents
and other established health risks. Whereas filtered cigarettes constituted 58%
of the market in 1963, they accounted for 96% of the market in 1991, having
risen steadily since the first surgeon general's report.[81] Currently, low-smoke
cigarettes are being introduced into the market. Philip Morris Superslim ads call
attention to 70% less smoke from the lit end of their product, a message likely to
be interpreted by many smokers in terms of lower health risks. The association
between low smoke and health is conjoined to an association between thinness
and health and beauty ideals. An ad for Carlton is provocative in establishing its
purported health benefits by juxtaposing ten packs of this lower-tar/nicotine cigarette to one pack of Marlboro and Camel with the line: "10 packs of Carlton has
less than 1 pack of these brands."

Analysis of the forms and styles of cigarette ads over the years reveals the
industry's responsiveness to consumer health concerns tied to public health
messages. The means of projecting healthiness has changed in response to regulatory efforts as well as insights from psychology-based consumer research. The
most dramatic change occurred in the late 1950s and early 1960s. Until then,
most health claims were made in direct verbal assertions, such as "more doctors
recommend" . . . "not a cough in a carload" . . . "Scientific studies prove . . ." In
the late 1950s, motivation researchers informed the industry that such ads drew
attention to health problems, cautioning that a more oblique approach to the

health issue would be beneficial. The new strategy replaced verbal statements with visual images in which healthiness was communicated through people and settings that were the very "pictures of health."[82]

A recent trend has been to appropriate the rhetoric of smoking cessation programs. For its low-tar brand Merit, Philip Morris launched an advertising campaign that features such rhetoric in slogans like "you can do it," subtly conveying the message that switching to low-tar cigarettes is a major health accomplishment associated with personal agency. In reality, once addicted, most smokers adjust their smoking habits to maintain their consumption of nicotine at an optimal psychophysiological level irrespective of the brand of cigarette smoked (see chapter 2).[83]

Ads playing up one's ability to down-switch to the lower-tar/nicotine brands gloss over the difficulties in giving up smoking once one is addicted to nicotine. Data from the Monitoring the Future Study reveal that the proportion of high school seniors who perceive "great risk" of physical harm from pack-a-day smoking has risen less than 6% since 1980 (to 69.5% in 1993).[84] Several studies have found that teenagers who smoke underestimate their chances of becoming addicted to nicotine and overestimate their ability to quit smoking at will.[85] Low-tar/nicotine cigarettes appeal to a growing segment of the youth market. Advertising and promotional activities that tend to convey a message that healthy smoking is feasible undermine smoking prevention messages aimed at youth.

The five themes described above appear not only in tobacco ads, but also in other ads and media images that foster tobacco use. For example, there are no restrictions on how smoking may be portrayed in ads for non-tobacco products in youth magazines. A study by the Health Education Authority in the United Kingdom found that in youth fashion and style magazines, many non-advertisement-driven scenes depict a glamorous model smoking.[86] *Rolling Stone* and other popular magazines for youths have featured interviews with stars of the popular teen television program, *Beverly Hills 90210*, who are all pictured with cigarettes dangling from their mouths. Recently, several major print advertisers whose products have nothing to do with tobacco have featured models who smoke; for example, Guess Jeans ran an ad in the October 1992 issue of *Esquire* showing their newest model in a sexy pose, holding a cigarette with a dangling ash. Pictures of popular people smoking who are not associated with a particular brand may be more likely to attract the attention of teens, than ads pitching name brands.[87] They are an indirect endorsement of smoking. The media have associated smoking with glamour, style, sophistication, sex appeal, street credibility, rebellion, independence, etc. Research is needed on the extent to which indirect promotion of tobacco use contributes to its appeal and may be countered by educational programs that teach youth to critically assess the enticement of commercial and noncommercial appeals.[88]

CRITICAL ASSESSMENT OF STUDIES ON ADVERTISING RECALL, ADVERTISING EXPENDITURES, AND TOBACCO CONSUMPTION

The surgeon general's report released in March of 1994, *Preventing Tobacco Use Among Young People*, thoroughly reviews the research literature on the impact of tobacco advertising and promotional activities on tobacco consumption by youths, and provides an historical account of cigarette advertising that highlights changes and continuity in cigarette advertising and promotional activities of tobacco and its likely impact on youths. The surgeon general's report summarizes the review in five conclusions:

1. Young people continue to be a strategically important market for the tobacco industry.

2. Young people are currently exposed to cigarette messages through print media (including outdoor billboards) and through promotional activities, such as sponsorship of sporting events and public entertainment, point-of-sale displays, and distribution of specialty items.

3. Cigarette advertising uses images rather than information to portray the attractiveness and function of smoking. Human models and cartoon characters in cigarette advertising convey independence, healthfulness, adventure-seeking, and youth activities—themes correlated with psychosocial factors that appeal to young people.

4. Cigarette advertisements capitalize on the disparity between an ideal and actual self-image and imply that smoking may close the gap.

5. Cigarette advertising appears to affect young people's perceptions of the pervasiveness, image, and function of smoking. Since misperceptions in these areas constitute psychosocial risk factors for the initiation of smoking, cigarette advertising appears to increase young people's risk of smoking.[89]

Readers who are interested in the details of the studies leading to those conclusions should refer to the surgeon general's report. The Committee does not repeat that review here, but instead focuses on methodological approaches to advertising research.

Studies of Advertising Recall

Several studies have shown a positive correlation between adolescents' ability to recall a particular advertisement, logo, or brand insignia and smoking intent, initiation, or level of smoking.[90] The key variable in such studies is *exposure* to cigarette ads. The concept of exposure has been applied in myriad ways, from environmental exposure to attention, physical exposure to psychological engagement.[91] Advertisement recall studies have consistently found that young people who maintain an interest in smoking retain more information from cigarette ads. In some cases this correlation has been used to imply that there is a causal link between consumption and exposure to advertising, as well as between recognition of ads and smoking behavior. This leap in the interpretation of the data is questionable. What can be said is that experimentation with cigarettes does affect the extent to which individuals recognize information presented in cigarette advertisements and that this may influence smoking-related behavior over time in a variety of ways.[92] For example, attentiveness to ads may reinforce smoking behavior by providing the smoker "evidence" of the values and benefits of smoking, such as reassurance that popular people use tobacco. What is not known at present is whether youths already interested in smoking become more attentive to advertisements or whether advertisements lead youths to become more interested in smoking. This is analogous to the issue of whether "peer pressure" leads youths to smoke or whether youths interested in smoking gravitate to peer groups (friends) who smoke. Studies of advertising recall, assessed independently of other data on smoking behavior, are insufficient to determine the direction of influence.

Econometric Studies of the Relationship Between Advertising and Consumption

Econometric studies of the relationship between advertising and tobacco use are prominent in debates between public health advocates and the tobacco industry. Econometric studies provide insights into the effects of general advertising trends, but are too imprecise to support firm conclusions about advertising's impact on the behavior of specific populations over time. It is unrealistic to expect that studies correlating trends in tobacco consumption with aggregate expenditures on advertising can provide meaningful insight about the influence of advertising on tobacco use by children and youths. The results, therefore, from numerous econometric studies do not provide a consistent picture regarding the impact of tobacco advertising on consumption. The mixed conclusions drawn from these studies should not be interpreted as evidence that advertising has little or no influence on tobacco use. Econometric methods are better suited to assessing the impact of governmental policies intended to restrict tobacco advertising or significantly increase the price of tobacco products, but even these studies are incapable of providing definitive information about how different population groups (for example, youths and ethnic groups) are likely to respond to advertising restrictions.

Studies of the Effects of Advertising Bans

Several studies have concluded that advertising bans have significantly reduced smoking prevalence in the population as a whole. In 1993 the Chief Economic Advisor of the Department of Health of the Government of Great

Britain reviewed the existing data and noted that advertising tends to increase consumption of tobacco products and that bans on tobacco advertising tend to decrease tobacco use beyond what would have occurred in the absence of such a ban. Focusing on the four countries with the most complete data—Norway, Finland, Canada, and New Zealand—the British report found that in all four countries, bans or restrictions on advertising resulted in an overall decrease in consumption.

The strongest evidence to date on the effect that legal restrictions of promotional activities have on tobacco consumption is drawn from a study of trends in 33 countries between 1970 to 1986, commissioned by the government of New Zealand. The 33 countries studied (24 free-market economies and 9 centrally planned East European economies) provide over 400 calendar years of observation of different tobacco prices, personal incomes, and advertising restrictions, including tobacco advertising bans. The methodology of this study was rigorous and examined adult tobacco consumption, accounting for income and tobacco price effects as well as health education effects. The overall finding of this study was that: ". . . the greater a government's degree of control over tobacco promotion, the greater the annual average fall in tobacco consumption and in the rate of decrease of smoking among young people."[93] Highlights of the report include the following (also see tables 4-1 and 4-2):

- "Total advertising bans for health reasons are, on average, accompanied by falls in tobacco consumption four times faster than in partial ban countries."
- "In countries where tobacco has been promoted virtually unrestricted in all media, consumption has markedly increased (+1.7% per year)."
- "In countries where advertising has been totally banned or severely restricted, the percentage of young people who smoke has decreased more rapidly than in countries where tobacco promotion has been less restricted."
- "When the results of this study of promotion/consumption trends in 33 countries between 1970 and 1986 are put alongside the evidence from econometric studies . . . it seems more likely than not that, other factors remaining unchanged, the elimination of tobacco promotion *causes* a reduction in tobacco consumption and smoking prevalence to a level below what it would have been otherwise."[94]

The report also concluded that comprehensive policies to reduce tobacco consumption are more effective than any single measure, for example:

- "Tobacco consumption increases when tobacco promotion is permitted and real price is allowed to fall; consumption declines markedly when promotion is totally banned and prices [are] raised."[95]

The three features deemed essential for an effective government policy to reduce the health consequences of tobacco use were (1) programs to educate the public

TABLE 4-1   Annual average rates of change in the percentage of adults smoking according to tobacco advertising restriction in force, 20 advanced economy countries, 1970-1986

Country (year of ban)	Age group	Years Begin	Years End	% Smokers Begin	% Smokers End	Annual % change Per country	Annual % change Per group
Enforced tobacco advertising ban							
Iceland (1972)	18-69	1985-1986		40.0	36.2	−9.5	Group
Finland (1978)[a]	15-64	1978-1986		25.8	25.5	−0.1	average
Norway (1975)	16-74	1973-1986		41.5	34.5	−1.1	−3.6
Portugal (1983)	na	1983-1984		na	23.5	na	
Tobacco promotion in few media							
Belgium	15+	1980-1987		41.5	32.0	−3.3	Group
France	15+	1976-1983		44	39.0	−1.6	average
Italy (enforced ban)	14+	1980-1983		34.9	31.1	−3.6	−2.5
New Zealand	15+	1976-1986		35.0	30.0	−1.4	
Singapore[b]	15+	1977-1984		23.0	19.0	−2.5	
Sweden[b]	16+	1976-1985		38.5	29.6	−2.6	
Tobacco promotion in most media							
Australia[b]	16+	1972-1983		38.0	33.5	−1.1	
Austria	15+	1972-1981		28.0	27.0	−0.4	
Belgium	15+	1970-1979		20.2	21.3	−0.6	
Canada	15+	1970-1986		45.0	32.0	−1.8	
Denmark	15+	1970-1979		57.9	48.9	−1.7	
France	15+	1970-1976		53.1	46.7	−2.0	
Ireland	15+	1973-1982		43.0	35.0	−2.1	
Netherlands	15+	1970-1986		58.5	38.0	−2.2	
Switzerland	15+	1972-1981		34.6	37.5	+0.9	
United Kingdom	16+	1972-1986		46.0	33.0	−2.0	
United States	17+	1970-1986		36.6	26.5	−1.7	
West Germany	15+	1970-1984		41.7	36.0	−1.0	
Tobacco promotion in all media							
Greece	15+	1985		na	21.5	na	
Japan	20+	1970-1986		46.6	37.6	−1.2	
Spain	15+	1970-1987		na	40.5	na	

[a]Average of two surveys.
[b]Male and female percentage averaged.

Sources: The following were cited by the Toxic Substances Board. *Health or Tobacco: An End to Tobacco Advertising and Promotion.* Wellington, New Zealand: Department of Health, 1989; Rothwell, K. and R. Masironi. *Cigarette Smoking in Developed Countries Outside Europe.* WHO, 1987; Rothwell, K., R. Masironi, and D. O'Byrne. *Smoking in Europe.* WHO, 1987.

TABLE 4-2   Annual average rates of change in the percentage of young people who smoke daily according to tobacco advertising restrictions in force, 18 advanced economy countries, 1970–1986

Country	Surveyed Age group	Years Begin End	% Smokers Begin End	Annual % change Per Survey	Per country	Per group
Tobacco promotion banned for health reasons						
Iceland	12-16	1974-1986	23	9	-5.1		
Iceland	17-18	1974-1986	34	29	-1.3	-3.0	
Iceland	19-20	1974-1986	41	29	-2.5		
Italy	15-18	1972	51	na	na		Group
Finland	16	1973-1985	35.5	26.5	2.6		average
Finland	18	1973-1985	47	29	-3.2		-2.7
Norway	16-24	1974-1986	41	28.5	-2.5	-2.5	
Portugal	20-24	1983	46	na	na		
	15-24	na	87	45	na		
Tobacco promotion in few media						
Belgium	17	1975-1981	44.5	28.5	-6.0	-3.0	
Belgium	18-24	1982-1984	44	44	0		
France	14-16	1976-1984	29	25.5	-1.5	-1.95	
France	18-24	1976-1983	66	55	-2.4		Group
Italy	15-24	1987		32.5	na		average
New Zealand	15-19	1976-1987	30	27.5	-0.8	-0.08	-2.7
Singapore	15-19	1984	na	4.8	na	na	
Sweden	16	1974-1984	38	19	-5.0	-5.15	
Sweden	16-24	1977-1986	41	21.5	-5.3		
Tobacco promotion in most media						
Australia	16-19	1974-1986	33.8	29.6	-1.0		
Austria	14-29	1972-1981	30.0	35.0	+1.8		
Canada	15-19	1972-1983	31.7	20.3	-3.3		Group
Denmark	17-19	1974-1980	38.1	33.0	-2.2		average
FR Germany	14-19	1976-1984	40.5	27.5	-4.0		-1.9
Ireland	18	1970-1980	39	36	-0.8	-2.4	
	16-24	1973-1982	48	31	-3.9		
Netherlands	15-19	1970-1986	56	22	-3.8		
Switzerland	15-24	1981		36.5	na		
United States	17-18	1968-1979	24.5	22.5	-0.7		
United Kingdom	16-19	1972-1986	41	30	-1.9		
Tobacco promotion in all media						Group
Japan	20-29	1970-1986	45	43.3	-0.2		average
Spain	15-24	1981-1987	53.5	55	+0.5		+0.1

NOTE: In all countries the rate given represents both sexes. In most countries female and male rates were averaged.

Sources: The following were cited by the Toxic Substances Board. *Health or Tobacco: An End to Tobacco Advertising and Promotion.* Wellington, New Zealand: Department of Health, 1989, Appendix 5; *International Digest of Health Legislation.* WHO; Aoki, M., S. Hisamichi, and S. Tominaga, eds. *Smoking and Health, 1987.* Elsevier Science Publishers. BV, 1988; *Smoking in Europe.* WHO, 1987; *Smoking in Developed Countries Outside Europe.* WHO, 1987.

about the dangers of tobacco use, (2) an increase in tobacco prices, and (3) a total ban on tobacco promotion.[96]

Currently, 18 countries have total bans on tobacco advertisements. Advertisement bans have been instituted as part of more comprehensive tobacco control efforts in Canada and New Zealand. In these countrires, ad bans have been complemented by aggressive antismoking activities and tax increases on tobacco. The rate of decline in Canada after implementation of an advertising ban was double that reported prior to the ban, and in New Zealand an ad ban was associated with an 11.3% decrease in smoking during a 6-month period. An assessment of the independent effect of each antismoking measure would be difficult, perhaps impossible, but the effect of the combination is clear.[97]

An important reason for calling attention to comprehensive approaches to reduce tobacco use is that single-factor approaches might have paradoxical effects on tobacco consumption. For example, *restrictions of advertising that are accompanied by a reduction in counter-advertising efforts may thwart prevention efforts.* In 1971, in the United States, the tobacco industry voluntarily removed from radio and television all cigarette advertising. Following this act, per capita cigarette consumption, which had been declining since the 1964 surgeon general's report, leveled off and then increased. This unexpected trend may be related to the fact that as the cigarette ads were removed from the airwaves, so too were the cigarette counter-ads in the form of public service announcements (PSAs). The PSAs, developed by the Public Health Service in the late 1960s, were designed to increase the public's knowledge about the dangers of smoking, and were pretested accordingly. These public service antismoking messages, which had appeared from July 1967 to January 1971 along with cigarette ads as a result of the FCC's Fairness Doctrine, apparently had been far more effective in reducing smoking than the pro-smoking ads in increasing it.[98] For this reason it was in the tobacco industry's best interest to remove ads from radio and television, and to shift marketing dollars to promotionals and giveaways.

RATIONALE FOR RESTRICTIONS

Over the decades, tobacco advertising and promotional efforts that reach children and youths have not diminished unless social or legal pressure was brought to bear on the tobacco industry or the advertising media. Criticism of the tobacco industry was widespread and strong in 1963, a year in which the average teenager viewed 100 cigarette commercials a month, and the average child viewed 70 due to airing of ads during programs commonly watched by youths. In 1965, in response, the tobacco industry adopted a voluntary code of conduct.[99] The voluntary code notwithstanding, a later analysis, in 1968, by the FTC revealed that the average teenager was exposed to 60 full-length cigarette commercials a month.[100]

The tobacco industry's self-regulatory code covered four areas of behavior:

advertising appealing to the young, advertising containing health representations, the provision of samples, and the distribution of promotional items to the young.[101] Notably, guidelines for following the code are lacking. For example, a specific stipulation of the voluntary code is that models used in ads should not appear to be younger than 25 years of age. Interpretation of what a model of 25 looks like is open to question. One study of cigarette ads found that 17% of models in cigarette ads were perceived (by persons 13 years old and older) to be younger than 25 years, that certain brands tend to employ younger-looking models, and that these models appeal to a broad audience.[102] In the wake of criticism, both from antismoking activists and from the advertising profession itself, that the Joe Camel campaign is especially appealing to those under 25, Philip Morris and R. J. Reynolds have responded by creating national advertising campaigns built around their commitment to "educate children" about smoking. The campaign is framed around smoking as an adult behavior and therefore the need for children to wait until they are of legal age before making decisions about smoking. A booklet entitled *Tobacco: Helping Youth Say No* has been widely distributed to governors, school boards, community groups, and parents who request it. The booklet makes no reference to the health and addictive effects of tobacco use. The educational impact of the campaign on youths has not been evaluated.

Another code stipulation states, "Cigarette *advertising* shall not depict as a smoker any person participating in, or obviously having just participated in, physical activity requiring stamina or athletic conditioning beyond that of normal recreation."[103] Nevertheless, ads routinely use imagery associated with athletics and physical activity, thereby linking smoking and vitality; Marlboro's Adventure Team of whitewater rafters, dirt bikers, and other adventure enthusiasts is a case in point. As currently framed, advertising and promotion of so-called "light" or "low-tar" cigarettes fail to convey accurate information regarding the hazards of smoking, and instead tend to foster the illusion of a "healthful" smoking alternative. Whether or not these product innovations reduce harm from smoking, they do address the marketing objective of reducing consumer concern; they are tools in a public relations approach to minimizing a major public health problem.[104] Furthermore, under self-regulation, many health issues are not presented to the public, issues such as the addictiveness of tobacco; risk of cancer, heart disease, and stroke; effects on nonsmokers; and risk from tobacco smoke constituents such as benzene and arsenic.

Public health groups contend that the industry's voluntary code is often inadequate in content and is inadequately enforced. They have therefore pressed for Congress to restrict tobacco promotion and advertising, arguing that the advertising and promotion of tobacco products on the scale and in the manner described in this chapter tend to increase the overall prevalence of tobacco consumption as well as increase the initiation of smoking by youths. In response, the tobacco industry argues that, among smokers, advertising and promotion affect market share, not the level of consumption. Moreover, the industry denies that advertising and promotion causally affect the decisions of young people to begin smoking.

Many of the participants in this ongoing debate seem to assume that a definitive finding of causality is a necessary predicate for legislative action restricting tobacco promotion and advertising. In the Committee's view, however, requiring definitive proof of causality on issues of this nature would unjustifiably stymie sensible public health regulation. Indeed, the history of public health successes, from vaccination to cholera prevention and injury control, suggest that detailed causal understanding is apt to *follow* an intervention, rather than be a precondition for it. If youth smoking fell *after* advertising and promotion were eliminated, this would corroborate a hypothesis for which there is already ample, suggestive evidence—that such advertising and promotion is an important factor in the initiation of tobacco use by youths. This seems to be the lesson from the experiences reviewed in the New Zealand report.

The inability to conduct case control studies in an environment free of tobacco marketing makes it impossible to discern the independent causal effect of advertising and promotion on tobacco consumption. It is difficult to disentangle the actual impact of marketing expenditures from the other social and cultural factors that affect tobacco use. Moreover, the influence of any of these environmental variables is mediated by, and interacts with, so many other variables affecting perceptions of and attitudes toward tobacco use that any statistical association between levels of promotional expenditures and levels of tobacco use is difficult to interpret. This is not to say that the relationship is *not* a causal one, only that any causal effect is inevitably obscured by layers of other factors, and that it is virtually impossible to quantify the causal effect in any definitive way. Indeed, when one takes into account the inherent difficulty of discerning a causal influence, the substantial convergent evidence that advertising and promotion increases tobacco use by youths is impressive and, in the Committee's view, provides a strong basis for legal regulation.

Having said this, the Committee does not think that the argument for restricting the advertising and promotion of tobacco products must rest on a definitive or unequivocal finding that such activities causally influence levels of consumption. It is enough that the advertising and promotional activities described above in this chapter have the natural tendency to encourage initiation and maintenance of smoking by children and adolescents. There can be no doubt that the tobacco companies aim to portray smoking in a favorable light and to communicate messages that link use of tobacco products to positive feelings, images, and experiences. Even if the primary objective of those marketing expenditures is to preserve or expand market share among existing smokers, youngsters are routinely exposed to messages that encourage them to smoke.

Tobacco advertising is characterized by images and themes that are especially appealing to adolescents, and some are appealing to children. In addition, a large proportion of promotional expenditures associate use of tobacco with activities and products that are attractive to children and youths. The sheer amount of expenditures for advertising and promotion assures that young people will be exposed to these messages on a massive scale. It is clear that society's efforts to discourage young people from smoking are obstructed—and perhaps fatally undermined—by the industry's efforts to portray their dangerous products in a positive light.[105]

In sum, portraying a deadly addiction as a healthful and sensual experience tugs against the nation's efforts to promote a tobacco-free norm and to discourage tobacco use by children and youths. This warrants legislation restricting the features of advertising and promotion that make tobacco use attractive to youths. The question is not, "Are advertising and promotion *the* causes of youth initiation?" but rather, "Does the preponderance of evidence suggest that features of advertising and promotion tend to encourage youths to smoke?" The answer is yes and this is a sufficient basis for action, even in the absence of a precise and definitive causal chain.

RECOMMENDATIONS

Policy Recommendations

The images typically associated with advertising and promotion convey the message that tobacco use is a desirable, socially approved, safe and healthful, and widely practiced behavior among young adults, whom children and youths want to emulate. As a result, tobacco advertising and promotion undoubtedly contribute to the multiple and convergent psychosocial influences that lead children and youths to begin using these products and to become addicted to them.

As already noted, the Committee believes that American society, through all organized social institutions, should take aggressive measures to discourage the use of tobacco products by children and youths. The message should be unequivocal—tobacco use is unhealthy and socially disapproved. In the context of this emergent social norm, the contradictory messages now conveyed by the tobacco industry can no longer be tolerated. The Committee therefore recommends a step-by-step plan to eliminate these commercial messages from the various media of mass communication. Realizing that implementation of this recommendation will require careful planning and a period of transition, the Committee proposes a sequential process for phasing in the necessary restrictions.

First, Congress should repeal the federal law preempting state regulation of tobacco promotion and advertising that occurs entirely within the states' borders. This should be accomplished by the end of 1995. The repeal will have the effect of stimulating local interest in tobacco regulation and community participation in reviewing tobacco data and in drafting legislation aimed at promotion, distribution, and use of tobacco products. Concordant with federal guidelines, a wide range of national experiments will take place, providing data on the effect of various programs.

State and local regulation of cigarette advertising to a large extent has been foreclosed by federal law, which expressly prohibits states and localities from imposing "any requirement or prohibition based on smoking and health . . . with respect to the advertising and promotion of any cigarettes" that meet federal labeling requirements.[106] To the extent that state and local regulation of tobacco advertising or promotion aims to promote public health objectives, it is curtailed by this sweeping federal preemption. It can be argued, however, that state and local governments retain the authority to ban advertising likely to reach a large audience of children because such action aims mainly to minimize violations of laws against youth access and is, therefore, not "based on smoking and health." Relying on this argument, transportation systems in the cities of Boston, Denver, Portland, New York, Seattle, and San Francisco, and in the state of Utah, have eliminated tobacco advertising on their vehicles.[107] Whether those actions are lawful remains unclear.

The communication and tobacco industries have legitimate interests in avoiding diverse and often incompatible state-by-state regulation of advertising and promotional activities occurring in national media. However, state and local governments should be free to circumscribe advertising and promotion that occur exclusively within the geographic boundaries of a single state in order to protect and promote the health and welfare of its citizens, subject only to the command of the first amendment. Therefore, Congress should modify the preemption provision so that the states have clear authority to restrict or ban advertising and promotion at the point of sale, on public transportation systems and vehicles, on billboards, in public arenas or sports facilities, or other locations located entirely within a state's boundaries.

Second, after state regulatory authority has been clarified and restored, states and localities should severely restrict the advertising and promotion of tobacco products on billboards and other outdoor media, on vehicles, in facilities of public transportation, in public arenas and sports facilities, and at the point of sale. States and localities should either ban tobacco advertising and promotion altogether or should restrict such messages to a "tombstone" format. Tombstone advertising would limit commercial messages to information about the product and would forbid the use of images and pictures. This approach is designed to eliminate all the images that imply that tobacco use is beneficial and make it attractive, and that encourage young people to use tobacco products. The most common concept of tombstone advertising would allow only text in an advertisement. A broader concept of tombstone advertising would permit the use of slogans, scenes, or colors in tobacco advertisements or on tobacco packaging. Specific decisions regarding the type of information that would be permitted should be made by a regulatory authority.

Third, Congress should enact comprehensive legislation establishing a timetable for gradual implementation of a plan for restricting tobacco advertising and promotion in interstate commerce. Essential components of this plan, which should be enacted by the end of 1996 and should become fully effective by the year 2000, include:

(a) restricting to a tombstone format the advertising of tobacco products in print media, including magazines and newspapers, or in other visual media, including videotape, videodisc, video arcade game, or film;

(b) banning the commercial use of the registered brand name of a tobacco product, trademark, or logo, or other recognizable symbol for such a product in any movie, music video, television show, play, video arcade game, or other form of entertainment, or on any other product; and

(c) banning the use of the registered brand name of a tobacco product, a trademark or logo, or other recognizable symbol for such a product, in any public place, or in any medium of mass communication for the purpose of publicizing, revealing, or documenting sponsorship of, or contribution to, any athletic, artistic, or other public event.

These proposals represent *essential* components of the regulatory plan. By recommending these steps, the Committee does not mean to exclude other restrictions or to disapprove more restrictive steps, such as banning advertising altogether. The Committee has endorsed the tombstone format because this approach is necessary to eliminate those features of advertising that tend to encourage tobacco use by children and youths. No less restrictive approach would accomplish the legislative objective. The Committee is confident that state and federal legislation implementing these recommendations will substantially further the nation's compelling interest in preventing tobacco use by children and youths and that such legislation would survive constitutional challenges brought by the affected media or by the tobacco industry.[108]

Research Recommendations

The Committee recommends:

Research should be conducted that attends to ethnic, gender, and social class differences; that is sensitive to youths' responses to advertising and promotional messages; and that assesses the success as well as the failure of advertising campaigns. The research question to date has primarily been, "What does advertising do to people?" Research should now ask, "What do people do with advertising (and counter-advertising)?"[109]

As a result of the types of research methods used and the research questions asked, much of the literature on tobacco use and advertising attributes little agency to the public in general and to youths in particular; the public is considered to be rather passive and easily manipulated. While there is some truth to this view, it hardly expresses a complete picture of this complex, interactive phenomenon. Required are longitudinal and ethnographic accounts of tobacco use that are responsive to local context, studies that are notably absent in the smoking literature. In need of consideration are the ways in which:

(a) advertising provides resources (images) for teen subgroup identity construction and social statement,

(b) advertising is responsive to existing and emergent social uses of smoking among various subgroups,

(c) tobacco use takes on meaning in response to anti-tobacco-use messages (generated by the tobacco industry as well as by public health advocates), that is, messages that are moralistic or focus attention on adult status, and

(d) imagery of tobacco use is appropriated and transformed by teens themselves.

REFERENCES

1. Federal Trade Commission. *Report to Congress for 1991: Pursuant to the Federal Cigarette Labeling and Advertising Act.* Washington, DC: Federal Trade Commission, 1994; Federal Trade Commission. *Report to Congress: Pursuant to the Comprehensive Smokeless Tobacco Health Education Act of 1986.* Washington, DC: Federal Trade Commission, 1993. 19, 26.

2. Centers for Disease Control and Prevention. *Preventing Tobacco Use Among Young People. A Report of the Surgeon General, 1994.* S/N 017-001-004901-0. Washington, DC: U.S. Government Printing Office, 1994. 175.

3. *Ibid.*, 65.

4. *Ibid.*, 58, 230.

5. Centers for Disease Control. "Differences in the Age of Smoking Initiation Between Blacks and Whites—United States." *Morbidity and Mortality Weekly Report* 40:44 (1991): 754-757.

6. Centers for Disease Control and Prevention. *Preventing Tobacco Use.* 74.

7. Johnston, Lloyd D., Patrick M. O'Malley, and Jerald G. Bachman. *Smoking, Drinking, and Illicit Drug Use Among American Secondary Students, College Students, and Young Adults, 1975-1991, Volume I.* NIH Pub. No. 93-3480. Rockville, MD: National Institute on Drug Abuse, 1992. 125.

8. Centers for Disease Control and Prevention. *Preventing Tobacco Use.* 230.

9. Johnston, Lloyd D., Patrick M. O'Malley, and Jerald G. Bachman. *National Survey Results on Drug Use from The Monitoring the Future Study, 1975-1992, Volume II.* NIH Pub. No. 93-3598 Rockville, MD: National Institute on Drug Abuse, 1993. 14, 163-165.

10. Federal Trade Commission, 1994. 20.

11. Hooker, K. "Developmental Tasks." In Lerner, R. M., A. C. Peterson, and J. Brooks-Gunn. eds. *Encyclopedia of Adolescence.* New York: Garland Publishing, 1991. 228-231.

12. All spending amounts are from the Federal Trade Commission report, 1994.

13. Kotler, P., and G. Armstrong. *Principles of Marketing.* Englewood Cliffs, NJ: Prentice Hall, 1991.

14. Gallup International Institute. *Teen-Age Attitudes and Behavior Concerning Tobacco.* GII 9104. Princeton, NJ: The George H. Gallup International Institute, Sept. 1992.

15. Roswell Park Cancer Institute. *Survey of Alcohol, Tobacco and Drug Use Among Ninth Grade Students in Erie County, 1992.* Buffalo, NY: Roswell Park Cancer Institute, 1993.

16. Slade, John. "Teenagers Participate in Tobacco Promotions." *9th World Conference on Tobacco and Health.* Paris. October 10-14, 1994. (Abstract.)

17. Comerford, Anthony W., and John Slade. "Selling Cigarettes: A Salesman's Perspective." Paper commissioned by the Committee on Preventing Nicotine Addiction in Children and Youths, 1994.

18. Roswell Park.

19. D'Onofrio, Carol N., and David G. Altman. "Children and Youths." In Houston, Thomas P., ed. *Tobacco Use: An American Crisis.* Washington, DC: American Medical Association, 1993. 32-42.

20. Comerford and Slade.

21. Schudson, M. *Advertising: The Uneasy Persuasion.* New York: Basic Books, 1984.

22. Comerford and Slade.

23. Freeman, Harold, Janet Delgado, and Clifford E. Douglas. "Minority Issues." In Houston, Thomas P., ed. *Tobacco Use: An American Crisis.* Washington, DC: American Medical Association, 1993. 43-47.

24. Fahey, Alison. "Outdoors Sets Limits." *Advertising Age* 61:26 (1990): 57.

25. *Advocacy Institute.* 5 Sept. 1990.

26. Mayberry, Robert M., and Patricia A. Price. "Targeting Blacks in Cigarette Billboard Advertising: Results From Down South." *Health Values* 17:1 (1993): 28-35.

27. "Other Side of the Billboard. III" News release. Washington, DC: Scenic America, November 1989.

28. Felgner, B. *U.S. Tobacco and Candy Journal* (28 December 1987): 16. Cited in Richards, John W., and Paul M. Fischer. *World Smoking and Health* 15:1 (March 1990): 12-14.

29. Blum, Alan. "The Marlboro Grand Prix: Circumvention of the Television Ban on Tobacco Advertising." *New England Journal of Medicine* 324:13 (28 Mar. 1991): 913-917.

30. Johnson, M. *Dallas Morning News.* (30 Dec. 1989). Cited in Richards, John W., and Paul M. Fischer. "Smokescreen: How Tobacco Companies Market to Children." *World Smoking and Health* 15:1 (Mar. 1990):12-14.

31. Slade, John. "Tobacco Product Advertising During Motorsports Broadcasts: A Quantitative Assessment." *9th World Conference on Tobacco and Health.* Paris, October 10-14, 1994. (Abstract.)

32. Meier, Kathryn S. "Tobacco Truths: The Impact of Role Models on Children's Attitudes Toward Smoking." *Health Education Quarterly* 18:2 (June 1991): 173-182; Aitken, P. P., D. S. Leathar, and S. I. Squair. "Children's Awareness of Cigarette Brand Sponsorship of Sports and Games in the United Kingdom." *Health Education Research* 1:3 (1986): 203-211; Ledwith, Frank. "Does Tobacco Sports Sponsorship on Television Act as Advertising to Children?" *Health Education Journal* 43:4 (1984): 85-88.

33. Slade, "Teenagers."

34. Warner, K. E., L. M. Goldenhar, and C. G. McLaughlin. "Cigarette Advertising and Magazine Coverage of the Hazards of Smoking: A Statistical Analysis." *New England Journal of Medicine* 326:5 (1992): 305-309.

35. Minkler, M., L. Wallack, and P. Madden. "Alcohol and Cigarette Advertising in Ms. Magazine." *Journal of Public Health Policy* (June 1987): 164-179; Whelan, Elizabeth M., M. J. Sheridan, K. A. Meister, and B. A. Mosher. "Analysis of Coverage of Tobacco Hazards in Women's Magazines." *Journal of Public Health Policy* 2:1 (Mar. 1981): 28-35.

36. Smith, R. C. "The Magazines' Smoking Habit." *Columbia Journalism Review* (Jan/Feb 1978): 29-31. In Roemer, Ruth. *Legislative Action to Combat the World Tobacco Epidemic.* 2nd ed. Geneva, Switzerland: World Health Organization, 1982. 28.

37. Pollay, Richard W., Jung S. Lee, and David Carter-Whitney. "Separate But Not Equal: Racial Segmentation in Cigarette Advertising." *Journal of Advertising* 21:1 (1992): 45-57.

38. Warner et al., 1992.

39. Bishofsky, Steven. "Magazines Uneasy about Accepting Anti-Smoking Ads." University of Washington: Office of News and Information, 1993. (Thesis.)

40. Ward, S. *Testimony in Tobacco Issues (Part 2)*. In Hearings Before the Committee on Energy and Commerce. House of Representatives. Serial No. 101-126. 1989. 302-308.

41. Centers for Disease Control. "Cigarette Smoking among Adults—United States, 1991." *Morbidity and Mortality Weekly Report* 42:12 (1993): 230-233; Tye, Joe B., Kenneth E. Warner, and Stanton A. Glantz. "Tobacco Advertising and Consumption: Evidence of a Causal Relationship." *Journal of Public Health Policy* (Winter 1987): 492-508.

42. Pollay, Richard W., and Anne M. Lavack. "The Targeting of Youths by Cigarette Marketers: Archival Evidence on Trial." In McAlister, Leigh, and Michael L. Rothschild. eds. *Advances in Consumer Research 20*. Provo, UT: Association for Consumer Research, 1993. 266-271.

43. Basil, Michael D., Caroline Schooler, David G. Altman, Michael Slater, Cheryl L. Albright, and Nathan Maccoby. "How Cigarettes Are Advertised in Magazines: Special Messages for Special Markets." *Health Communication* 3:2 (1991): 75-91; Warner, Kenneth E. *Selling Smoke: Cigarette Advertising and Public Health.* Washington, DC: American Public Health Association, 1986; Krupka, L. R., and A. M. Vener. "Gender Differences in Drug (Prescription, Non-Prescription, Alcohol and Tobacco) Advertising: Trends and Implications." *The Journal of Drug Issues* 22:2 (1992): 339-360; and Hutchings. "A Review of the Nature and Extent of Cigarette Advertising in the United States." In *Proceedings of the National Conference on Smoking and Health: Developing a Blueprint for Action*. New York: American Cancer Society, 1981. 249-262.

44. Pierce, John P., Lora Lee, and Elizabeth Gilpin. "Smoking Initiation by Adolescent Girls, 1944 Through 1988." *Journal of the American Medical Association* 271:8 (23 Feb. 1994): 608-611.

45. DiFranza, Joseph R., John W. Richards, Paul M. Paulman, Nancy Wolf-Gillespie, Christopher Fletcher, Robert Jaffe, David Murray. "RJR Nabisco's Cartoon Camel Promotes Cigarettes to Children." *Journal of the American Medical Association* 266:22 (1991): 3149-3153.

46. Dubow, Joel. "Was Joe Camel Framed?" *Food and Beverage Marketing* (July 1993): 28ff.

47. Pierce, John P., A. Farkas, N. Evans, C. Berry, W. Choi, B. Rosbrook, M. Johnson, and D. G. Bal. *Tobacco Use in California 1992. A Focus on Preventing Uptake in Adolescents*. Sacramento, CA: California Department of Health Services, 1993.

48. Reed, O. Lee, and D. Whitman. "A Constitutional and Policy-Related Evaluation of Prohibiting the Use of Certain Nonverbal Techniques in Legal Advertising." *Brigham Young University Law Review* 2 (1988): 265-338.

49. Batra, Rajeev, and M. L. Ray. "How Advertising Works at Contact." In Alwitt, Linda, and A. Mitchell, eds. *Psychological Processes and Advertising Effects.* Hillsdale, NJ: L. Erlbaum Assoc., 1985; and Zajonc, R. B. "Feeling and Thinking: Preferences Need No Inferences." *American Psychologist* 35:2 (1980): 151-175.

50. Fishbein, Martin, and Icek Ajzen. *Belief, Attitude, Intention and Behavior: An Introduction to Theory and Research*. Reading, MA: Addison Wesley, 1975.

51. Donohue, Thomas R., Lucy L. Henke, and William A. Donohue. "Do Kids Know What TV Commercials Intend?" *Journal of Advertising Research* 20:5 (Oct. 1980): 51-57.

52. Fishbein, Martin. "Consumer Beliefs and Behavior with Respect to Cigarette Smoking: A Critical Analysis of the Public Literature." Report prepared for the Federal Trade Commission, May 1977.

53. Bandura, Albert. *Social Foundations of Thought and Action: A Social Cognitive Theory*. Englewood Cliffs, NJ: Prentice-Hall, 1986; Bandura, Albert. "Social Cognitive Theory of Mass Communication." In Bryant, Jennings, and D. Zillmann, eds. *Media Effects: Advances in Theory and Research*. Hillsdale, NJ: Lawrence Erlbaum, 1994. 61-92.

54. Comerford et al., 8.

55. Goldman, R. *Reading Ads Socially*. London: Rouledge, 1992; Wernick, Andrew. *Promotional Culture: Advertising, Ideology, and Symbolic Expression*. London: Sage Publications, 1991.

56. Wong-McCarthy, William J., and Ellen R. Gritz. "Preventing Regular Teenage Cigarette Smoking." *Pediatric Annals* 11:8 (1982): 683-689; Chassin, Laurie, Clark C. Presson, Steven J. Sherman, Eric Corty, and Richard W. Olshavsky. "Predicting the Onset of Cigarette Smoking in Adolescents: A Longitudinal Study." *Journal of Applied Social Psychology* 14:3 (1984): 224-243.

57. DiClemente, C. Carlo, Scott K. Fairhurst, and Nancy A. Piotrowski. "The Role of Self-Efficacy in the Addictive Behaviors." In Maddux, James, ed. *Self-Efficacy, Adaptation, and Adjustment: Theory, Research, and Application.* New York: Plenum, 1994. (In press.)

58. Elkind, David, and R. Bowen. "Imaginary Audience Behavior in Children and Adolescents." *Developmental Psychology* 15:1 (1979): 38-44.

59. Chassin, Laurie, Clark C. Presson, Steven J. Sherman, Eric Corty, and Richard W. Olshavsky. "Self-Images and Cigarette Smoking in Adolescence." *Personality and Social Psychology Bulletin* 7:4 (Dec. 1981): 670-676; Grube, Joel W., Ivan L. Weir, Shelly Getzlaf, and Milton Rokeach. "Own Value System, Value Images, and Cigarette Smoking." *Personality and Social Psychology Bulletin* 10:2 (1984): 306-313.

60. Chassin, Laurie, C. C. Presson, and S. J. Sherman. "Social Psychological Contributions to the Understanding and Prevention of Adolescent Cigarette Smoking." *Personality and Social Psychology Bulletin* 16:1 (1990): 133-151; McCarthy, W. J., and E. R. Gritz. "Teenagers, Cigarette Smoking and Reactions to Selected Cigarette Ads." Los Angeles, CA: Western Psychological Association Meeting, April 16, 1984; and Grube et al.

61. Chassin et al., 1981.

62. Greenberg, Jeff, and Tom Pyszczynski. "Compensatory Self-Inflation: A Response to the Threat to Self-Regard of Public Failure." *Journal of Personality and Social Psychology* 49:1 (1985): 273-280.

63. Schudson, Michael. "Symbols and Smokers: Advertising, Health Messages, and Public Policy." In Rabin, Robert L., and Stephen D. Sugarman. *Smoking Policy: Law, Politics, and Culture.* New York: Oxford University Press, 1993. 216.

64. Pollay and Lavack, 268-269.

65. *Ibid.*

66. Chassin, Laurie, Clark C. Presson, and Steven J. Sherman. "'Constructive' vs. 'Destructive' Deviance in Adolescent Health-Related Behaviors." *Journal of Youth and Adolescence* 18:3 (1989): 245-262.

67. Jessor, Richard, and Shirley L. Jessor. *Problem Behavior and Psychosocial Development: A Longitudinal Study of Youth.* New York: Academic Press, 1977; Moshbach, Peter, and H. Leventhal. "Peer Group Identification and Smoking: Implications for Intervention." *Journal of Abnormal Psychology* 97:2 (1988): 238-245; Sussman, Steve, Clyde W. Dent, Alan W. Stacy, Catherine Burciaga, Anne Raynor, Gencie E. Turner, Ventura Charlin, Sande Craig, William B. Hansen, Dee Burton, and Brian R. Flay. "Peer-Group Association and Adolescent Tobacco Use." *Journal of Abnormal Psychology* 99:4 (1990): 349-352.

68. Moshbach and Leventhal.

69. Pollay, 1990.

70. Basil et al.

71. Blum, Alan, and Matt Myers. "Tobacco Marketing and Promotion." In Houston, Thomas P., ed. *Tobacco Use: An American Crisis* (1993): 63-71.

72. Aitken, P. P., D. S. Leathar, F. J. O'Hagan, and S. I. Squair. "Children's Awareness of Cigarette Advertisements and Brand Imagery." *British Journal of Addiction* 82 (1987): 615-622.

73. Glantz, Stanton A. "Removing the Incentive to Sell Kids Tobacco. A Proposal." *Journal of the American Medical Association* 269:6 (1993): 793-794.

74. Pollay and Lavack.

75. *Ibid.;* and Altman, David G., Michael D. Slater, Cheryl L. Albright, and Nathan Maccoby. "How an Unhealthy Product Is Sold: Cigarette Advertising in Magazines, 1960-1985." Journal of Communication 37:4 (1987): 95-106.

76. Burnett, L. *Communications of an Advertising Man.* Chicago: Burnett, 1961.

77. Pollay and Lavack, 1993.

78. Pollay, 1990. 24.

79. Wong-McCarthy and Gritz; and Gritz, E. R. "Cigarette Smoking by Adolescent Females: Implications for Health Care and Behavior." *Women and Health* 9:2/3 (1984): 103-115.

80. Pollay, 1990. 9.

81. Federal Trade Commission, 1994. 12.

82. Pollay, 1990. 9, 27.

83. Centers for Disease Control. *The Health Consequences of Smoking: Nicotine Addiction. A Report of the Surgeon General, 1988.* USDHHS Pub No. (CDC) 88-8406. Washington, DC: U.S. Department of Health and Human Services, 1988.

84. Johnston, Lloyd D., Jerald G. Bachman, and Patrick M. O'Malley. "Monitoring the Future Study." Press release. The University of Michigan, Ann Arbor. (27 January 1994.)

85. Allen, Karen, Abigail Moss, Gary A. Giovino, Donald R. Shopland, and John P. Pierce. "Teenage Tobacco Use: Data Estimates From the Teenage Attitudes and Practices Survey, United States, 1989." *Advance Data* 224 (1 Feb. 1993): 1-20.

86. Amos, Amanda. "Youth and Style Magazines: Hooked on Smoking?" *Health Visitor* 66:3 (1993): 91-93.

87. *Ibid.*

88. McKenna, Jeffrey W., and K. N. Williams. "Crafting Effective Tobacco Counter-advertisements: Lessons from a Failed Campaign Directed at Teenagers." *Public Health Reports* 108:S1 (1993): 85-89.

89. Centers for Disease Control and Prevention. *Preventing Tobacco Use*, 195.

90. Aitken et al., 1987; Goldstein, Adam O., Paul M. Fischer, John W. Richards, and Deborah Creten. "Relationship Between High School Student Smoking Recognition of Cigarette Advertisements." *Journal of Pediatrics* 110:3 (1987): 488-491; Pierce et al., 1994; and Pierce, John P., Elizabeth Gilpin, David M. Burns, Elizabeth Whalen, Bradley Rosbrook, Donald Shopland, and Michael Johnson. "Does Tobacco Advertising Target Young People to Start Smoking?" *Journal of the American Medical Association* 266:22 (1991): 3154-3158.

91. For a review of exposure as an ambiguous construct, see: Klitzner, Michael, Paul J.. Greunewald, and Elizabeth Bamberger. "Cigarette Advertising and Adolescent Experimentation with Smoking." *British Journal of Addiction* 86 (1991): 287-298.

92. Aitken, P. P., D. R. Eadie, G. B. Hastings, and A. J. Haywood. "Predisposing Effects of Cigarette Advertising on Children's Intentions to Smoke When Older." *British Journal of Addiction* 86 (1991): 383-390.

93. New Zealand Toxic Substances Board. *Health or Tobacco: An End to Tobacco Advertising and Promotion.* Wellington, New Zealand: Department of Health, 1989. xxix.

94. *Ibid.*, xxiii, xxiv, 76.

95. *Ibid.*, 76.

96. *Ibid.*, 103.

97. Action on Smoking and Health. *Tobacco Advertising: The Case for a Ban.* London: ASH, 1991. Cited in Amos, Amanda. "Cigarette Advertising and Marketing Strategies." *Tobacco Control* 1 (1992): 3-4.

98. Warner, K. "Clearing the Airwaves: The Cigarette Ban Revisited." *Policy Analysis* 5:4 (1979): 435-450.

99. Pollay, Richard W. "The Major Minor Issue: Children, Cigarettes and Advertising Self-Regulation in the Sixties." In Thorson, Esther, ed. *Proceedings of the American Academy of Advertising.* Columbia: University of Missouri, 1993. 2-11.

100. Federal Trade Commission. *Report to Congress: Pursuant to the Federal Cigarette Labeling and Advertising Act.* Washington, DC: Federal Trade Commission, 1968.

101. U.S. Congress. *Hearings on HR2248 Before the Committee on Interstate and Foreign Commerce.* House of Representatives, 89th Congress, 1st Session. Serial No. 89-11. Washington, DC: U.S. Government Printing Office, 1965.

102. Mazis, Michael B., Debra J. Ringold, Elgin S. Perry, and Daniel W. Denman. "Perceived Age and Attractiveness of Models in Cigarette Advertisments." *Journal of Marketing* 56:1 (Jan. 1992): 22-37.

103. Tobacco Industry. "Cigarette Advertising Code." 5.

104. Comerford and Slade.

105. Pollay, 1990. 33-35.

106. 15 U.S.C. Par. 1334, cited in Shiffrin, Steven H. "Alcohol and Cigarette Advertising: A Legal Primer." *Adolescent Medicine* 4:3 (1993): 627.

107. *Ibid.*

108. See, for example, Gostin, Lawrence O. and Allan M. Bandt. "Criteria for Evaluating a Ban on the Advertisement of Cigarettes." *Journal of the American Medical Association* 269 (17 February 1993): 904-909.

109. Chapman, S. "The Limitations of Econometric Analysis in Cigarette Advertising Study." *British Journal of Addiction* (1989): 1267-1274.

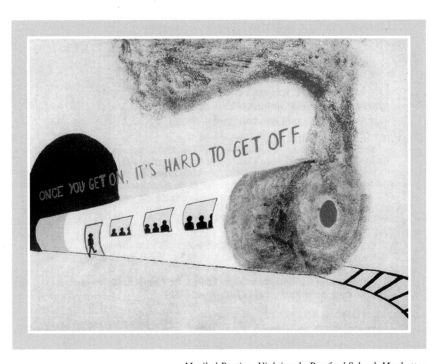

Maribel Bastian, Nightingale-Bamford School, Manhattan

CONTENTS

5

PREVENTION AND CESSATION OF TOBACCO USE

RESEARCH-BASED PROGRAMS

PREVENTION OF SMOKING

School-Based Smoking Prevention Research

In the absence of a comprehensive national children's health policy, the responsibility for preventing adolescent tobacco use has fallen primarily on individual school districts, often guided by their state legislatures or departments of education, which may mandate general health education goals. Schools are the only place where virtually all young people can be reached. This universal access enables health promotion programs to address variations in ethnicity, age, socioeconomic status, and cultural factors, all of which may contribute to tobacco use within the structure of the schools. School settings afford easy access to youth peer groups, access that is critical for affecting peer social interactions related to initiation and use of tobacco. Moreover, the purpose of schooling—to prepare young people for future productive adult roles—is compatible with the goal of health promotion.

However, many schools are ill-equipped to conduct effective smoking prevention programs and unmotivated to do so, and only a few preventive efforts have been mounted by the schools themselves. The major impetus for prevention of tobacco use has been largely external to school systems, driven by federally funded research and voluntary health agencies concerned with the magnitude of health problems caused by tobacco use and the continued high prevalence of adolescent smoking. These programs have worked under severe constraints within the school system, including time restrictions (hours available of class time and for training sessions), limited qualified personnel, and lack of material resources. Because health promotion may not be seen as central to the school's mission, the development and implementation of smoking prevention programs have had to contend with many obstacles.

Despite these impediments, significant knowledge of how to prevent young people's tobacco use has been gained over the past two decades. School-based research programs have explored a variety of approaches, which have helped identify the most useful program elements. School-based smoking prevention efforts have also been made more effective when reinforced by broad-based community programs. Moreover, these methods are now being applied with success to preventing smokeless tobacco use.

Recent publication of the Centers for Disease Control and Prevention's Guidelines for School Health Programs to Prevent Tobacco Use and Addiction[1] and reviews calling for a national agenda for school health promotion[2] give further impetus to supporting schools as the locus for tobacco prevention efforts. Comprehensive prevention and health promotion programs that prevent the initiation and use of tobacco products can assist in attaining Healthy People 2000 objectives.[3] A review of school-based tobacco prevention programs and programs that integrate prevention into the context of a community effort to reduce tobacco use is a useful basis for developing the model for a comprehensive policy to prevent addiction to tobacco among children and youths.

Approaches to School-Based Prevention Research

Following the publication of the surgeon general's report in 1964, development of school-based programs to prevent tobacco use by youths grew incrementally, theoretical approach by theoretical approach, program concept by program concept, for two reasons. First, the limitations of behavioral research techniques made it difficult to measure the effect of more than one intervention component at a time. Second, prevention as a lifestyle behavioral concept was a new approach to public health. During this time, however, the most successful components were identified and, as the capacity to conduct multicomponent research among large populations advanced with experience and technology, the best behavioral approaches and program components were combined into more effective interventions. The following section highlights the promising approaches and their components for school-based prevention programs that are reinforced by community-based programs.

Information-Deficit Model. The 1964 surgeon general's report provided evidence to the public health community and to the general public that smoking contributes to mortal diseases. A significant percentage of adults acted on that information by quitting smoking. The information, however, had not been designed to reach children and youths. Public health professionals and educators assumed that youths who smoked would quit using tobacco if they were exposed to information about the health risks of smoking. Behavioral scientists tested "information-deficit models" to determine whether providing students with information about the health risks of smoking would get them to stop smoking or never initiate smoking.

Informational programs were designed and implemented using most forms of educational media available: books, pamphlets, posters, films, and lectures. The images and messages were explicit: smoking increases the risk for numerous serious physical consequences throughout life, including premature death from heart disease or cancer. The message often was presented in a manner intended to arouse fear. Comprehensive reviews of the programs conducted in the 1970s based on the information-deficit model showed that the model had not deterred the adoption of cigarette smoking by youths.[4] Providing knowledge of the health consequences of smoking is a basic and necessary step, but it is not sufficient to change the behavior of most youths, for three reasons. First, the information-deficit model does not address the complex relationship between knowledge acquisition and subsequent behavior. Second, the model does not consider the addictive nature of tobacco use. Third, the model does not address risk factors such as peer use and approval of tobacco and perceived prevalence of peer tobacco use.

Affective Education Model. When the shortcomings of the information-deficit model became apparent, behavioral scientists turned their attention to personal factors that mediate cognitive factors, for example, beliefs, attitudes, intentions, and perceived norms. Another approach, known as affective education or motivational education, was developed during the 1970s to change smoking behavior among youths. The approach was based on the assumption that adolescents use tobacco because their self-perceptions are somehow compatible with that health-compromising behavior.[5] The affective education approach focused on increasing the students' sense of self-worth or self-esteem by helping them learn general skills such as assertiveness, communication, and problem solving. Educators and counselors hypothesized that since smoking and other problem behaviors, such as low motivation to achieve, school absenteeism, and antisocial behavior, were often related, a focus on increasing self-worth could positively affect all of these behaviors. The questions asked, therefore, by researchers were (1) If adolescents' sense of self-worth were increased, would they establish a health-related value system that would preclude tobacco use? and (2) If an adolescent were helped to change his or her attitudes about school, family, or community, would various problem behaviors, including tobacco use, be prevented?

Research on the affective education model reported that this approach was no more successful than the information-deficit model at preventing youths from smoking. In fact, an unintended effect of the programs, suggested but not conclusively proven by several studies, might be the elicitation of interest in the very behaviors that are being discouraged.[6]

Social Influences Resistance Model. A third approach to prevention of tobacco use was developed after evaluations of the earlier interventions demonstrated two critical deficiencies. First, interventions had largely been used among
high school and college students. Although smoking is heavier and more prevalent among these students than among younger students, the development of
smoking behavior actually begins early, when students are in the sixth or seventh
grade.[7] Therefore, prevention of smoking initiation and early use necessarily
must target students at an age when most initiation occurs. Second, the programs were designed on a universal basis of intervention. It became apparent
that tobacco use typically develops in a series of phases, progressing gradually to
more addicted behavior. Children progress from experimental, to occasional, to
regular tobacco use.[8] The time span and the progression through phases of
smoking behavior imply that influences beyond just information or affective
factors must be considered as determinants of adolescent tobacco use. By the
early 1980s, researchers understood those factors to be socio-demographic, environmental, behavioral, personal, and pharmacologic.[9] Essentially, the earlier
programs had not taken into account the extent to which social environmental
factors influence adolescent tobacco use.

The third approach, resisting social influences, recognized the importance of
the social environment as an influence of tobacco use, and researchers posed the
question: If adolescents were to develop skills that allow them to identify and
resist social influences, would they refrain from using tobacco? The assumption
was that adolescents who smoke lack the skills to counteract (a) the misperception that most people smoke, (b) the appeal of image advertising and
promotional activities, and (c) the desire to behave as their tobacco-using role
models, peers, or family members behave. Therefore, most programs based on
the resisting-social-influences model include training components that foster general assertiveness, decision making, and communication skills that are clearly
linked with smoking.[10] The skills-based interventions avoided the earlier scare
tactics of the information-deficit model and instead focused on the detrimental
short-term social consequences of smoking, on understanding the techniques of
tobacco advertising, and on the social advantages of being a nonsmoker.

Although the theory underlying the skills approach derives from the knowledge that multiple factors influence tobacco use, the knowledge is limited to
broad understandings of these factors. There are major gaps in the knowledge
about factors influencing tobacco use. These factors are multidimensional by
nature, and current theories conflict on the psychological routing of those factors. A theory that attempts to describe that complexity is the theory of "triadic
influence," which considers three types of influence that flow through three
levels or tiers from ultimate to distal to proximal. Flay and Petraitis review 13
theories to account for the initiation and use of tobacco by youth, and identify
gaps in each of them.[11] Their approach considers distal causes, such as behavior
of family members and genetic inheritance of traits, as indirect influences on

behavior, through their effects on more proximal or direct predictors (such as social skills, motivations, and expectancies). Causes at one level could be said to be "mediated" by causes at another level. Factors of one type of influence could also "moderate" or affect the influence at another level. In analysis of research studies of multiple factors, this is known as the statistical interaction effect, and it is difficult to interpret how this combination of factors works to affect smoking behavior. To date, no single theory comprehensively encompasses all of the factors or accounts for a large proportion of the variance in smoking behavior. Prevention programs have targeted social influences that are most proximal to smoking behavior, but these interventions have not affected more distal factors. The following section describes several structural and content components in current skills programs, and highlights programs that have most successfully applied those components.

Most programs based on a skills-resisting model incorporate several components:

- information about the short-term negative consequences of tobacco use (for example, bad breath, yellow teeth, reduced blood circulation, or vasoconstriction);
- an exploration of inaccurate beliefs about tobacco use (for example, that students usually overestimate the percentage of peers who smoke);
- an examination of the many reasons students smoke (for example, peer acceptance and image seeking); and
- practice of strategies for resisting the influences of tobacco use (for example, refusal skills).

An example of a large-scale randomized trial that incorporates all of the above components is the Waterloo Smoking-Prevention Program, implemented with sixth graders in six 1-hour weekly sessions. The program was effective in preventing the onset of experimental smoking through the end of the eighth grade.[12]

Format variations are, in most cases, minor among the numerous approaches to developing skills to resist social influences to smoke.[13] Most programs rely on classroom teachers to implement these programs, although variations include using trained health teachers and science teachers.[14] Some intervention variations have used a combination of trained teachers with same-age student peer leaders.[15] Peer leaders from high school have helped junior high school students develop the skills needed to resist social pressures to smoke by identifying social pressures and then rehearsing and modeling the strategies for coping with the pressures.[16] A prototypical peer-led social influences intervention reduced the incidence of daily and weekly smoking 35-50% more than an adult-led program emphasizing health consequences. These effects had dissipated at the 5- and 6-year follow-ups.[17] College undergraduate students have also served as leaders to young adolescents, both in the classroom and over the telephone, in booster calls, when students left middle schools.[18]

Other interventions have used media supplements and have involved the students' parents. For example, five different 5-minute video segments were aired on a local television station and coordinated with a classroom program in Los Angeles, and a significant number of youths got their parents to view the segments.[19] Another program used homework activities to involve parents and other family members in role playing in order to reinforce a social influences program taught by health, science, and social studies teachers.[20] A slightly different approach to enlist parental support was mailing to parents a set of four messages designed to reinforce classroom activities and urging parents to establish family policies regarding smoking.[21] The media and parent interventions have attempted to broaden the social context for components on peer pressure and resistance skills training.

Videotapes of nonsmoking peers were used to impart information and to teach skills needed to resist social influences in a program described as "social inoculation" developed in the mid-1970s.[22] Another variation of the social-skills training approach adds components on self-control, decision making, problem solving, and self-reward. By this problem-solving approach, students learn self-control skills for smoking prevention coupled with self-reward for personal successes.[23]

Numerous programs implementing an approach of personal and social skills training based on various aspects of cognitive-behavioral theory have been successful in reducing experimental smoking and initiation of smoking, and in reducing regular smoking. The general goal of the program is to enhance students' self-esteem, self-mastery, and self-confidence in order to decrease their susceptibility to indirect social pressures to smoke and to prepare students to cope with anxiety induced by social situations. The life skills approach focuses on knowledge, capabilities, and skills to enact pertinent behaviors, such as not smoking around peers. The approach, which may involve up to twenty classroom sessions, includes resistance skills, behavioral research, role playing, self-control, decision making, problem solving, and self-reward, as well as components devoted to increasing self-esteem, self-confidence, autonomy, and assertiveness.[24]

Effectiveness of School-Based Smoking Prevention Programs

Research on smoking prevention has by its nature had to contend with various threats to validity posed by methodologic issues of mixed units of analysis (individual student versus school or classroom), attrition of the subject (student) population, quality of implementation, and homogeneity of the subject population.[25] To a large extent, most recent research studies have been designed to deal with these methodologic obstacles and have consistently found moderately strong prevention effects. These factors have been assessed in four important meta-analytic studies published since 1980.

Program Content Components. Tobler examined 143 studies of drug-use prevention programs for sixth- through twelfth-grade students and found that these programs do have an effect on behavior, skills, and knowledge. Peer-led programs and programs dealing with social influences were more effective than other models.[26] Tobler later confirmed these findings with more rigorous analytic methods.[27] The Rundall and Bruvold meta-analysis of 47 studies of school-based smoking intervention programs examined knowledge, attitude, and behavioral outcomes of social influence programs versus traditional programs; the social influence programs were more likely to affect attitudes and behavior.[28] Rooney examined 90 school-based tobacco use prevention programs conducted from 1974 through 1989 that sought to develop skills to resist social influences. The meta-analysis took into account the clustering of students in schools and used the school as the unit of analysis. Results indicated that smoking prevalence was 4.5% lower among students in the social influence programs than among students in control conditions. The social influence programs that were most effective at 1-year follow-up had the following components: they were delivered to sixth-grade students, used booster sessions, concentrated the program in a short time period, and used an untrained peer to present the program. Under these more optimal conditions, long-term smoking prevalence was about 25% lower.[29]

Bruvold's meta-analysis included 94 separate interventions from the 1970s and 1980s. The intervention programs were categorized as rational (providing factual information), developmental (increasing self-esteem and decision-making skills), social-norms-oriented (providing alternatives and reducing alienation), and social-reinforcement-oriented (developing skills to deal with social pressures to smoke). The meta-analysis showed that the rational approach had very little impact on smoking behavior, that the developmental and social norms approaches had equivalent and intermediate effects on smoking behavior, and that the social reinforcement approach had the greatest effect on smoking behavior.[30]

The results of several individual studies suggest that the initial positive impacts of school-based interventions may dissipate over time,[31] particularly if intervention activities and booster sessions do not extend throughout middle school, junior high, and high school.[32] School-based programs may also be strengthened by supplementary intervention activities that extend beyond the school context into the community.[33] (See section below on community interventions.)

Efforts have been made to test the generalizability of the social influence model of prevention program with ethnic groups and special populations. Some studies have yielded comparable results with African-American and Hispanic-American adolescents.[34] A specific program has been suggested for American Indians.[35] However, reports with ethnic populations are relatively few, and more research is clearly warranted. These studies must address the group-specific social factors that affect smoking onset that research has begun to identify[36] and the cultural norms and values that are an essential part of culturally appropriate interventions.[37]

The meta-analyses described above do not distinguish between smoking prevention programs implemented in the context of wider drug use prevention programs and those that focus on tobacco alone. Most research on smoking prevention has been conducted on programs that focus solely on tobacco use. Programs that are multi-behavioral and target several drug use behaviors (such as life skills programs) can be effective if adequate time is allocated to social reinforcement components such as resistance skills specific to tobacco use.

Program Structural Elements. Eight structural elements are considered both necessary and sufficient for effective school-based smoking prevention programs. These features were identified by a National Cancer Institute (NCI) panel of experts who analyzed 15 intervention trials conducted by NCI.[38] These essential elements, listed below, were confirmed in Rooney's meta-analysis of research studies 1974-1989.[39]

1. Classroom sessions should be delivered at least five times per year in each of two years in the sixth through eighth grades.

2. The program should emphasize the social factors that influence smoking onset, short-term consequences, and refusal skills.

3. The program should be incorporated into the existing school curricula.

4. The program should be introduced during the transition from elementary school to junior high or middle school (sixth or seventh grades).

5. Students should be involved in the presentation and delivery of the program.

6. Parental involvement should be encouraged.

7. Teachers should be adequately trained.

8. The program should be socially and culturally acceptable to each community.

Of critical importance is the integrity of implementation and the fidelity of instruction.[40] The programs should be adopted by schools and used in a manner that is close to the way they were evaluated.

In addition to the above eight elements, an effective component is the establishment of school policies restricting tobacco use and compliance with the policy by students. States such as Minnesota and California report widespread support and adoption of tobacco-free policies; enforcement of these policies can have a significant impact on reducing tobacco use. A study of the impact of smoking policies on over 5,000 adolescents in 23 schools in 2 California counties found that schools with comprehensive policies (restricting smoking on and near school grounds and including educational programs) had significantly lower smoking rates than schools with less comprehensive policies.[41]

The CDC Guidelines for School Health Programs to Prevent Tobacco Use and Addiction recommend that the above-mentioned essential elements be implemented in the context of broader policy support.

1. Develop and enforce a school tobacco-free policy.

2. Provide instruction about the short- and long-term negative physiologic and social consequences of tobacco use, social influences on tobacco use, peer norms regarding tobacco use, and refusal skills.

3. Provide intensive tobacco-use prevention education during early adolescence (sixth grade), in junior high or middle school, and reinforce the program in high school.

4. Provide program-specific training for teachers.

5. Involve parents or families in support of school-based programs to prevent tobacco use.

6. Support cessation efforts among students and all school staff who use tobacco.

7. Assess the tobacco-use prevention program at regular intervals.[42]

Dissemination. To date, the dissemination and diffusion of prevention programs have been documented, but there are no data on their impact on smoking rates. In Minnesota, 81 schools were invited to receive one of four recommended smoking prevention programs and to participate in a study. Seventy percent of contacted schools agreed to participate in the study, and 96% of all schools applied for and received tobacco use prevention funds from the State of Minnesota.[43] The study demonstrates the feasibility of a large-scale adoption of a smoking prevention program by schools.

Community-wide Programs to Prevent Smoking

Although schools offer a number of pragmatic and practical advantages for launching a preventive effort, there are limitations to what they can accomplish. Schools have limited time and resources for meeting routine educational demands. In addition, they are only one of the settings in which social influences on smoking operate. In fact, while the results of more than 20 research studies have shown that school-based prevention programs alone have consistently delayed onset of smoking, lasting effects have only been demonstrated at 2-year follow-up.[44] The concept of reciprocal determinism would argue that successful interventions should target the major elements of the dynamic person-environment interaction that school-based interventions may not be capable of reaching, much less influencing.[45] These more wide-ranging determinants include community influences, environmental regulations, legislative initiatives concerning the pricing and promotion of tobacco products, and other types of societal interventions described elsewhere in this report. Recent research has begun to add community intervention components that explicitly target the social environment to help adolescents remain nonsmokers. The term "community interventions" has been used in a variety of ways. These efforts vary and include using print and electronic media to reach a broad community, using specific targeted programs (smoking cessation), and targeting community leaders and organizations to change community practices in specific ways to reduce tobacco use (for example, enforcing age restrictions on sale of tobacco in local stores). All community programs share a focus on altering the social environment or social context in which tobacco products are obtained or consumed. The components all share the goal of making the social environment supportive of non-use or cessation, and therefore could increase the effects of a school-based program by creating a social context for the program that enhances the effects of its messages.[46] Also, community programs can reach adolescents who are missed by school-based programs, either because they have dropped out of school, are absent during the intervention, or are not influenced by the school program. School-based prevention programs report a higher attrition rate among smokers (at pretest) and a much higher smoking prevalence among absentees and dropouts (over 70%); thus, students most at risk may be missing either from the intervention or the follow-up. Community programs, however, report equivalent reductions in tobacco use for youths at different levels of risk.[47]

Community interventions can also help change community norms or practices that are relevant to adolescent tobacco use (for example, enforcement of age restrictions on the sale of tobacco) and that make repeated interventions necessary.[48] Evidence for the efficacy of community interventions comes from both large-scale multicommunity studies of heart disease prevention and large-scale studies that focus explicitly on smoking and drug use. Three studies have shown consistent effects on reducing tobacco use by teens, each using experimental designs that have overcome some, but not all, of the methodologic problems of school-based prevention programs. In fact, because the community is the unit of assignment, the small number of communities in each of the studies precludes a true experiment.

The Class of 1989 Study, a part of the Minnesota Heart Health Program, tested the efficacy of a smoking prevention intervention within the larger program to reduce heart disease in entire communities. The study used cohort and cross-sectional analyses to compare two matched communities over a 7-year period. One community received a school-based smoking prevention program for 3 years. In addition to the school intervention, this community participated in a population-wide intervention that included risk-factor screening, adult smoking cessation, and consideration of new smoking ordinances at school and other community components. At the follow-up assessment, the smoking rates for adolescents in the intervention (educated) community were 40% lower than in the reference community, which did not receive the intervention.[49] A significant reduction in smoking rates was maintained over a 6-year period, even with the school, not the individual student, as the unit of analysis. At the end of high school, the smoking rates for students in the intervention community remained 40% lower than in the reference community.[50]

The North Karelia Youth Project in Finland, a comprehensive community program to reduce cardiovascular risk factors, also reports lower smoking rates immediately after, 2 years after, and 8 years after classroom interventions taught to 13- to 15-year-old students. The difference is attributed to the context of the community program in which specific school interventions were implemented.[51]

The Midwestern Prevention Project is a 6-year longitudinal intervention study that varied the interventions and grade levels (grades six and seven). The project was implemented in 50 middle/junior high schools in the Kansas City and Indianapolis areas. The project included schools, media, parent and community organizations, and health policy programs that focused on resistance skills training and environmental support for nonsmoking and non-drug use. The program first targeted the most proximal influences on youth initiation of smoking (school and parents) and subsequently the more distal influences (community organization and policy changes). Media were used in all years to promote and reinforce other components. Results, adjusted for race and grade, showed a significant effect of the program on reducing cigarette smoking. A pattern maintained (though not as strongly) at 2-year follow-up. At 2 years, the rate of increase of smoking in control schools was 1.5 times the rate in program schools.[52]

The results of the Midwestern Prevention Project, the North Karelia Youth Project, and Class of 1989 Study demonstrate the potential impact of a broad community prevention program. In all cases a strong school-based prevention intervention was embedded in a community-wide program. These programs appear to have enhanced the effects of school-based interventions, and the positive effects endured; however, experimental designs examining the effects of school-based and community-based programs administered separately and jointly are needed to verify these suggestive findings. Current randomized community interventions will provide further evaluation of the degree to which community-wide programs enhance or extend the effects of school-based programs on adolescent smoking.

Researchers have debated whether smoking prevention programs should be integrated into drug prevention programs or stand alone as independent interventions. Evaluations of smoking prevention programs that were integrated into comprehensive drug use prevention programs have been inconclusive. Some researchers have reported positive results,[53] whereas others have reported only short-term effects on smoking[54] or no effects.[55] The results may have to do with the amount of time provided for exposure to smoking and to creating a clear norm about nonsmoking. Preventive programs targeting multiple drugs may not provide adequate instruction on how to manage social influences to use tobacco products.

Community-based prevention studies have not included economic analyses in their reports. Overall effects are modest in terms of the percentage of students not going on to regular smoking, about 6.4%;[56] nevertheless, prevention of even moderate (monthly or weekly) use of cigarettes during adolescence may translate to a substantial effect in terms of the long-term health care and social cost savings. An assessment of potential cost savings and maintenance of preventive effects is needed to determine the economic basis for integrating school-based prevention with a community effort to reduce tobacco use.

Summary Points

Most reviews of the smoking-prevention research consistently have come to the same conclusions, summarized as follows:

1. School-based prevention programs that identify the social influences prompting youths to smoke and that teach skills to resist such influences have demonstrated consistent and significant reductions or delays in adolescent smoking. These programs usually target youths in the seventh to ninth grades, when smoking experimentation and initiation is foremost. The effects of these prevention programs dissipate with time, but can be enhanced with booster sessions or further application of the program. The difference in smoking rates or initiation between treatment and nontreatment student groups ranges from 25% to 60% and persists from 1 to 4 years (although few studies include more than a 1-year follow-up).

2. The effectiveness of school-based programs appears to be strengthened by community-wide programs involving parents, school policies, mass media and youth access, and mobilizing community organizations. The tendency for positive intervention effects to dissipate over time has been particularly evident in school-based intervention studies that included little or no emphasis on booster sessions, few (if any) community-wide activities or policy interventions, or few (if any) mass-media-based components.

3. A school-based prevention program alone has inherent limitations in impact and scope. Any effort to prevent adolescent tobacco initiation or dependence must address the social context for tobacco use. Initial studies suggest that the combination of school and community tobacco use prevention programs can enhance the short-term impact of the school-based programs by providing a longer-term, multi-pronged approach that complements or is synergistic with school-based programs. Given the number of studies, the variability in program format and scope, the various communities and subcultures in which these studies were implemented, and the potential threats to internal and external validity in school-based research, the consistency in overall reductions in smoking prevalence across all these studies is all the more remarkable. Still, while current studies have demonstrated that adolescents from different environments and cultural backgrounds are generally responsive to social influence programs, an as-

sessment is needed of programs tailored to ethnic groups, particularly for African-American, Hispanic, and Asian youths.

PREVENTION OF SMOKELESS TOBACCO USE

During the past several years, approximately 11% of high school seniors have reported using smokeless tobacco (SLT) within the past 30 days and about 4% have reported daily use.[57] The publication of the surgeon general's report in 1986 on the health consequences of using smokeless tobacco and subsequent reports of widespread smokeless tobacco use by children and adolescents[58] resulted in the publication of a wide range of written and media materials on the risks of using SLT.[59] The objective of these materials, which have been made available to school personnel and parents, is to counter the perception of SLT as "a safe alternative to smoking." Materials and programs have been produced and widely distributed by federal agencies, such as the National Cancer Institute and the National Institute of Dental Research; voluntary nonprofit groups, such as the American Cancer Society; and professional organizations, such as the American Dental Association and the American Academy of Otolaryngology. However, their impact on SLT use by youths aged 12-18 has not been evaluated. Unique aspects of SLT use and a review of prevention programs are presented below.

Unique Aspects of Smokeless Tobacco Use

Five unique aspects of smokeless tobacco use should be considered in the development and evaluation of prevention and cessation programs. First, children or youths can use moist snuff without other people being aware of it (this is also true for chewing tobacco, though less so). This potential for surreptitious use of snuff provides some difficulty in monitoring its use and allows for use in situations where use is not permitted, for example, in school classrooms or during sports activities. Second, smokeless tobacco causes oral lesions, which are direct physical evidence of detrimental health effects from using snuff or chewing tobacco. Third, up to 30% of regular users of chewing/spitting tobacco also report use of cigarettes.[60] Fourth, smokeless tobacco is perceived as a safe product to use: 81% of youths regard smokeless tobacco to be "much safer than cigarettes."[61] One study reports that only 40% of junior and senior high students believe that SLT is "very harmful."[62] This inaccurate perception of SLT as "safe" may lead adolescents to start using tobacco products and parents to allow this behavior. Furthermore, adolescents perceive SLT to be more socially acceptable to adults than smoking.[63] Parents' acceptance of their child's chewing or dipping contributes, in turn, to the perception that this behavior is safe and encourages continued use. And fifth, unlike cigarettes, chewing tobacco products are generally not packaged in individual doses; therefore, self-monitoring of use and accurate measurement of use are difficult.[64]

Evaluation of SLT Prevention Programs

Use of smokeless tobacco by youths is a relatively recent phenomenon; therefore, evaluation of prevention efforts is in a developmental phase, and few SLT prevention programs have been evaluated for either short- or long-term efficacy. Those that have been evaluated are either single components embedded in broad tobacco prevention programs, or single programs whose impact is evaluated on both cigarette smoking and smokeless tobacco use. Seldom have SLT prevention programs been implemented independently of other substance use prevention efforts or more general tobacco use prevention efforts. The rationale for this integration is that smokeless tobacco products are used primarily by males, prevalence may be lower for SLT than for cigarette use, and concern about use of snuff or chewing tobacco is often less than for hard drugs and cigarette smoking. Although logical, inclusion of smokeless tobacco prevention in other prevention efforts renders the evaluation of the smokeless tobacco component problematic.

NIH has funded eight research grants to develop interventions to prevent the initiation or regular use of smokeless tobacco by youths and to help youths quit using SLT. Most of these projects have been school-based activities, with the primary focus on middle school students and students in grades six, seven, and eight. A few SLT programs have been implemented in non-school settings, for example, in 4-H clubs, Little League baseball clubs, and Native-American community centers. Smokeless tobacco prevention has also been included in more comprehensive drug use prevention curricula such as the Comprehensive Health Education Foundation's "Here's Looking at You, 2000," and in community-based interventions to reduce drug use.

School-Based Programs

Studies of two curricula in which adolescents received a preventive curriculum targeting both smoking and smokeless tobacco use report positive outcomes. A multicomponent social influence intervention program of seven class periods was delivered by regular classroom teachers and same-age peer leaders to classes in randomly assigned middle and high schools in Oregon. The intervention focused on sensitizing students to overt and covert pressures to use tobacco, and on developing effective skills to respond to these pressures (refusal skills), especially through role playing. The physical and social consequences of SLT use were highlighted in a video, *Big Dipper*. An effort to involve parents included mailing of three brochures with "parent messages" designed to reinforce refusal skills and encourage parents to discuss their standards and expectations on tobacco use. Follow-up of 1,768 students 1 year later confirmed that there was less of an increase in the use of SLT by middle school boys in the intervention than by control students and a reduction in smokeless tobacco use by high school boys. Parallel analysis of the intervention did not show any positive effect of the intervention on cigarette smoking. The results are encouraging, since only two of the seven class periods of the intervention were devoted to SLT information and activities.[65]

The Toward No Tobacco Use (TNT) project has had a positive effect in reducing SLT use. The TNT project implements four different prevention curricula independent of one another. The curricula address: (1) peer norms for using tobacco (normative social influence); (2) incorrect social information about tobacco use (informational social influence aid); (3) misperceptions and lack of knowledge about physical consequences resulting from tobacco use; and (4) the effects of combined social and physical consequences. In each curriculum, trained health educators deliver ten lessons to seventh grade students. The evaluation of TNT included a control, or usual care, group that offered health education by school personnel. Seventh-grade classes in 48 schools in southern California were randomized to the four curricula and the control group. The outcome variables were changes in reported tobacco use, smokeless tobacco, and cigarettes, at 1-year follow-up (eighth grade). All program curricula except for the informational social influence approach resulted in a significant reduction in smokeless tobacco use and experimentation. The curriculum on combined consequences was superior to all other program curricula for reducing initial and weekly use of smokeless tobacco and cigarettes. The results indicate that learning about the physical consequences of SLT use can be as successful as a social influence program (refusal skills) and that a combination of both is probably best for deterring use of SLT.[66]

The Southern California and Oregon studies suggest that a tobacco prevention program can be successful in reducing SLT use by embedding the smokeless program in a school-based tobacco prevention intervention provided to seventh and ninth grade students. Other school-based interventions, however, have not been as successful in deterring adolescents' use of SLT. Project SHOUT (Students Helping Others Understand Tobacco) was evaluated in 22 junior high schools in San Diego County (California). Trained undergraduate group leaders delivered ten intervention sessions to seventh, eighth, and ninth graders. The curriculum focused on health consequences of tobacco use, celebrity endorsements of non-use, social consequences of use, rehearsal of methods to resist peer pressure, and decision making. The eighth grade curriculum also included community action projects designed to mobilize the students as anti-tobacco activists. The intervention had a significant effect on cigarette use, smokeless tobacco use, and combined use of cigarettes and smokeless tobacco at the 3-year follow-up. The low prevalence of smokeless tobacco use in the sample (5.2% in control subjects and 2.7% for intervention subjects in the ninth grade) made it difficult to assess the impact of the program on SLT use.[67]

Non-School-Based Programs

Non-school-based SLT prevention programs implemented at 4-H clubs, to Little League teams, and on American-Indian reservations may reach subgroups of children and adolescents who are most likely to use smokeless tobacco products. Chewing tobacco and snuff have long been used by baseball players,[68] and several gum products provide youths with look-alike products (for example, "Big League Chew"). The focus of a prevention program on youngsters who play organized baseball in Little League provides a unique early opportunity to provide information on health roles of SLT use and counter or negate some of the positive image youngsters may hold for using SLT "like the pros do." Observations of televised broadcasts of the World Series in 1987 documented 24 minutes of viewing time of professional sports heroes chewing.[69] Later observations, in 1989, reported a decrease in televised spitting tobacco use by these sports idols during the broadcast of the World Series; however, the World Series still represents significant visibility of tobacco use by sports stars.[70] The results of a recent large-scale prevention intervention with youngsters playing organized Little League baseball are not yet available.

A program to reduce SLT use by children ages 10-14 was developed and implemented in 72 4-H clubs in 24 California counties. Five tobacco-related outcome variables were evaluated: knowledge, attitudes, perceived social influences, intentions, and behaviors. In the program, five sessions of tobacco education were provided at the monthly club meetings by volunteers (41 adults and 26 teens) trained to deliver the program in their locales. The 1-year follow-up showed that the program had a significant effect on knowledge of harmful effects of SLT use and intentions to smoke, but no effect on actual use of SLT. The 2-year follow-up showed no difference between program and control 4-H clubs. The authors concluded that, despite the difficulty of managing a tobacco prevention program through 4-H clubs because of time constraints on club meetings, the program is a useful complement to school-based programs to change social norms.[71]

Smokeless tobacco use by American-Indian youths on reservations is higher than by other groups. American-Indian and Native-Alaskan children use snuff and chewing tobacco early, frequently, and heavily. Girls use these products at levels almost equal to boys.[72] Programs being implemented on reservations are characterized by sensitivity to the unique aspects of tobacco use by Native Americans, especially its role in sacred rites. Native Americans present these programs, which adapt materials to specific tribal groups. These programs have not yet been evaluated.

Summary Points

1. Smokeless tobacco prevention programs have modest effects on reducing SLT initiation and use by middle school and high school boys.

2. Smokeless tobacco prevention programs have been modeled after cigarette smoking interventions and have similar components. Most SLT programs focus on social influence components and include information about the detrimental health effects of regular SLT use.

3. Children and adolescents perceive smokeless tobacco as a safe alternative to cigarette smoking, and this belief should be countered in any prevention program. Adolescents erroneously believe that they can easily quit using smokeless tobacco; thus, the addictive potential of snuff and chewing tobacco should be emphasized in any program.

4. Preventive interventions targeting high-risk youth or special populations require tailored interventions and alternative channels of community delivery. These programs have not been evaluated.

ADOLESCENT CESSATION OF SMOKING

Data on Smoking Cessation

Few studies have been conducted on adolescent cessation of tobacco use, and those vary considerably in scientific quality; many are anecdotal. Therefore, at this time, no effective means are known for helping youths to quit using tobacco or to remain abstinent once they have attempted to quit.

Four sources of data on adolescent smoking cessation are available: (1) national probability surveys on patterns of adolescent attempts to quit, (2) convenience sample surveys on self-initiated quit attempts by adolescents, (3) reports from adolescent prevention projects on treatment effects on youth who were smokers at baseline, and (4) programs that explicitly try to recruit adolescent smokers into cessation programs. The data available show that adolescent smokers do make repeated attempts to quit smoking, but usually fail. Two large national population surveys provide data on a few aspects of adolescent smoking cessation: the High School Seniors Survey (sponsored by the National Institute on Drug Abuse) and the Youth Risk Behavior Survey. Both surveys sample high school classrooms, and therefore do not include school dropouts (who have much higher smoking rates).[73] Data from the High School Seniors Survey since 1976 show that 42-47% of smokers want to stop smoking (They answer yes to the question, "Do you want to stop now?") In the more recent (1985-1989) surveys, in response to the question "Have you ever tried to quit and found that you could not?", 27.8% of those smoking at all and 39.4% of those smoking more than 1 cigarette in the past month answered affirmatively.[74] In the 1989 Teenage Attitudes and Practices Survey, 74% of 12- through 18-year-old smokers reported that they had seriously thought about quitting, 64% that they had tried to quit smoking, and 49% that they had tried to quit during the previous 6 months.[75]

The strength of chemical dependency, or addiction, to nicotine is evident in that over half of adolescents who try to quit smoking experience withdrawal symptoms, the same symptoms reported by adult smokers. (See chapter 2.) The use of nicotine replacement therapy has not been evaluated with adolescent smokers, but has been consistently efficacious with adult smokers.[76] Some older adolescent smokers might be appropriate candidates for nicotine reduction therapy, although this is currently contraindicated and does not have FDA approval. In a survey of adolescents going to primary care facilities, 29% of adolescent smokers (mean age = 16.4) checked "medication to make quitting easier" as a suggestion for smoking cessation, whereas only 8% checked "stop smoking class or program."[77]

Cessation Intervention Programs

Although the primary goal of smoking prevention programs, reviewed earlier in this chapter, is to prevent smoking initiation and the progression from experimentation to regular smoking, occasionally an added effect is that some smokers participating in these programs reduce the amount of cigarettes they smoke.[78] Nevertheless, the impact of prevention programs on students who are experimental or regular smokers is small and inconsistent.[79] Furthermore, smoking prevention programs typically are implemented for middle-school children, and the small number of regular smokers in this population tends to preclude meaningful cessation analyses.[80]

Cessation Interventions in Schools

A number of smoking cessation programs and materials have been developed and implemented in schools, but evaluation has typically been anecdotal or descriptive. Two school-based cessation programs evaluated in 1983, one using trained peer leaders[81] and one using a cognitive behavioral group approach,[82] reported no quits. The largest and most systematic school-based cessation study recruited students in 16 rural and suburban high schools in two states. At the 3-month follow-up, there was no effect from the intervention; 6.8% of clinic participants and 7.9% of controls were abstinent. Attrition was high: 48.4% from session one to session five, and an additional 60.8% from session five to the 3-month follow-up. The negative results in the study are especially noteworthy because the investigators used input from 31 focus groups with adolescents to develop the recruitment strategies and the content of the intervention.[83] (This study also treated smokeless tobacco users.)

One program did have some success: four sessions on immediate physiological effects of smoking and social cues influencing adoption of the habit implemented in tenth grade health classes in three California high schools (n = 477) resulted in a significantly greater percentage of subjects reporting abstinence than in the control group.[84] A follow-up study that evaluated the efficacy of individual components of the program found no significant differences.[85]

Adolescent smokers are reluctant to participate in multisession quit programs. Several factors may underlie the pervasive difficulty in recruiting adolescent smokers to school-based quit programs. Adolescents may worry that parents or teachers will learn that they smoke (since parental consent would be required for participation). Adolescents may not be highly motivated to quit, because long-term health consequences are less salient for them. Possibly, the population of smokers at schools, and therefore the recruitment base, is small. Or, the methods of recruitment might not be effective. Participants are usually recruited through school channels such as newsletters and class and public address announcements. One study found that intensive, face-to-face recruitment is better than public address and other announcements and posters.[86] When the participants are referred by school authorities for infractions of school smoking policies, quit rates are likely not to be high. For example, in one program, in which over half the participants enrolled because they had been caught smoking on school property, only 13.5% (n = 30) were abstinent (by self-report) at the end of the program. Though minimally successful, programs for rule-breaking smokers are likely to be more in demand, as some states such as Oregon have made smoking (or possession of tobacco products) a misdemeanor for persons under age 18 and thereby force school authorities to take action against students caught smoking on school grounds.

Non-School-Based Interventions

Although recruitment was more successful in an HMO-based smoking cessation program, the outcome was not.[87] Adolescents between 14 and 17 years of age who were members of a large health maintenance organization (HMO) were screened and recruited by mail and phone; 325 girls (46%) and 168 boys (37.2%) agreed to participate and were randomly assigned to either an intervention or a no-treatment control group. The intervention consisted of a counseling session with a nurse practitioner at a convenient HMO clinic, encouragement for the adolescent to set a quit date, provision of strategies for successful quitting, and telephone follow-up. At the 1-year follow-up, there were no significant effects of the intervention. The intervention was modeled on interventions for adult smokers that usually yield positive results, but this was clearly not the case for adolescent smokers.

Some success was obtained with boys but not girls in a program that awarded money for achieving target carbon monoxide levels in expired air samples. Eleven "hard core" smokers, ages 13 to 18, in an alternative school participated. Five of the six boys successfully reduced smoking and carbon monoxide levels during the reduction and quit phases with four maintaining abstinence during a 5-month fading, follow-up phase. In contrast, all five girls dropped out during the program and were unsuccessful. The authors speculate that the girls were less responsive than the boys to monetary rewards, and possibly would be more influenced by social consequences.[88]

Intervention Program Concepts

Clearly, there is a need for cessation programs for adolescent smokers. More than half of adolescent smokers want to quit, try to quit, and fail to quit. A survey by the Gallup Organization reported that 38% of youths ages 12 to 17 had some interest in youth-targeted smoking cessation programs.[89] Research is needed to discover from youths the kinds of assistance they will respond to and some of the barriers that keep them from seeking assistance in quitting tobacco use. For example, since youths spend much time with computers, watching television and or movies, and talking on the telephone, might these media, singly or in combination, be effective vehicles for cessation interventions? Interactive computer programs for adolescents are already developed for health education and health promotion and could be adopted for smoking cessation.[90] There are numerous videos on smoking and health, and even on smoking cessation, but these have not been specifically developed for youths; specially developed videos informed by focus groups might be a useful way of reaching adolescents, especially the high-risk smokers who are not comfortable with written materials. Finally, telephone counseling has been shown to be a useful and effective treatment channel for adult smokers and might be a useful way of reaching adolescents as well.[91] Telephone counseling can be a cost-effective way to provide personalized assistance that complements written or video materials.[92]

Summary Points

Because the addictive quality of nicotine is powerful, there is a strong need to evaluate whether the use of techniques for quitting tobacco use by adults can be beneficial to adolescents. It is reasonable to assume that if adolescent tobacco users are addicted at adult levels (for example, if they smoke a pack a day), the use of nicotine replacement should prove to be an effective adjunct to behavioral treatment in cessation.

The following conclusions are supported by the research base:

1. Adolescent smoking cessation has been the subject of very little systematic research. Adolescents who are regular smokers experience the same withdrawal symptoms as adults when they attempt to quit.

2. Adolescents frequently express interest in quitting and report making numerous, usually unsuccessful quit attempts, but they tend not to participate or remain in formal cessation programs.

3. Cessation programs for adolescents have not resulted in significant quit rates.

4. Once a person becomes a regular smoker, he or she finds it difficult to quit; few adolescents succeed in quitting.

CESSATION OF SMOKELESS TOBACCO USE

Desire to Quit Using Smokeless Tobacco

Three types of evidence indicate that snuff and chewing tobacco users are interested in quitting their use of SLT products. First, users respond to ads for cessation programs. In recruiting adults for a study, Boyle reported that he received 675 phone calls in 11 weeks in response to newspaper and radio ads for a cessation program.[93] It is less clear that adolescent SLT users will readily volunteer for cessation programs: only modest success has been reported in soliciting adolescent male volunteers for school-based SLT clinic programs.[94] A program in Tennessee reported poor response to flyers and ads in papers, but was able to recruit 130 subjects from 11 post-secondary schools in Tennessee by having coaches and health educators contact SLT users directly.[95] Second, users report interest in quitting or their intention to quit. In a survey, 68% of SLT users reported that they had tried to quit, with an average of four attempts each, and 54% reported that they would make a quit attempt in the subsequent year.[96] Third, users report prior quit attempts. In one study, more than one-third of current male adolescent SLT users reported unsuccessful quit attempts.[97] In a national probability sample, 39% of adult SLT users reported having made unsuccessful attempts to quit.[98] Given the addictive nature of nicotine, reversing the trend of SLT use requires the development of interventions to first motivate youths to quit using snuff and chewing tobacco, then to help them stop using tobacco.

Studies of Cessation of Smokeless Tobacco Use

Despite the evidence of negative health consequences from use of SLT, research on cessation of smokeless tobacco use has been minimal; to date, only a few studies have been reported in the scientific literature. One of the barriers to conducting research on cessation of SLT use is the lack of standardized methods for assessing levels of SLT use (as discussed in chapter 2). Furthermore, just as interventions for smoking cessation have not been transferred successfully to youths, neither are interventions for cessation of SLT use likely to be transferable. For example, the American Cancer Society's Fresh Start Adult Smoking Cessation Program was adapted for youths 18 to 22 years of age using SLT, but the program was ineffective.[99] An intervention that has not been adapted for youths but was successful with adult men involved four components: cue extinction, setting a target date for quitting, the use of a buddy system, and relapse prevention. Cue extinction involved identifying two or three situations most strongly associated with SLT use and breaking the associations by refraining from taking a dip for 30 minutes or more. Eight men (with a mean age of 32 years and who had used SLT on average for 9 years) participated in 8 1-hour behavioral treatment sessions over a period of 7 weeks in small groups of 3 subjects each. Of the 7 men completing the program, 6 remained abstinent at the 9-month follow-up.[100]

Studies of Users Recruited from Schools

Three recent studies are informative about school-based interventions for cessation of SLT use. An intervention in high schools in Eugene, Oregon, had modest success with daily SLT users. The study recruited 25 boys, ages 14-18, 11 of whom constituted a comparison group by receiving delayed treatment. This behavioral treatment consisted of three 1-hour small-group meetings with counselors, for example, focusing on coping skills for cessation (e.g., "The 4-As": Avoid, Alter, Alternatives, and Activities). Of the 21 boys completing the program, 9 were successful in quitting their SLT use at the end of treatment. At 6-month follow-up only 3 (12%) were still abstinent. However, participants not achieving abstinence reported reduction of 45% in their daily use of SLT from baseline levels. The participants reported that in addition to the group sessions, the telephone calls and support by the counselor were key elements in their quitting.[101]

The study, conducted in 16 high schools in Illinois and California, described above in the smoking cessation section, also included a component for cessation of SLT use. The attrition rate was high, about half. Of the 16 SLT users who participated in the 5 sessions, 7 (43.8%) reported quitting at the end of treatment, whereas none of the 5 SLT subjects in the wait-group reported quitting. At 3-month follow-up, 3 (15.2%) of the subjects randomized to treatment were confirmed as still abstinent. It appears that a school-based multi-session clinic can result in modest cessation rates for volunteering adolescents; however, attrition is high.[102]

Non-nicotine substitutes for snuff were used as a cessation intervention for 83 boys recruited from 6 high schools in rural Illinois. Two schools each were randomized to either the mint snuff substitute, chewing gum, or a lecture only. Of the 70 boys in the program, 30 were in the mint snuff groups, 15 in the gum groups, and 25 in the lecture-only groups. At the end of treatment (session two was 30 days later), there was no difference in quit rates for the 3 groups, but the self-reported reductions of SLT use by those using the mint snuff substitute were significantly higher than for the other 2 groups. There were no follow-up data provided about maintenance or relapse.[103]

Self-Help Program

A self-help guide produced by the American Cancer Society combined with modest counselor assistance was effective in getting 12% of participating young adult SLT users to quit. One hundred thirty participants, ages 18 to 27, were recruited from 11 postsecondary schools in the Memphis, Tennessee, area. Subjects were randomized into 2 groups; one group met for 2 sessions, the other met for 4 sessions. There was a 15.4% attrition rate, with 110 subjects completing treatment. At 90-day follow-up, the cessation rate was 10.6% for the 2-session group and 14.1% for the 4-session group, for an overall quit rate of 12.3%.[104] The modest quit rate is consistent with other self-help minimal interventions for tobacco use. To date, no other self-help programs for smokeless users have been evaluated.

Nicotine Replacement Therapy

The use of nicotine replacement therapy for SLT users has been studied in adults only. One hundred smokeless users were randomized to receive active (2 mg) nicotine gum or placebo (0 mg) nicotine gum as an adjunctive aid in a five-session group counseling program. Fifty percent of the subjects in the active nicotine gum condition were verified abstinent at the end of treatment, and 40% of the subjects receiving placebo were abstinent; the differences were not statistically significant. Nevertheless, the study demonstrates that adult SLT users, even those on placebo, can be successful in quitting SLT use. At 6- and 12-month follow-up the biochemically confirmed quit rates were 16% and 14% with no difference between groups.[105] There are no published reports to date on the use of nicotine skin patches as an adjunct to behavioral treatment for users of smokeless tobacco.

Clinic-Based Interventions

Given that most smokers do not go to cessation programs to quit but many respond to a prompt from a health care provider,[106] health care settings might be an attractive avenue for promoting cessation of SLT use. One example is a low-cost intervention conducted at seven prepaid dental clinics in the Portland, Oregon, area. Men who use moist snuff and/or chewing tobacco (n = 576) were identified by a questionnaire in clinic waiting rooms; participants were randomized to either usual care or an intervention. The intervention consisted of a routine oral exam; an explanation of the health risks of using SLT, including pointing out any lesions or other effects of SLT identified during the exam; advice to stop using tobacco; a 9-minute videotape; and a self-help manual. The differences between the groups in self-reported abstinence at 3 months were statistically significant, furthermore, the quit rates were significant for subjects reporting abstinence from SLT at both 3 and 12 months (18.4% for the intervention group and 12.5% for the usual care group).[107] The results are modest in terms of overall quit rate, but the impact of having dentists, hygienists, nurses, and physicians counseling patients to quit their use of smokeless tobacco could have significant impact on prevalence in the longer term. Programs for adolescents conducted in the context of regular visits to dentists or to other health care providers have not been studied. The identification of oral lesions could be a natural entry to raise the issue of SLT use, since many daily users have an identifiable lesion—one study reported that 79% of SLT users had observable lesions.[108]

Co-use of SLT and Cigarettes

The Monitoring the Future Project, 1985-1989, reports that 43% of high school seniors who use SLT also smoke cigarettes, and 32.5% of smokers use SLT. Studies report co-use of SLT and cigarettes at prevalences between 12% and 30% for all regular SLT users.[109] Since the addictive element in tobacco is nicotine, individuals who quit using snuff or chewing tobacco might increase their use of cigarettes, and vice versa. For adolescents who use both substances, a decrease in the use of one tobacco product may lead to a direct increase in their use of the other tobacco product.[110] There is no net gain in the health risk status of those individuals. Tobacco cessation rates among men who use both cigarettes and SLT are significantly lower than those who use SLT exclusively.[111]

Summary Points

Little is known about cessation of smokeless tobacco use, and the evidence available must be considered cautiously. Additionally, research is needed on the psychosocial factors that may affect both cessation and relapse. The small sample sizes, self-selective nature of subjects, lack of control groups, and lack of long-term follow-up render the few studies reported inconclusive. Research is needed to (1) describe the factors that accompany cessation, for example, use levels and patterns and relapse rates, and (2) test the effectiveness of various kinds of interventions, for example, nicotine replacement, self-help quitting, physician or health professional's advice, environmental restrictions, and increased product cost.

The following conclusions are supported by the research base:

1. Smoking cessation materials can be adapted and used to help people quit their use of smokeless tobacco. Preliminary evidence from clinical studies with adults shows modest quit rates that are comparable to smoking cessation (15% quit rates at 1-year follow-up).

2. There have been few studies with adolescents of cessation of smokeless tobacco use. The results have been both negative and positive. The cessation rates at follow-up are modest: 12% to 16% confirmed at 3- to 6-month follow-up. Response by adolescents to school-based cessation programs is modest; dropout rates are high.

3. There is a need to provide cessation aids to SLT users, as a significant number of users have made unsuccessful quit attempts or report interest in quitting.

4. Smokeless tobacco users are as addicted to nicotine as regular smokers and experience the same withdrawal symptoms. Nicotine replacement therapy (use of gum or patches) may be appropriate as an adjunct to behavioral therapy, as it has consistently proven beneficial with adult smokers.

RECOMMENDATIONS

Over the past 20 years, school-based prevention programs have evolved a focus on the social influences that are most proximal to a young person's decision to initiate and use tobacco products. Research has consistently demonstrated that a brief school intervention that focuses on social influences and teaches refusal skills can have a modest but significant effect in reducing onset and level of tobacco use. Multiple-grade interventions and more intensive interventions can increase this effect. Community programs that include parent involvement, school rules and regulations with regard to tobacco use, community organizations, and use of media can increase the effectiveness of school-based programs. Some community components have also focused on reducing youth access to tobacco by educating store clerks or conducting sting operations at convenience stores known to be lax in checking the age of purchasers (see chapter 7).

To be most effective, school-based programs must target youths before they initiate tobacco use or drop out of school. School programs offer the opportunity to prevent the initiation of regular tobacco use and help persons avoid the difficulties of trying to stop after they are addicted. School-based programs to prevent tobacco use can also contribute to preventing the use of illicit drugs such as marijuana and cocaine, especially if the programs are designed to prevent the use of these substances. The Centers for Disease Control and Prevention's *Guidelines for School Health Programs to Prevent Tobacco Use and Addiction* offer specific program recommendations for meeting the tobacco use prevention objectives of the nation for the year 2000.

Although the Committee concludes that prevention of tobacco use is the better public health approach to the health consequences of tobacco use, it also recognizes that many adolescents have already become regular users, and in some cases heavy daily users, of tobacco products. Many of these youths want to quit using tobacco and need help with their addiction problem. There is a paucity of research on how to reach, motivate, and treat adolescents addicted to cigarettes or smokeless tobacco products.

To prevent the addiction of children and youths to tobacco products, and thereby to prevent the associated health consequences, the Committee recommends:

1. **Under federal leadership, the United States should develop a national child health policy that gives high priority to the prevention of tobacco use by youths.** This policy should provide the mechanisms to guide and support multifaceted health promotion programs for children and youths.

2. **All schools should adopt and implement the CDC guidelines to prevent tobacco use and addiction.** To ensure the greatest impact, schools should implement all seven recommendations.

3. **Already proven models of school-based prevention programs should be systematically implemented into a comprehensive approach to reducing tobacco use by children and youths.** The comprehensive approach should embrace prevention programs that include broader social networks of influences (that is, parents, community, and media) set in the context of a community effort. A comprehensive program to reduce tobacco use is not a new idea. The Committee recognizes that most schools and communities do not have comprehensive tobacco prevention programs in place. Without significant resources it is unlikely that schools would be in a position to implement the CDC guidelines listed above. School prevention programs without the support of community efforts are less successful in reducing adolescent tobacco use.

4. **Tobacco prevention should be integrated into any drug prevention program aimed at youth.**

5. **Systematic research should be conducted on the optimal way to disseminate and implement tobacco use prevention programs on a large scale.**

6. **Research should be conducted on the development and evaluation of programs to help children and youths who are regular tobacco users to quit their habitual use of cigarettes, snuff, or chew.** Research is needed to determine whether or not nicotine replacement therapies as an adjunct to behavior therapies contribute to achievement of enduring cessation.

7. **Research should be conducted to identify the need for, and to develop and evaluate, prevention programs aimed at reducing tobacco use among specific ethnic groups.**

REFERENCES

1. Centers for Disease Control and Prevention. "Guidelines for School Health Programs to Prevent Tobacco Use and Addiction." *Morbidity and Mortality Weekly Report* 43:RR-2 (25 Feb. 1994): 1-18.

2. Lavin, Alison T., G. R. Shapiro, and K. S. Weill. "Creating an Agenda for School-Based Health Promotion: A Review of Selected Reports." *Journal of School Health* 62:6 (1992): 212-228.

3. U.S. Department of Health and Human Services. Public Health Service. *Healthy People 2000: National Health Promotion and Disease Prevention Objectives.* USDHHS Publication No. (PHS) 91-50212, 1990.

4. Thompson, Eva L. "Smoking Education Programs 1960-1976." *American Journal of Public Health* 68:3 (1978): 250-257; and Goodstadt, Michael S. "Alcohol and Drug Education: Models and Outcomes." *Health Education Monographs* 6:3 (1978): 263-279.

5. Durell, Jack, and W. Bukoski. "Preventing Substance Abuse: The State of the Art." *Public Health Reports* 99:1 (1984): 23-31.

6. Kinder, Bill N., N. E. Pape, and S. Walfish. "Drug and Alcohol Education Programs: A Review of Outcome Studies." *The International Journal of the Addictions* 15:7 (1980): 1035-1054; Schaps, Eric, R. DiBartolo, J. Moskowitz, C. S. Palley, and S. Churgin. "A Review of 127 Drug Abuse Prevention Program Evaluations." *Journal of Drug Issues* (Winter 1981): 17-43; Hansen, William B., C. A. Johnson, B. R. Flay, J. W. Graham, and J. Sobel. "Affective and Social Influences Approaches to the Prevention of Multiple Substance Abuse Among Seventh Grade Students: Results from Project SMART." *Preventive Medicine* 17 (1988): 135-154.

7. Leventhal, Howard, and Paul D. Cleary. "The Smoking Problem: A Review of the Research and Theory in Behavioral Risk Modification." *Psychological Bulletin* 88:2 (1980): 370-405; Stern, Robert A., J. O. Prochaska, W. F. Velicer, and J. P. Elders. "Stages of Adolescent Cigarette Smoking Acquisition: Measurement and Sample Profiles." *Addictive Behaviors* 12 (1987): 319-329.

8. Chassin, Laurie A., C. C. Presson, and S. J. Sherman. "Stepping Backward in Order to Step Forward: An Acquisition-Oriented Approach to Primary Prevention." *Journal of Consulting and Clinical Psychology* 53:5 (1985): 612-622.

9. Evans, Richard I. "A Social Inoculation Strategy to Deter Smoking in Adolescents." In Matarazzi, J. D., S. M. Weiss, J. A. Herd, N. E. Miller, and S. M. Weiss, eds. *Behavioral Health: A Handbook of Health Enhancement and Disease Prevention.* New York: John Wiley, 1984; McAlister, Alfred L., J. A. Krosnick, and M. A. Milburn. "Causes of Adolescent Cigarette Smoking: Test of a Structural Equation Model." *Social Psychology Quarterly* 47:1 (1984): 24-36; and Chassin, Laurie, C. Presson, and S. J. Sherman. "Cigarette Smoking and Adolescent Psychosocial Development." *Basic and Applied Social Psychology* 5:4 (1984): 295-315.

10. Botvin, Gilbert J., and E. M. Botvin. "Adolescent Tobacco, Alcohol, and Drug Abuse: Prevention Strategies, Empirical Findings, and Assessment Issues." *Developmental and Behavioral Pediatrics* 13:4 (1992): 290-301.

11. Flay, Brian R., and J. Petraitis. "A Review of Theory and Prospective Research on the Causes of Adolescent Tobacco Onset." Unpublished paper for the Robert Wood Johnson Foundation. (9 November 1993.)

12. Best, J. Allan., S. J. Thomson, S. M. Santi, E. A. Smith, and K. S. Brown. "Preventing Cigarette Smoking Among School Children." *Annual Review of Public Health* 9 (1988): 161-201.

13. *Ibid.*

14. Biglan, Anthony, R. Glasgow, D. W. Ary, R. Thompson, H. H. Severson, E. Lichtenstein, et al. "How Generalizable Are the Effects of Smoking Prevention Programs? Refusal Skills Training and Parent Messages in a Teacher-Administered Program." *Journal of Behavioral Medicine* 10:6 (1987): 613-628.

15. Perry, Cheryl L., K.-I. Klepp, and C. Sillers. "Community-wide Strategies for Cardiovascular Health: The Minnesota Heart Health Program Youth Program." *Health Education Research* 4:1 (1989): 87-101; and Arkin, Rise M., H. F. Roemhild, C. A. Johnson, R. V. Luepker, and D. M. Murray. "The Minnesota Smoking Prevention Program: A Seventh-Grade Health Curriculum Supplement." *The Journal of School Health* (November 1981): 611-616.

16. McAlister, Alfred L., C. Perry, J. Killen, L. A. Slinkard, and N. Maccoby. "Pilot Study of Smoking, Alcohol and Drug Abuse Prevention." *American Journal of Public Health* 70:7 (1980): 719-721.

17. Murray, David M., M. Davis-Hearn, A. I. Goldman, P. Pirie, and R. V. Luepker. "Five- and Six-Year Follow-Up Results from Four Seventh-Grade Smoking Prevention Strategies." *Journal of Behavioral Medicine* 12:2 (1989): 207-218.

18. Young, Russell L., C. de Moor, M. B. Wildey, S. Gully, M. F. Hovell, and J. P. Elder. "Correlates of Health Facilitator Performance in a Tobacco Use Prevention Program: Implications for Recruitment." *Journal of School Health* 60:9 (November 1990): 463-467; and Elder, John P., M. Wildey, C. de Moor, J. F. Sallis, Jr., L. Eckhardt, C. Edwards, et al. "The Long-Term Prevention of

Tobacco Use Among Junior High School Students: Classroom and Telephone Interventions." *American Journal of Public Health* 83:9 (1993): 1239-1244.

19. Flay, Brian R., W. B. Hansen, C. A. Johnson, L. M. Collins, C. W. Dent, K. M. Dwyer, et al. "Implementation Effectiveness Trial of a Social Influences Smoking Prevention Program Using Schools and Television." *Health Education Research* 2:4 (1987): 385-400.

20. Pentz, Mary A., J. H. Dwyer, D. P. MacKinnon, B. R. Flay, W. B. Hansen, E. Y. I. Wang, and C. A. Johnson. "A Multicommunity Trial for Primary Prevention of Adolescent Drug Abuse." *Journal of the American Medical Association* 261:22 (1989): 3259-3266.

21. Biglan, Glasgow, et al.

22. Evans, Richard I., B. E. Raines, and J. G. Getz. "Applying the Social Inoculation Model to a Smokeless Tobacco Use Prevention Program with Little Leaguers." In National Cancer Institute. *Smokeless Tobacco or Health: An International Perspective.* NIH Pub. No. 92-3461. Washington, DC: NCI, 1992. 260-276.

23. Schinke, Steven P., L. D. Gilchrist, R. F. Schilling II, W. H. Snow, and J. K. Bobo. "Skills Methods to Prevent Smoking." *Health Education Quarterly* 13:1 (1986): 23-27.

24. Botvin, Gilbert J. "Substance Abuse Prevention Research: Recent Developments and Future Directions." *Journal of School Health* 56:9 (November 1986): 369-374.

25. Flay, Brian R. "Psychosocial Approaches to Smoking Prevention: A Review of Findings." *Health Psychology* 4:5 (1985): 449-488; Biglan, Anthony, H. Severson, D. Ary, C. Faller, C. Gallison, R. Thompson, R. Glasgow, and E. Lichtenstein. "Do Smoking Prevention Programs Really Work? Attrition and the Internal and External Validity of an Evaluation of a Refusal Skills Training Program." *Journal of Behavioral Medicine* 10:2 (1987): 159-171; and Murray, David M., and P. J. Hannan. "Planning for the Appropriate Analysis in School-Based Drug-Use Prevention Studies." *Journal of Consulting and Clinical Psychology* 58:4 (1990): 458-468.

26. Tobler, Nancy S. "Meta-analysis of 143 Adolescent Drug Prevention Programs: Quantitative Outcome Results of Program Participants Compared to a Control or Comparison Group." *Journal of Drug Issues* 16:4 (1986): 537-567.

27. Tobler, Nancy S. "Drug Prevention Programs Can Work: Research Findings." *Journal of Addictive Diseases* 11:3 (1992): 1-28.

28. Rundall, Thomas G., and W. H. Bruvold. "A Meta-analysis of School-Based Smoking and Alcohol Use Prevention Programs." *Health Education Quarterly* 15:3 (1988): 317-334.

29. Rooney, Brenda. *A Meta-analysis of Smoking-Prevention Programs After Adjustment for Study Design.* Minneapolis-St. Paul: University of Minnesota, 1992. (Dissertation).

30. Bruvold, William H. "A Meta-analysis of Adolescent Smoking Prevention Programs." *American Journal of Public Health* 83:6 (1993): 872-880.

31. Kozlowski, Lynn T., R. B. Coambs, R. G. Ferrence, and E. M. Adlaf. "Preventing Smoking and Other Drug Use: Let the Buyers Beware and the Interventions Be Apt." *Canadian Journal of Public Health* 80 (1989): 452-456; and Flay, Brian R., D. Koepke, S. J. Thomson, S. Santi, J. A. Best, and K. S. Brown. "Six-Year Follow-Up of the First Waterloo School Smoking Prevention Trial." *American Journal of Public Health* 79:10 (1989): 1371-1376.

32. Botvin and Botvin. "Adolescent Tobacco," 1992.

33. Perry, Cheryl L., K.-I. Klepp, and J. M. Shultz. "Primary Prevention of Cardiovascular Disease: Communitywide Strategies for Youth." *Journal of Consulting and Clinical Psychology* 56:3 (1988): 358-364; and Perry, Cheryl L., S. H. Kelder, D. M. Murray, and K.-I. Klepp. "Communitywide Smoking Prevention: Long-Term Outcomes of the Minnesota Heart Health Program and the Class of 1989 Study." *American Journal of Public Health* 82:9 (1992): 1210-1216.

34. Botvin, Gilbert J., H. W. Batson, S. Witts-Vitale, V. Bess, E. Baker, and L. Dusenbury. "A Psychosocial Approach to Smoking Prevention for Urban Black Youth." *Public Health Reports* 104:6 (1989): 573-582; Botvin, Gilbert J., L. Dusenbury, E. Baker, S. James-Ortiz, and E. M. Botvin. "Smoking Prevention Among Urban Minority Youth: Assesssing Effects on Outcome and Mediating Variables." *Health Psychology* 11:5 (1992): 290-299; and Sussman, Steve, C. W. Dent, A. W. Stacy,

P. Sun, S. Craig, T. R. Simon, D. Burton, and B. R. Flay. "Project Towards No Tobacco Use: 1-Year Behavior Outcomes." *American Journal of Public Health* 83:9 (1993): 1245-1250.

35. Schinke, Steven P., M. A. Orlandi, R. F. Schilling II, G. J. Botvin, L. D. Gilchrist, and C. Landers. "Tobacco Use by American Indian and Alaska Native People: Risks, Psychosocial Factors, and Preventive Intervention." *Journal of Alcohol and Drug Education* 35:2 (1990): 1-12.

36. Sussman, Steve, C. W. Dent, B. R. Flay, W. B. Hansen, and C. A. Johnson. "Psychosocial Predictors of Cigarette Smoking Onset by White, Black, Hispanic, and Asian Adolescents in Southern California." *Morbidity and Mortality Weekly Report* 36:4S (1987): 11S-16S.

37. Marin, Gerardo. "Defining Culturally Appropriate Community Interventions: Hispanics as a Case Study." *Journal of Community Psychology* 21 (April 1993): 149-161.

38. Glynn, Thomas J. "Essential Elements of School-Based Smoking Prevention Programs." *Journal of School Health* 59:5 (May 1989): 181-188.

39. Rooney.

40. Flay, Brian R. "Social Psychological Approaches to Smoking Prevention: Review and Recommendations." *Advances in Health and Education Promotion* 2 (1987): 121-180.

41. Pentz, Mary A., B. R. Brannon, V. L. Charlin, E. J. Barrett, D. P. MacKinnon, and B. R. Flay. "The Power of Policy: The Relationship of Smoking Policy to Adolescent Smoking." *American Journal of Public Health* 79:7 (1989): 857-862.

42. Centers for Disease Control and Prevention, "Guidelines," 1994.

43. Perry, Cheryl L., D. M. Murray, and G. Griffin. "Evaluating the Statewide Dissemination of Smoking Prevention Curricula: Factors in Teacher Compliance." *Journal of School Health* 60:10 (1990): 501-504.

44. Botvin, Gilbert J., 1986.

45. Bandura, Albert. *Social Foundations of Thought and Action: A Social Cognitive Theory.* Englewood Cliffs, NJ: Prentice Hall, 1986.

46. Flay, Brian R. "What We Know About the Social Influences Approach to Smoking Prevention: Review and Recommendations." In Bell, Catherine S. and R. Gatjes, eds. *Prevention Research: Deterring Drug Abuse Among Children and Adolescents.* NIDA Research Monographs 63. Rockville, MD: National Institute on Drug Abuse, 1985.

47. Biglan, Severson, et al.; Pirie, Phyllis L., D. M. Murray, and R. V. Luepker. "Smoking Prevalence in a Cohort of Adolescents, Including Absentees, Dropouts, and Transfers." *American Journal of Public Health* 78:2 (1988): 176-178.; Johnson, C. Anderson, M.A. Pentz, M.D. Weber, et al. "Relative Effectiveness of Comprehensive Community Programming for Drug Abuse Prevention with High-Risk and Low-Risk Adolescents." *Journal of Consulting and Clinical Psychology* 58:4 (1990):447-456.

48. Mittelmark, Maurice B., R. V. Luepker, D. R. Jacobs, N. F. Bracht, R. W. Carlaw, R. S. Crow, et al. "Community-wide Prevention of Cardiovascular Disease: Education Strategies of the Minnesota Heart Health Program." *Preventive Medicine* 15 (1986): 1-17.

49. Perry, Klepp, and Sillers, 1989; Pentz, Dwyer et al., 1989; and Vartianen, Erkki, U. Fallonen, A. L. McAlister, and P. Puska. "Eight-Year Follow-Up Results of an Adolescent Smoking Prevention Program: The North Karelia Youth Project." *American Journal of Public Health* 80:1 (1990): 78-79.

50. Perry, Kelder et al., 1992.

51. Vartianen et al.

52. Pentz, Mary, D. P. MacKinnon, J. H. Dwyer, E. Y. I. Wang, W. B. Hansen, B. R. Flay, and C. A. Johnson. "Longitudinal Effects of the Midwestern Prevention Project on Regular and Experimental Smoking in Adolescents." *Preventive Medicine* 18 (1989): 304-321.

53. Pentz, Mary A., J. H. Dwyer, D. P. MacKinnon, et al. "A Multicommunity Trial for Primary Prevention of Adolescent Drug Abuse." *Journal of the American Medical Association* 261:22 (1989): 3259-3266; and Errecart, Michael T., H. J. Walberg, J. G. Ross, R. S. Gold, J. L. Fiedler, and L. J. Kolbe. "Effectiveness of Teenage Health Teaching Modules." *Journal of School Health* 61:1 (1991): 26-30.

54. Ellickson, Phyllis L., R. M. Bell, and K. McGuigan. "Preventing Adolescent Drug Use: Long-Term Results of a Junior High Program." *American Journal of Public Health* 83:6 (June 1993): 856-861.

55. Clayton, R. R., A. Cattarello, L. E. Day, and K. P. Walden. "Persuasive Communication and Drug Prevention: An Evaluation of the DARE Program." In Donhew, L., H. E. Sypher, and W. J. Bukoski, eds. *Persuasive Communication and Drug Abuse Prevention.* Hillsdale, NJ: Lawrence Erlbaum Associates, 1991.

56. Pentz, MacKinnon, Dwyer, et al., 1989.

57. Johnston, Lloyd, J. Bachman, P. O'Malley. "Monitoring the Future Study." Press release. The University of Michigan, Ann Arbor. (27 January 1994.)

58. Boyd, Gayle, et al. "Use of Smokeless Tobacco Among Children and Adolescents in the United States." *Preventive Medicine* 16 (1987): 402-421; and Office of the Inspector General. *Youth Use of Smokeless Tobacco: More Than a Pinch of Trouble.* Washington, DC: OIG, Office of Analysis and Inspections, 1986.

59. Wilson, Mark G., and K. M. Wilson. "Strategies and Materials for Smokeless Tobacco Education." *Journal of School Health* 57:2 (1987): 74-76; and Laflin, Molly, E. D. Glover, and J. F. McKenzie. "Resources for Smokeless Tobacco Education." *Journal of School Health* 57:5 (1987): 191-194.

60. Severson, Herbert H. "Enough Snuff: ST Cessation from the Behavioral, Clinical, and Public Health Perspectives." *Smoking and Tobacco Control Monograph 2.* NIH Publication No. 92-3461. Bethesda, MD: National Cancer Institute, 1992. 279-290; and Chassin et al., 1985.

61. Office of the Inspector General.

62. Schaefer, Steven D., A. H. Henderson, E. D. Glover, and A. G. Christen. "Patterns of Use and Incidence of Smokeless Tobacco Consumption in School-Age Children." *Archives of Otolaryngology* 111 (October 1985): 639-642.

63. Chassin et al., 1985.

64. Severson, Herbert H. "Smokeless Tobacco: Risks, Epidemiology, and Cessation." In Orleans, C. Tracy, and John Slade, eds. *Nicotine Addiction: Principles and Management.* New York: Oxford University Press, 1993. 262-278.

65. Severson, Herbert H., R. Glasgow, R. Wirt, P. Brozovsky, L. Zoref, C. Black, et al. "Preventing the Use of Smokeless Tobacco and Cigarettes by Teens: Results of a Classroom Intervention." *Health Education Research* 6:1 (1991): 109-120.

66. Sussman, Steve, C. W. Dent, A. W. Stacy, et al. "Project Towards No Tobacco Use: 1-Year Behavior Outcomes." *Journal of Public Health* 83:9 (1993): 1245-1250.

67. Elder et al.

68. Connolly, Gregory N., C. T. Orleans, and M. Kogan. "Use of Smokeless Tobacco in Major-League Baseball." *New England Journal of Medicine* 318:9 (1988): 1281-1285; and Ernster, Virginia L., D. G. Grady, J. C. Greene, et al. "Smokeless Tobacco Use and Health Effects Among Baseball Players." *Journal of the American Medical Association* 264:2 (1990): 218-224.

69. Jones, Rhys B. "Use of Smokeless Tobacco in the 1986 World Series." *New England Journal of Medicine* 316:15 (1987): 952.

70. Sussman, Steve, and M. Barovich. "Smokeless Tobacco: Less Seen at 1988 World Series." *American Journal of Public Health* 79 (1989): 521-522. (Letter.)

71. D'Onofrio, C., J. Moskowitz, and M. Braverman. Unpublished data cited in Centers for Disease Control. *Preventing Tobacco Use Among Young People. A Report of the Surgeon General.* Washington, D.C.: U.S. Department of Health and Human Services, 1994. 237.

72. Schinke, Steven P., R. F. Schilling II, L. D. Gilchrist, M. R. Ashby, and E. Kitajima. "Native Youth and Smokeless Tobacco: Prevalence Rates, Gender Differences, and Descriptive Characteristics." *Smokeless Tobacco Use in the United States. Monographs No. 8.* Bethesda, MD: National Cancer Institute, 1989. 39-42.

73. Pirie et al.

74. Centers for Disease Control and Prevention. *Preventing Tobacco Use,* 1994. 78.

75. Allen, Karen, A. J. Moss., G. A. Giovino, D. R. Shopland, and J. P. Pierce. "Teenage Tobacco Use: Data Estimates From the Teenage Attitudes and Practices Survey, United States, 1989." *Advance Data* 224 (1 Feb. 1993): 1-20.

76. Foulds, J. "Does Nicotine Replacement Therapy Work?" *Addiction* 88 (1993): 1473-1478; Hughes, John R. "Combined Psychological and Nicotine Gum Treatment for Smoking: A Critical Review." *Journal of Substance Abuse* 3:3 (1991): 337-350; Fagerström, Karl-Olov, R. D. Hurt, U. Sawe, and P. Tonnesen. "Therapeutic Use of Nicotine Patches: Efficacy and Safety." *Journal of Smoking-Related Diseases* 3 (1992): 247-261.

77. Tuakli, Nadu, M. A. Smith, and C. Heaton. "Smoking in Adolescence: Methods for Health Education and Smoking Cessation. A MIRNET Study." *Journal of Family Practice* 31:4 (1990): 369-374.

78. Murray et al.

79. Best, J. Allan, C. L. Perry, B. R. Flay, K. S. Brown, S. M. J. Towson, M. W. Kersell, K. B. Ryan, and J. R. D'Avernas. "Smoking Prevention and the Concept of Risk." *Journal of Applied Social Psychology* 14:3 (1984): 257-273; Johnson, C. Anderson, W. B. Hansen, L. M. Collins, and J. W. Graham. "High School Smoking Prevention: Results of a Three-Year Longitudinal Study." *Journal of Behavioral Medicine* 9:5 (1986): 439-452; and Biglan, Severson, et al., 1987.

80. Best et al., 1984.

81. St. Pierre, Richard W., R. E. Shute, and S. Jaycox. "Youth Helping Youth: A Behavioral Approach to the Self-Control of Smoking." *Health Education* (Jan./Feb. 1983): 28-31.

82. Lotecka, Llynn, and M. MacWhinney. "Enhancing Decision Behavior in High School 'Smokers.'" *The International Journal of the Addictions* 18:4 (1983): 479-490.

83. Sussman, Steve, D. Burton, A. W. Stacy, and B. R. Flay. *School-Based Adolescent Tobacco Use Prevention and Cessation Research.* Newbury Park, CA: Sage Publications. (In press.)

84. Perry, Cheryl, J. Killen, M. Telch, L. A. Slinkard, and B. G. Danaher. "Modifying Smoking Behavior of Teenagers: A School-Based Intervention." *American Journal of Public Health* 70:7 (July 1980): 722-725.

85. Perry, Cheryl L., M. J. Telch, J. Killen, A. Burke, and N. Maccoby. "High School Smoking Prevention: The Relative Efficacy of Varied Treatments and Instructors." *Adolescence* 18:71 (1983): 561-566.

86. Peltier, Bruce, M. J. Telch, and T. J. Coates. "Smoking Cessation with Adolescents: A Comparison of Recruitment Strategies." *Addictive Behaviors* 7 (1982): 71-73.

87. Hollis, Jack F., T. M. Vogt, V. Stevens, A. Biglan, H. Severson, and E. Lichtenstein. "The Tobacco Reduction and Cancer Control (TRACC) Program: Team Approaches to Counseling in Medical and Dental Settings." In National Cancer Institute, *Tobacco and the Clinician: Interventions for Medical and Dental Practice. Smoking and Tobacco Control Monograph No. 5.* NIH Pub. No. 94-3693. USDHHS, 1994. 143-185.

88. Weissman, Wendy, R. Glasgow, A. Biglan, and E. Lichtenstein. "Development and Preliminary Evaluation of a Cessation Program for Adolescent Smokers." *Psychology of Addictive Behaviors* 1:2 (1987): 84-91.

89. Gallup International Institute. *Teen-Age Attitudes and Behavior Concerning Tobacco.* Princeton, NJ: The George H. Gallup International Institute, Sept. 1992.

90. Hawkins, Robert P., D. H. Gustafson, B. Chewning, K. Bosworth, and P. M. Day. "Reaching Hard-To-Reach Populations: Interactive Computer Programs as Public Information Campaigns for Adolescents." *Journal of Communication* 37:2 (1987): 8-28.

91. Orleans, C. Tracy, V. J. Schoenbach, E. H. Wagner, D. Quade, M. A. Salmon, D. C. Pearson, J. Fiedler, C. Q. Porter, and B. H. Kaplan. "Self-Help Quit Smoking Interventions: Effects of Self-Help Materials, Social Support Instructions, and Telephone Counseling." *Journal of Consulting and Clinical Psychology* 59:3 (1991): 439-448.

92. Elder et al.

93. Boyle, Raymond. *Smokeless Tobacco Cessation with Nicotine Replacement: A Randomized Clinical Trial*. Eugene, OR: University of Oregon, 1992. (Dissertation.)

94. Eakin, Elizabeth, H. Severson, and R. E. Glasgow. "Development and Evaluation of a Smokeless Tobacco Cessation Program: A Pilot Study." *NCI Monographs 8* (1989): 95-100; Sussman, Burton, et al., in press; and Chakravorty, Bonnie J. *A Product Substitution Approach to Adolescent Smokeless Tobacco Cessation*. Chicago, IL: University of Illinois, 1992. (Thesis.)

95. Williams, Nancy J. *A Smokeless Tobacco Cessation Program for Postsecondary Students*. Memphis State University, May 1992. (Thesis.)

96. Severson, Herbert H., E. G. Eakin, E. Lichtenstein, and V. J. Stevens. "The Inside Scoop on the Stuff Called Snuff: An Interview Study of 94 Adult Male Smokeless Tobacco Users." *Journal of Substance Abuse* 2 (1990): 77-85.

97. Ary, Dennis V., E. Lichtenstein, and H. H. Severson. "An In-Depth Analysis of Male Adolescent Smokeless Tobacco Users: Interviews with Users and Their Fathers." *Journal of Behavioral Medicine* 12:5 (1989): 449.

98. Novotny, Thomas E., J. P. Pierce, M. C. Fiore, and R. M. Davis. "Smokeless Tobacco Use in the United States: The Adult Use of Tobacco Surveys." *National Cancer Institute Monographs 8* (1989): 25-28.

99. Glover, Elbert D. "Conducting Smokeless Tobacco Cessation Clinics." Letter. *American Journal of Public Health* 76:2 (1986): 207.

100. DiLorenzo, Thomas M., T. G. Kern, and R. M. Pieper. "Treatment of Smokeless Tobacco Use Through A Formalized Cessation Program." *Behavior Therapy* 22 (1991): 41-46.

101. Eakin et al.

102. Sussman, Burton, et al., in press.

103. Chakravorty.

104. Williams.

105. Boyle, Raymond, H. H. Severson, E. Lichtenstein, and J. Gordon. "Smokeless Tobacco Cessation with Nicotine Reduction: A Placebo-Controlled Trial." Presentation. American Public Health Association. San Francisco, 25 Oct. 1993.

106. Ockene, Judith K. "Clinical Perspectives: Physician-Delivered Interventions for Smoking Cessation: Strategies for Increasing Effectiveness." *Preventive Medicine* 16 (1987): 723-737.

107. Stevens, Victor J., H. H. Severson, E. Lichtenstein, S. J. Little, and J. Leben. "Making the Most of a Teachable Moment: Smokeless Tobacco Intervention in the Dental Office Setting." *American Journal of Public Health*. (In press.)

108. Little, Sally J., V. J. Stevens, P. A. LaChance, H. H. Severson, M. H. Bartley, E. Lichtenstein, and J. R. Leben. "Smokeless Tobacco Habits and Oral Mucosal Lesions in Dental Patients." *Journal of Public Health Dentistry* 52:5 (1992): 269-276.

109. Centers for Disease Control and Prevention, *Preventing Tobacco Use*. 87.

110. Benowitz, Neal L. "Pharmacology of Smokeless Tobacco Use: Nicotine Addiction and Nicotine-Related Health Consequences." In *Smokeless Tobacco or Health. An International Perspective. Smoking and Tobacco Control Monograph 2*. NIH Pub. No. 92-3461. Bethesda, MD: National Cancer Institute, 1992. 219-228.

111. Stevens et al.

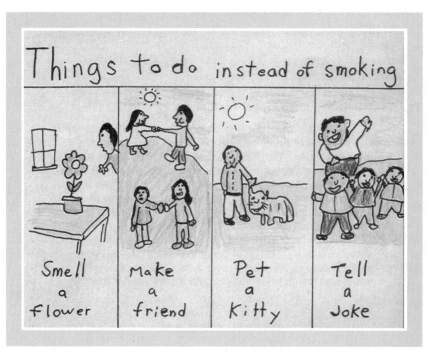

Ismael Zayas, C.S. 44, Bronx

CONTENTS

6 | TOBACCO TAXATION IN THE UNITED STATES

In the United States, tobacco is taxed by federal, state, and local governments. Tobacco products are taxed in two ways: the unit tax, which is based on a constant nominal rate per unit (that is, per pack of cigarettes), and the ad valorem tax, which is based on a constant fraction of either wholesale or retail price. Currently, federal taxes on cigarettes, small cigars, and smokeless tobacco products are unit taxes; federal taxes on large cigars are ad valorem taxes. In 1993, all states and most localities used a unit tax for taxing cigarettes and ad valorem taxes for non-cigarette tobacco products. In 1993, consumer excise taxes on tobacco generated more than $12 billion in tax revenue, 98% of which was derived from taxes on cigarettes.[1]

Historically, governments have levied tobacco taxes to generate revenues. Increasingly, however, taxation of tobacco products is being recognized as an effective strategy to discourage tobacco use and enhance public health.[2] This chapter of the report reviews the history of tobacco taxation in the United States, compares tobacco tax policy in the U.S. with policies in other industrialized countries, and reviews evidence regarding the impact of tobacco taxation on overall consumption and on tobacco use by adolescents specifically. The chapter concludes with a discussion of arguments for and against using tobacco taxes as a strategy to discourage adolescent tobacco use in the United States.

TOBACCO TAXES IN THE UNITED STATES

Federal Tobacco Taxes

Tobacco was one of the first consumer goods to be taxed in North America, first by the British and then by the newly independent republic in the early

1790s. Federal taxes on tobacco have been part of the federal tax system since the Civil War. Between 1864 and 1983, the federal tax on cigarettes has fluctuated in response to the revenue requirements of the government, corresponding mainly to alternating periods of war and peace.[3] In 1951, the federal cigarette excise tax was increased from 7 cents to 8 cents per pack to help finance the Korean War. The federal cigarette tax was not increased again until 1983, when it was doubled to 16 cents per pack. In January 1992 the federal tax on cigarettes was increased from 16 to 20 cents per pack, with another 4 cents per pack added in January 1993. In 1985, the federal government levied a tax of 24 cents per pound on snuff, 8 cents per pound on chewing tobacco, and 45 cents per pound on pipe tobacco. As of 1993, federal taxes on snuff, chewing tobacco, and pipe tobacco are 36, 12, and 67.5 cents per pound, respectively.[4]

State and Local Tobacco Taxes

All 50 states, the District of Columbia, and 440 cities, towns, and counties levy taxes on cigarettes.[5] (See table 6-1.) In addition, 40 states impose taxes on tobacco products other than cigarettes. In 1921, Iowa became the first state to tax cigarettes; in 1969, North Carolina was the last state to enact a cigarette excise tax.[6] In addition to the excise tax on cigarettes, 43 states have general sales taxes that apply to cigarettes. In all but 4 of these 43 states, the sales tax base includes the excise tax, adding between 6 cents and 14 cents to the price of a pack of cigarettes.[7]

With few exceptions, the imposition of, and increases in, state tobacco taxes are the result of the need to raise revenues. However, the level of tax imposed appears to be influenced by how dependent a state is on tobacco production. For example, in 1992, the average cigarette tax in non-tobacco-producing states was 19 cents higher than in large tobacco-producing states.[8] Recently, public health advocates in several states have attempted to increase tobacco taxes through ballot initiatives. In November 1988, California voters passed Proposition 99, which increased the state cigarette excise tax from 10 cents to 35 cents per pack and earmarked 20% of the additional revenue raised for a statewide antismoking campaign.[9] Similarly, in November 1992, voters in Massachusetts passed an initiative to increase the tax on cigarettes by 25 cents per pack and on chewing tobacco by 25%.

In addition to state excise taxes, over 440 local jurisdictions in 9 states also levy taxes on tobacco products. In 1993, 440 cities and counties imposed taxes on cigarettes, while 82 cities and counties levied taxes on non-cigarette tobacco products.[10]

Differences in cigarette tax rates among states and localities can create problems in the enforcement of tax laws. A 1977 report by the Advisory Commission on Intergovernmental Relations identified a variety of tax evasion strategies including casual smuggling (that is, individuals buying cigarettes in neighboring

TABLE 6-1 State cigarette excise tax rates (as of November 1993)

State	Tax per pack (cents)	State	Tax per pack (cents)
DC	65.0	NH	25.0
HI	60.0	KS	24.0
NY	56.0	DE	24.0
WA	54.0	OH	24.0
MA	51.0	OK	23.0
MN	48.0	SD	23.0
CT	47.0	NM	21.0
ND	44.0	LA	20.0
TX	41.0	CO	20.0
NJ	40.0	AZ	18.0
RI	37.0	MT	18.0
ME	37.0	MS	18.0
IA	36.0	VT	18.0
MD	36.0	ID	18.0
CA	35.0	WV	17.0
NV	35.0	AL	16.5
AR	34.5	IN	15.5
FL	33.9	MO	13.0
PA	31.0	TN	13.0
IL	30.0	WY	12.0
AK	29.0	GA	12.0
OR	28.0	SC	7.0
NE	27.0	NC	5.0
UT	26.5	KY	3.0
MI	25.0	VA	2.5

states with lower taxes), purchase of cigarettes through tax-free outlets such as military stores and American-Indian reservations, commercial smuggling for resale, and illegal diversion of cigarettes within the traditional distribution system by forging tax stamps and underreporting. During the late 1960s and early 1970s, as the differential between state cigarette tax rates increased, organized smuggling and illegal diversion of cigarettes from the legal distribution system also increased.[11] In response to this problem, the Federal Cigarette Contraband Act was enacted. This law prohibits the transportation, receipt, shipment, possession, distribution, or purchase of more than 60,000 cigarettes not bearing the indicia of the state in which the cigarettes were found. A 1985 study by the Advisory Commission on Intergovernmental Relations concluded that the Cigarette Contraband Act had markedly reduced organized interstate smuggling of cigarettes.[12] However, the casual smuggling of cigarettes from neighboring states and the purchasing of cigarettes from tax-free outlets continues to be a problem for many states with high cigarette taxes.[13] A recent analysis of tobacco product sales at U.S. military stores found that sales are strongly influenced by the price gap between nonmilitary retail outlets and military stores.[14]

Trends in Cigarette Prices, Taxes, and Affordability

Figure 6-1 shows the federal and state cigarette taxes (actual costs) and pack prices between 1955 and 1993 in the United States. This figure illustrates the growing discrepancy between taxes and pack price. In 1955, the average price of a pack of cigarettes was 23 cents, of which 11 cents (48%) was due to taxes. As of November 1, 1993, the average price per pack of cigarettes was $1.79, of which 53 cents was due to taxes (30%). Figure 6-1 also shows that the average state excise tax on cigarettes has increased by more (3 cents to 29 cents) than the federal tax (8 cents to 24 cents) since 1955.

Because excise taxes on cigarettes in the United States are unit rather than ad valorem taxes, inflation reduces the real value of the tax relative to the price. Figure 6-2 shows trends in cigarette taxes and pack prices adjusted for inflation.

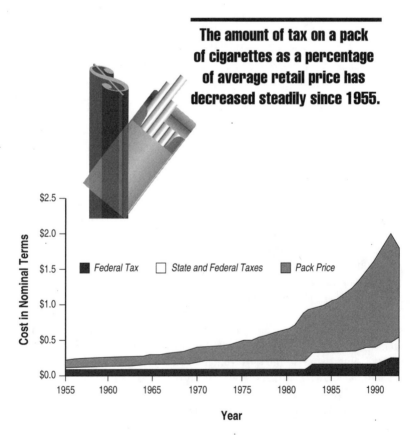

The amount of tax on a pack of cigarettes as a percentage of average retail price has decreased steadily since 1955.

FIGURE 6-1 Source: Tobacco Institute. *The Tax Burden on Tobacco.* Washington, D.C.: Tobacco Institute, 1994.

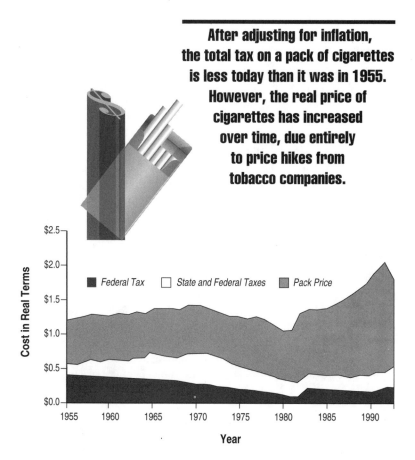

After adjusting for inflation, the total tax on a pack of cigarettes is less today than it was in 1955. However, the real price of cigarettes has increased over time, due entirely to price hikes from tobacco companies.

Cost in Real Terms

■ *Federal Tax*   □ *State and Federal Taxes*   ■ *Pack Price*

Year

FIGURE 6-2   Source: Tobacco Institute. *The Tax Burden on Tobacco.* Washington, D.C.: Tobacco Institute, 1994.

Overall, taxes today have failed to keep pace with inflation and therefore are less, in real value, than they were in 1955. As seen in figure 6-2, although the actual tax amount increased by 16 cents from 1955 to 1993, the *real value* of the federal tax on cigarettes in 1993 is only worth about 56% of what it was in 1955. Overall, the combined real value of federal and state taxes amounts to 88% of what they were in 1955. Interestingly, the real *price* of a pack of cigarettes is about 43% higher today than in 1955; thus, the higher price of cigarettes today is the result of price increases from tobacco manufacturers, not taxes.

In order to appreciate economic incentives or disincentives to use tobacco products, one must consider not only price changes but also price affordability. Over the past half century, tobacco has become increasingly more affordable to consumers in the United States because of rising income.[15]   Table 6-2 shows changes in the affordability of cigarettes in the United States between 1955 and 1990, using 1955 as the base year. Until the 1980s, the affordability of cigarettes increased because of the declining real price of cigarettes. Between 1985 and 1990, tobacco manufacturers increased cigarette prices in excess of the rate of inflation and consumer income. Thus, there was a sharp decline in the affordability of cigarettes, although prices remained more affordable than in 1955. The lower affordability of cigarettes in the 1980s corresponds with a decline in consumption. As illustrated in table 6-2, the lower cigarette affordability since 1985 had little to do with government taxes; total taxes on a pack of cigarettes were no less affordable in 1990 than in 1980. More significantly, total taxes were 60% more affordable in 1990 than in 1955. In 1993, cigarette manufacturers, led by Philip Morris, Inc., implemented major price cuts on premium brand cigarettes, significantly increasing their affordability.

Trends in Cigarette Tax Revenues and Sales

The dollar amount of tobacco tax revenue (combined federal and state) increased from $2 billion in 1955 to $12 billion in 1993. However, when these figures are adjusted for inflation they show a decline: federal tobacco tax revenues have fallen dramatically, from a peak of $9.5 billion (expressed in 1993 dollars) in 1963 to $5.5 billion in 1993. The decline in revenues from tobacco taxes partly reflects a steady drop in per capita cigarette consumption since the mid-1970s. However, the primary reason for the declining revenues is the fail-

TABLE 6-2 Changes in the affordability of a pack of cigarettes in the United States between 1955 and 1990, using 1955 as the base year

	% Change in affordability relative to 1955		
Year	Federal taxes	State and federal taxes	Average pack price
1955	0%	0%	0%
1960	+14%	−1%	+4%
1965	+33%	+2%	+13%
1970	+51%	+15%	+17%
1975	+67%	+43%	+32%
1980	+80%	+61%	+45%
1985	+71%	+57%	+35%
1990	+78%	+60%	+23%

Note: "+" indicates an increase in affordability relative to 1955; "−" indicates a decrease in affordability relative to 1955.

Source: Non-smoker's Rights Association of Canada, 1992.

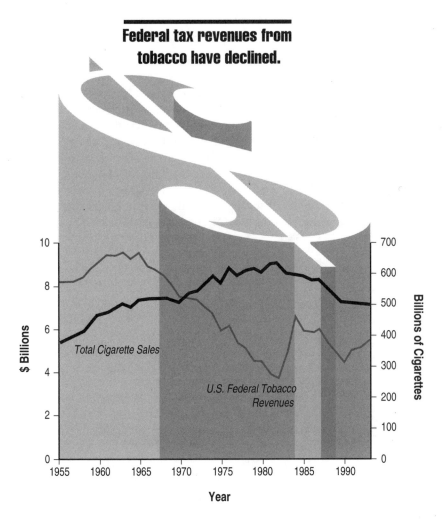

Federal tax revenues from tobacco have declined.

FIGURE 6-3 Source: Tobacco Institute. *The Tax Burden on Tobacco.* Washington, D.C.: Tobacco Institute, 1994.

ure of the federal government to adjust cigarette tax rates to keep pace with inflation. For example, figure 6-3 shows that the decline in federal tobacco tax revenues occurred despite the fact that total cigarette sales were nearly identical in 1993 and 1963. As a result of inflation, declining consumption, and identification of other revenue sources, tobacco taxes at both the federal and state levels now account for a significantly smaller share of total revenues compared to 40 years ago.[16]

TAX RATES IN OTHER
INDUSTRIALIZED COUNTRIES

Among industrialized countries of the world, the United States has one of the lowest tax rates on cigarettes (see table 6-3). In two countries, taxes are now above $3 per pack—Denmark ($3.48) and Norway ($3.11). In the United States, the average combined federal and state tax on cigarettes in 1993 was 53 cents per pack. The combination of lower cigarette taxes and a higher standard of living (that is, more money to spend on goods) makes cigarettes much more affordable for Americans than for persons in nearly all other industrialized countries.

TABLE 6-3   Average retail selling price, total taxes, and percentage tax of average retail price for a pack of 20 cigarettes in 24 selected countries as of December 1, 1993

Country	Total taxes (U.S.$)	Average retail price (U.S.$)	Tax (% of retail price)
Denmark	$3.48	$4.11	85
Norway	$3.11	$4.55	68
Canada	$2.90	$4.22	69
United Kingdom	$2.85	$3.68	77
Ireland	$2.68	$3.55	75
Sweden	$2.43	$3.33	73
Finland	$2.28	$3.08	74
Germany	$2.04	$2.86	71
New Zealand	$1.93	$2.85	68
France	$1.70	$2.33	75
Belgium	$1.70	$2.31	73
Netherlands	$1.65	$2.28	72
Hong Kong	$1.50	$2.78	54
Japan	$1.21	$2.02	60
Luxemburg	$1.19	$1.76	68
Portugal	$1.17	$1.48	79
Italy	$1.16	$1.60	73
Switzerland	$1.04	$2.07	50
Argentina	$0.96	$1.37	70
Greece	$0.78	$1.13	69
Taiwan	$0.62	$1.31	47
United States	**$0.56**	**$1.89**	**30**
Korea	$0.45	$0.74	60
Spain	$0.42	$0.63	66

Source: Non-Smokers' Rights Association of Canada, 1993.

EFFECT OF EXCISE TAXES ON CONSUMPTION

It is well recognized in economic theory, as well as in everyday life, that purchasing decisions are influenced by price.[17] Economists use a particular measure, termed "price elasticity," to judge the degree to which the demand for a product is responsive to its price. The price elasticity of demand is defined as the percentage change in consumption that results from a 1% change in price; for example, a price elasticity of –0.5 implies that a 10% increase in price would reduce consumption by 5%.

Because of the addictive qualities of tobacco, some researchers have speculated that consumption of cigarettes will be insensitive to price changes at least in the short run.[18] However, numerous studies, using a variety of methodologies, have shown that overall consumption of cigarettes is responsive to price changes.[19] Estimates of the price effect vary, but generally speaking a 10% increase in the real price reduces consumption by around 4%.[20] Decreases in consumption occur both because some people choose not to smoke and because some smokers choose to smoke fewer cigarettes. Studies estimate that approximately two-thirds of the decreased consumption is the result of people choosing not to smoke at all.[21] Conversely, a decline in the real price of tobacco leads to increased consumption. An analysis of Finland's cigarette consumption between 1960 and 1987 found that the demand for cigarettes was twice as sensitive to falling prices as to rising prices.[22]

An estimate of the impact of tax increases on consumption must account for the extent to which taxes are incorporated into the price of cigarettes, since cigarette taxes account for only a share of the total retail price of cigarettes. Increases in excise taxes are usually passed on to consumers.[23] Thus, to determine the effect of a tax change, the price elasticity of demand must be multiplied by the percent change in price resulting from the tax change. In addition to taxes, the retail price of tobacco products is determined by the manufacturer's costs and profits and wholesale and retail markups. For example, Harris argues that most of the decline in U.S. cigarette consumption during the mid-1980s resulted from increases in the wholesale prices of cigarettes because of markups from manufacturers, not from increases in federal and state taxes.[24]

While numerous studies have investigated the impact of cigarette taxes on consumption, only a few studies have attempted to estimate the impact of increased cigarette taxes on the consumption of non-cigarette tobacco products. In Finland, Pekurinen found that the most important factor influencing demand for pipe tobacco was the price of cigarettes.[25] Similarly, in Canada consumption of fine-cut tobacco (used to make roll-your-own cigarettes) increased in relationship to the widening price gap between cigarettes and fine-cut tobacco.[26] It is possible that the increased popularity of smokeless tobacco seen among male adolescents in the United States during early 1980s may have resulted in part from higher cigarette prices. In other words, at least for male adolescents, there may be a significant degree of substitutability between cigarettes and smokeless tobacco; however, no studies have actually tested this hypothesis.

The Canadian Experience

The Canadian experience with raising tobacco taxes during the past decade provides a useful model for predicting the impact of tobacco tax increases in the United States.[27] Canada, like the United States, has a federal system of government; in both countries the national and state/provincial governments levy taxes on tobacco products.

In the early 1980s, federal taxes on tobacco products in Canada were modest, not unlike the current tax rate in the United States. Since 1985, there have been three significant increases in the federal cigarette tax in Canada, raising the tax from 32 cents (U.S. dollars) in 1984 to $1.45 (U.S. dollars) per 20 cigarettes in 1992. During the same period, provincial governments also dramatically increased taxes on tobacco, raising the combined average federal and provincial tax to close to $3 ($2.91 in U.S. dollars as of December 1993) and the average price of 20 cigarettes to over $4 ($4.22 in U.S. dollars as of December 1993).[28] In addition to increases in cigarette taxes, federal and provincial governments implemented other measures to limit smoking, including banning smoking in public buildings and prohibiting tobacco advertising on billboards, at the point of purchase, and at sporting events.[29]

Between 1982 and 1992, total per capita cigarette consumption in Canada, adjusted for estimates of tobacco smuggling, fell by 38%.[30] An analysis comparing the slope of the decline in per capita tobacco consumption in the United States and Canada reveals that during the 1980s consumption dropped 30% faster in Canada than in the United States.[31] A 1991 independent investment research report on Imperial Tobacco, the largest of the three Canadian tobacco manufacturers, concluded that a large share of the reduction in cigarette consumption in Canada between 1982 and 1990 could be attributed to price increases in cigarettes, primarily from higher federal and provincial taxes.[32] The report also concluded that prices still are a major determinant of levels of smoking and that there is no indication that consumption was less responsive to price increases in 1991 than in 1980. Declines in cigarette smoking prevalence have mirrored trends in per capita sales. Between 1979 and 1991, prevalence of regular smoking among Canadians over age 14 decreased from 38% to 26%.[33]

The most recent analysis of Canadian price sensitivity for tobacco, prepared by the Canadian Department of Finance, reports an increasing elasticity as prices have increased. The findings from this study are of interest for several reasons. First, the price elasticity of demand for tax-paid cigarettes was significantly higher than found in most other studies. In 1991, it was estimated that a 10% increase in the real price of cigarettes would lead to a short-term 9% decline in consumption.[34] Second, contrary to the findings of other economic studies,[35] the price elasticity of demand for cigarettes tended to be more inelastic in the long run (–0.7) than in the short run (–0.9), although the level is still higher than found in most other studies (range –0.2 to –0.5). The report speculates that Canadian smokers may have initially reacted to price increases either by reducing the amount smoked or by quitting. However, over time, the addictive nature of tobacco leads some of these individuals to return to their past consumption levels. Third, the study found a significant degree of substitutability between cigarettes and fine-cut tobacco. Since 1980, both price and tax increases have widened the price differential between cigarettes and fine-cut tobacco. As a result, some smokers have switched from cigarettes to cheaper, fine-cut (roll-your-own) tobacco products. The analysis estimates that a 10% increase in the price of cigarettes led to a 13% increase in the sales of tax-paid fine-cut tobacco. Fourth, exports and smuggling of cigarettes increased as a result of tax hikes. Between 1985 and 1991 there was a large increase in the number of seizures of illicitly imported tobacco products, indicating that smuggling had become a problem in Canada. In February 1994, the Canadian government announced plans to cut the tax on tailor-made cigarettes by 30% and increase the export tax as a way of reducing illegal smuggling of cigarettes from the United States into Canada. Finally, the study found that tobacco taxes were particularly important in discouraging younger Canadians from smoking. A comparison of the smoking habits of teenagers and adults showed that younger Canadians were more sensitive to price changes than adults. Overall, the study concluded that "On balance, federal tax increases since 1985 have resulted in a net decline in overall tobacco consumption in Canada."[36]

Adolescents' Sensitivity to Price

The issue of whether adolescents respond differently than adults to changes in tobacco prices is of interest for several reasons. First, as noted in chapter 1, the vast majority of adult smokers began their smoking careers before they turned 21; therefore, there is a good chance that persons who have not started smoking by age 20 will never smoke. Second, preventing people from starting to smoke is likely to be the most effective approach in the long term for reducing the health problems associated with tobacco use. Finally, there is good reason to expect that adolescents are more price sensitive than adults because they are less addicted to smoking (that is, they smoke fewer cigarettes per day) and have less disposable income (that is, cigarettes are less affordable for them).[37] A teenager in a focus group conducted under the auspices of the Committee illustrated the effect of a tax increase on cigarettes as follows: "Major . . . Sure, they'll buy them every once in a while, and they start thinking: running out of money. No money to go to the movies, no money for gas or whatever."

Only a few studies have examined the question of whether cigarette price increases affect teenagers differently than adults.[38] In the United States, three studies have investigated adolescents' sensitivity to cigarette prices. The largest of these studies utilized data from Cycle III of the Health Examination Survey conducted between 1966 and 1970 to study the effects of cigarette prices, advertising restrictions, and sociodemographic factors on the cigarette smoking behavior of 5,308 teenagers between the ages of 12 and 17. The study found that cigarette prices had a significant effect on the smoking behavior of teenagers.[39] Moreover, the estimated price elasticity of demand observed among teenagers of –1.4 was roughly three times higher than that estimated for adults in a separate study conducted by Lewit and Coate.[40]

Results from a study[41] utilizing national surveys on drug abuse conducted between 1974 and 1979 to estimate the effects of cigarette price on adolescent smoking behavior confirmed the 1981 finding by Lewit and colleagues[42] that the smoking behavior of teenagers is negatively related to the price of cigarettes. The summary price elasticity of demand of –0.76 observed for teenagers in this study is also higher than that usually found for adults, implying that teenagers are more responsive to price than adults.

However, a more recent study, utilizing data collected in the Second National Health and Nutrition Examination Survey (1976-1980), failed to find a statistically significant effect of cigarette prices on cigarette smoking by youths aged 12 through 17.[43] The authors speculate that one reason for the lack of association between price and consumption was the inclusion in their cigarette demand model of an index that captured state regulations limiting smoking in public locations; this regulation index highly correlated with price. The index measuring state antismoking regulations was found to have a significant effect on cigarette consumption by teenagers, leading the authors to conclude that restrictions on indoor smoking may have a greater impact on preventing youths from initiating smoking than do increases in cigarette prices. However, critics of this study point out that antismoking regulations are not likely to have any direct impact on youths because youths spend most of their time in school; instead, the regulation may merely reflect the level of antismoking sentiment in a region.[44] Other critics point out that the study did not take into account the rapid market growth of discount cigarettes in the United States during the late 1970s and 1980s, which offered price-sensitive consumers a range of very cheap products.[45] Because of the wide differential in price between discount and premium brands, average retail price (used in the study to measure price) may not be an accurate indicator of actual price, since price-sensitive consumers would presumably gravitate toward lower-priced products.[46] However, while this argument may be valid for adults, it is not likely to hold true for teenagers in the United States, 90% of whom report smoking one of three premium cigarette brands: Marlboro, Newport, or Camel.[47] The conflicting results of the few U.S. studies that have examined the impact of cigarette prices on consumption by adolescents, including possible substitution of smokeless tobacco products in response to higher cigarette prices, reinforce the need for new research to assess the potential for using higher tobacco taxes to deter adolescent tobacco use.

The Canadian experience in raising tobacco taxes during the 1980s provides useful data for comparing the price sensitivity of teenagers and adults. An analysis comparing the cigarette smoking prevalence and average daily consumption of Canadian teenagers (ages 15-19) and the total population (over age 15) between 1980 and 1989 found that the decline in smoking prevalence among teenagers was steeper than for the total population.[48] Teenage smoking declined by 52%, from 45% to 22% between 1980 and 1989, while smoking in the total population age 15 and older declined by only 23% (from 41% to 31%). Figure 6-4 illustrates the price sensitivity of Canadian teenagers by juxtaposing teenage smoking trends between 1979 and 1991 with changes in the average retail price for 20 cigarettes.

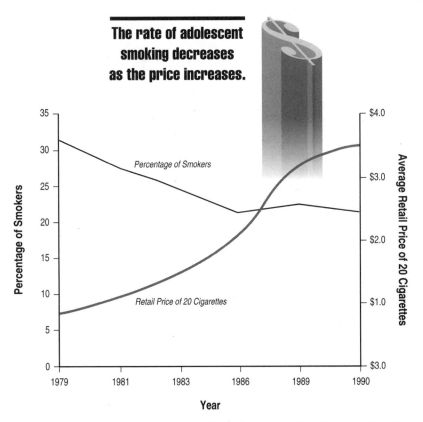

FIGURE 6-4   Source: Sweanor, David T., L. R. Martial, and J. B. Dossetor. *The Canadian Tobacco Tax Experience: A Case Study.* Ottawa, Ontario: The Non-Smokers' Rights Association of Canada and the Smoking and Health Foundation of Canada, 1993.

In addition to changes in the proportion of teenagers smoking, there has been a dramatic change in the pattern of smoking by Canadian teens. From 1979 to 1991, there has been a 62% decline (from 42% to 16%) in the percentage of 15- to 19-year-olds who report daily (or regular) smoking. Conversely, there has been an increase in the percentage of young Canadians who report smoking occasionally.[49] It appears that many of Canada's young people have reduced tobacco use in response to the comprehensive set of tobacco control measures, which have included large increases in cigarette taxes. However, Sweanor and colleagues caution that reductions in tobacco prices or increases in personal income may result in many occasional smokers becoming regular smokers in the future, and argue that ". . . the trend toward occasional smoking makes a strong case for continued tax increases and ancillary tobacco control strategies."[50]

A 1992 study attempted to evaluate teenagers' perceptions of the impact that cigarette price increases would have on their smoking behavior.[51] Approximately 8,000 14- and 15-year-olds located in Erie County, New York, were asked to indicate what impact increases of 10 cents and of $1 in the price of cigarettes would have on their decision to smoke. Not surprisingly, a 10-cent increase in the price of a pack of cigarettes was perceived not to be a large deterrent to smoking, especially among current daily smokers. However, over one-third of the teenagers reported that a $1 increase in the price of a pack of cigarettes would make them less likely to smoke. Interestingly, those most at risk of becoming regular smokers (that is, nonsmokers who said they expect to smoke in the next year and those who already report smoking occasionally) were most likely to report that a $1 price increase would make it less likely that they would smoke. The findings from this study suggest that teenagers themselves perceive sizable price increases on tobacco products to be an important deterrent to tobacco use. This perception was also confirmed in focus groups conducted under the Committee's auspices. The following statement by one teen represents the opinion expressed by many of the teens:

"A $2 increase in the price would definitely stop a lot of teens from smoking. Kids have better ways to spend $5 than on cigarettes. A 50-cent increase wouldn't make any difference."

ARGUMENTS FOR AND AGAINST
HIGHER TOBACCO TAXES

The data from research on the relationship between cigarette prices and cigarette consumption support the conclusion that substantial increases in cigarette excise taxes will reduce cigarette smoking.[52] The higher price of tobacco products would encourage individuals to stop smoking or to smoke less, and would discourage children and youths from initiating smoking. Despite the fact that only a few studies have actually examined the relationship between cigarette prices and smoking by youths, most health economists conclude that the price responsiveness of adolescents is likely to be at least as high as for adults, if not higher.[53] Therefore, it is reasonable to suppose that raising tobacco taxes in the United States to the levels current in areas such as Canada, Scandinavia, and the United Kingdom could significantly reduce tobacco consumption and related disease in future generations. For example, it has been estimated that if Congress were to raise the federal cigarette tax by $2 per pack and maintain this tax in real terms, tobacco use would decrease by 23% (approximately 7 million fewer smokers).[54]

In addition to the health benefit, other potential benefits support the argument for large increases in tobacco taxes in the United States. Because tobacco taxes are relatively low, higher taxes would generate large increases in revenue even while smoking rates decline. The United States could raise an additional $35 billion annually from tobacco taxes before consumption rates would drop to a point where tax revenues would begin to decline.[55] Obviously, while no tax is desirable, the simple fact is that governments need money to operate, and they acquire that money through taxation. Some taxes can have undesirable effects; for example, income taxes might discourage working, and investment taxes might discourage savings. However, high taxes on tobacco products are desirable because they would discourage use of the nation's leading cause of preventable death.[56] Opinion polls and the recent successful ballot initiatives in California and Massachusetts indicate that the public is willing to support substantial increases in tobacco taxes.[57] The level of public support for higher tobacco taxes tends to increase when revenues from those taxes are earmarked for specific purposes such as deficit reduction or health care financing.[58] In 1992, seven states were using cigarette tax revenues to finance tobacco-related public health programs.[59]

Opponents of tobacco taxes argue that these taxes are undesirable because they unfairly affect the poor. A 1990 report by the Congressional Budget Office supports the widely held belief that tobacco taxes are regressive. Data from the 1984-1985 Consumer Expenditure Survey were used to relate expenditures for tobacco products with income. Results showed that families in the lowest income quintile spend 4% of their post-tax income on tobacco, whereas families in the highest quintile spend only 0.5% of their post-tax income on tobacco.[60] Only a few studies have attempted to evaluate differences in price elasticity of demand for tobacco between income groups. A study in the United Kingdom found a greater sensitivity to cigarette prices among people with lower incomes.[61] A recent study in the United States, however, failed to find a significant relationship between price elasticity and income, but did show that the estimated income elasticities have changed in this country over time from positive to negative; that is, cigarette consumption tends to be lower at higher income levels.[62] The growth of discount cigarette brands in the United States during the past decade, mentioned above, may be masking differences between income groups in response to price changes.[63] The regressiveness of tobacco taxes is a valid concern. On the other hand, the burden of illness and death caused by tobacco is borne to a greater extent by the poor.[64] For the poor as a class, the hardship imposed by steep increases in tobacco prices produced by higher tobacco taxes is arguably outweighed by the reduction in suffering and premature death resulting from lower consumption of tobacco. Moreover, revenues generated through higher tobacco taxes could be earmarked for health care for the indigent, thus offsetting the regressivity of tobacco taxes.[65]

Loss of tobacco-related jobs and the potential economic consequences of such job loss on the economy is another argument used to oppose increases in tobacco taxes.[66] However, of the 2.3 million jobs claimed by the Tobacco Institute to be dependent on tobacco,[67] only 11% are directly involved in growing, warehousing, manufacturing, or wholesaling tobacco products. The remaining 2 million jobs are in sectors of the economy (retailing, supplier jobs) that have no relation at all to tobacco.[68] Money not spent on tobacco products because of a tax increase would not disappear from the economy, but would be redirected to non-tobacco goods and services, creating employment and tax benefits in other sectors of the economy.[69] Even in tobacco-growing states, such as North Carolina, the economic impact of a tobacco tax increase is likely to be fairly small as a share of total economic activity.[70]

CONCLUSIONS AND RECOMMENDATIONS

The consumption of tobacco products is strongly related to their affordability. If tobacco is made less affordable by higher prices resulting from higher taxes or other reasons, consumption will tend to decline, especially among children and youths, whose smoking habits are not firmly established. Therefore, policymakers have an effective means available to them—increasing the real price of tobacco by increasing excise taxes—to reduce the consumption of tobacco by youths and thereby to reduce the health toll of tobacco use in future years.

Despite the rather obvious relationship between consumption and affordability, the federal government and most state governments have given little attention to the role of pricing in controlling tobacco consumption. Evidence from Canada,[71] New Zealand,[72] and the United Kingdom[73] lead the Committee to the conclusion that pricing policy is perhaps the single most important element of an overall comprehensive strategy to reduce tobacco use, and particularly to reduce use among children and youths. This evidence leads the Committee to make the following five recommendations for changing how tobacco products are taxed in the United States:

1. Tobacco tax policies at the federal and state levels should be linked to the national objectives for reducing tobacco use. In other words, government policymakers should use tobacco taxes as an intervention to accomplish these health goals.

2. The excise tax on cigarettes should be increased to a level comparable with that in other major industrialized countries. A reasonable target would be to increase the federal cigarette tax by $2 by 1995. Accomplishing this objective would also have the added benefit of reducing illegal smuggling of tobacco products between Canada and the United States.

3. All tobacco products should be taxed on an equivalent basis. For example, when cigarette taxes are increased, taxes on non-cigarette tobacco products should also be increased on an equivalent basis to discourage substitution of one harmful form of tobacco for another (such as smokeless tobacco).

4. The real value of tobacco taxes should be maintained to account for inflation over time. Optimally, tobacco tax policy should take into consideration the affordability of tobacco products to prevent tobacco from becoming more affordable.

5. Tobacco products in U.S. military stores should be priced at the same rate that exists in the surrounding community. This policy change would have an effect on the smoking behavior of military personnel, many of whom are young adults. Also by eliminating the price differential between military and nonmilitary retail outlets, the incentive for illegal smuggling of tobacco products out of military bases would be eliminated.

While the Committee feels that the empirical evidence is sufficiently developed to make these five recommendations, at the same time the Committee acknowledges the need for additional research to understand better the impact of tobacco pricing on consumption by youths and the benefits of various taxation policies. For this reason, **the Committee recommends that the National Institutes of Health should allocate resources to support research on tobacco tax questions.** A summary discussion of research issues on tobacco taxation policy, and of priority areas for future research, is presented in a 1992 report by a study group formed as a result of meetings convened on the topic of tobacco policy research.[74]

REFERENCES

1. Tobacco Institute. *The Tax Burden on Tobacco.* Washington, DC: Tobacco Institute, 1993.

2. Lewit, Eugene M., and Douglas Coate. "The Potential for Using Excise Taxes to Reduce Smoking." *Journal of Health Economics* 1 (1982): 121-145; Warner, K. E. "Cigarette Taxation: Doing Good by Doing Well." *Journal of Public Health Policy* 5 (1984): 312-319; National Cancer Institute. Cancer Control Science Program, Division of Cancer Prevention and Control. *The Impact of Cigarette Excise Taxes on Smoking Among Children and Adults. Summary Report of a National Cancer Institute Expert Panel.* 1993; and Sweanor, David, and K. E. Warner. "The Role of the Federal and State Excise Taxes." In Houston, T.P., ed. *Tobacco Use: An American Crisis. Final Conference Report.* Chicago: American Medical Association, 1993. 59-62.

3. Lewit, Eugene M. "U.S. Tobacco Taxes: Behavioral Effects and Policy Implications." *British Journal of Addiction* 84 (1989): 1217-1234.

4. Centers for Disease Control and Prevention. *Preventing Tobacco Use Among Young People.*

A Report of the Surgeon General. S/N 017-001-00491-0. Washington, DC: U.S. Government Printing Office, 1994. 265.

5. Tobacco Institute, 1993.

6. Centers for Disease Control and Prevention. *Preventing Tobacco Use.* 265.

7. Tobacco Institute, 1993.

8. Centers for Disease Control and Prevention. *Preventing Tobacco Use.* 265.

9. Breslow, Lester, and Michael Johnson. "California's Proposition 99 on Tobacco, and its Impact." *Annual Reviw of Public Health* 14 (1993): 585-604.

10. Tobacco Institute, 1993.

11. Advisory Commission on Intergovernmental Relations. *Cigarette Bootlegging. A State and Federal Responsibility.* Washington, DC: ACIR, 1977.

12. Advisory Commission on Intergovernmental Relations. *Cigarette Tax Evasion. A Second Look.* Washington, DC: ACIR, 1985.

13. Lewit.

14. Office of the Surgeon General, U.S. Navy. "Tobacco and the Military." Internal document. 1993.

15. Non-Smokers' Rights Association of Canada. *The Tax Burden on Tobacco? An Analysis of Tobacco Taxation Policy in the United States.* Ottawa, Ontario: Non-Smokers' Rights Association of Canada, 1992.

16. Lewit.

17. Watson, Donald S. *Price Theory and Its Uses.* Boston, MA: Houghton Mifflin Co., 1972.

18. Becker, Gary S., and K. M. Murphy. "A Theory of Rational Addiction." *Journal of Political Economy* 96 (1988): 675-699.

19. Lewit, Eugene M., Douglas Coate, and Michael Grossman. "The Effects of Government Regulation on Teenage Smoking." *Journal of Law and Economics* 24 (1981): 545-569; Lewit and Coate; Grossman, M. "The Demand for Cigarettes." (Editorial.) *Journal of Health Economics* 10 (1991): 101-103; Bishop, John A., and J. H. Yoo. "Health Scare: Excise Taxes and Advertising Ban in the Cigarette Demand and Supply." *Southern Economic Journal* 52 (1985): 402-411; Baltagi, Badi H., and D. Levin. "Estimating Dynamic Demand for Cigarette Using Panel Data: The Effects of Bootlegging, Taxation and Advertising Reconsidered." *Review of Economics and Statistics* 68 (1986): 147-155; Pekurinen, Markuu "The Demand for Tobacco Products in Finland." *British Journal of Addiction* 84 (1989): 1183-1192; Simonich, William L. *Government Antismoking Policies.* New York: Peter Lang, 1991; Wasserman, J., W. G. Manning, J. P. Newhouse, and J. D. Winkler. "The Effects of Excise Taxes and Regulations on Cigarette Smoking." *Journal of Health Economics* 10 (1991): 43-64; Peterson, Dan E., S. Zeger, P. L. Remington, and H. A. Anderson. "The Effects of State Cigarette Tax Increases on Cigarette Sales, 1955 to 1988." *American Journal of Public Health* 82:1 (1992): 94-96; Department of Finance Canada. *Tobacco Taxes and Consumption.* Ottawa, Ontario: Department of Finance Canada, 1993; Emont, Seth L., Won S. Choi, Thomas E. Novotny, and Gary A. Giovino. "Clean Indoor Air Legislation, Taxation, and Smoking Behaviour in the United States: An Ecological Analysis." *Tobacco Control* 2:1 (1993): 13-17; and Keeler, Theodore E., Teh-Wei Hu, Paul G. Barnett, and Willard G. Manning. "Taxation, Regulation, and Addiction: A Demand Function for Cigarettes Based on Time-Series Evidence." *Journal of Health Economics* 12 (1993): 1-18.

20. See for example: Lewit; Centers for Disease Control. *Reducing the Health Consequences of Smoking: 25 Years of Progress. A Report of the Surgeon General.* DHHS Publication No. (CDC) 89-8411, 1989. 533-540; and Centers for Disease Control. *Smoking in the Americas. A 1992 Report of the Surgeon General, in Collaboration With the Pan American Health Organization.* DHHS Publication No. (CDC) 92-8419, 1992.

21. Lewit and Coate.

22. Pekurinen.

23. Harris, J. E. *The 1983 Increase in the Federal Cigarette Tax.* In Summers, L. H. ed. *Tax Policy and the Economy, Vol. I.* Cambridge, MA: MIT Press, 1987.

24. *Ibid.*

25. Pekurinen.

26. Department of Finance Canada.

27. Ferrence, Roberta G., J. M. Garcia, K. Sykora, N. E. Collishaw, and L. Farinan. *Effects of Pricing on Cigarette Use Among Teenagers and Adults in Canada, 1980-1989.* Toronto, Ontario: Addiction Research Foundation, 1991; Kaiserman, Murray J., and Byron Rogers. "Tobacco Consumption Declining Faster in Canada Than in the US." *American Journal of Public Health* 81:7 (July 1991): 902-904; Department of Finance Canada; Sweanor, David T., L. R. Martial, and J. B. Dossetor. *The Canadian Tobacco Tax Experience: A Case Study.* Ottawa, Ontario: The Non-Smokers' Rights Association of Canada and the Smoking and Health Foundation of Canada, 1993; and Sweanor and Warner.

28. Sweanor et al., 1993.

29. *Ibid.*

30. *Ibid.*

31. Kaiserman and Rogers.

32. Burns and Fry, Ltd. *Imasco Limited—Investment Highlights. Burns Fry Limited Investment Research.* Toronto, Ontario: 26 Sept. 1991.

33. Sweanor et al., 1993.

34. Department of Finance Canada.

35. Becker, Gary S., M. Grossman, and K. M. Murphy. Working Paper No. 3322. *An Empirical Analysis of Cigarette Addiction.* Cambridge, MA: National Bureau of Economic Research, 1990; and Chaloupka, Frank "Rational Addictive Behavior and Cigarette Smoking." *Journal of Political Economy* 99:4 (1991): 722-742.

36. Department of Finance Canada.

37. U.S. General Accounting Office. *Teenage Smoking, Higher Excise Tax Should Significantly Reduce the Number of Smokers.* GAO Publication No. GAO/HRD 89-119, 1989; and Non-Smokers' Rights Association of Canada. *Average Retail Selling Price and Total Tax Incidence for a Pack of 20 Cigarettes in Various Countries as of December 1, 1993.* Ottawa, Ontario: Non-Smokers' Rights Association of Canada, 1993.

38. Lewit et al.; Ferrence et al.; Wasserman et al.; Department of Finance Canada; and Grossman, M., D. Coate, E. M. Lewit, and R. A. Shakotko, *Economic and Other Factors in Youth Smoking. Final Report.* Washington, DC: National Science Foundation, 1983. Grant No. SES-8014951.

39. Lewit et al.

40. Lewit and Coate.

41. Grossman et al.

42. Lewit et al.

43. Wasserman et al.

44. Grossman et al.

45. Sweanor et al., 1993.

46. Maxwell, John C. "Maxwell Report: U.S.A: Philip Morris Takes Stronger Lead," *Tobacco Reporter* (April 1992):12-22. Cited in Federal Trade Commission. *Report to Congress for 1991 Pursuant to the Federal Cigarette Labeling and Advertising Act.* 1994. 14-15.

47. Centers for Disease Control. "Comparison of the Cigarette Brand Preference of Adult and Teenage Smokers—United States 1989, and 10 U.S. Communities, 1988 and 1990." *Morbidity and Mortality Weekly Report* 41 (1992): 169-173, 179-181.

48. Ferrence et al., and Department of Finance Canada.

49. Sweanor et al., 1993.

50. *Ibid.*

51. Roswell Park Cancer Institute. Department of Cancer Control and Epidemiology. *Survey of Alcohol, Tobacco and Drug Use Among Ninth Grade Students in Erie County, 1992.* Buffalo, NY: Roswell Park Cancer Institute, 1993.

52. Lewit; National Cancer Institute; Sweanor and Warner; Centers for Disease Control, *Reduc-*

ing the Health Consequences, 1989. 533-540; and Centers for Disease Control and Prevention, *Preventing Tobacco Use.* 269-274

53. Lewit; Department of Finance Canada; National Cancer Institute; Sweanor and Warner; and Centers for Disease Control and Prevention, *Preventing Tobacco Use.* 271-272

54. Coalition on Smoking OR Health. *Saving Lives and Raising Revenue: The Case for Major Increases in State and Federal Tobacco Taxes.* Washington, DC: Coalition on Smoking OR Health, 1993.

55. Sweanor and Warner.

56. *Ibid.*

57. Gallup Organization. *The Public's Attitudes Toward Cigarette Advertising and Cigarette Tax Increases.* Princeton, NJ: The Gallup Organization, Inc., April 1993; and Marttila & Kiley, Inc. Survey *Highlights from an American Cancer Society Survey of U.S. Voter Attitudes Toward Cigarette Smoking.* Boston, MA: Marttila & Kiley, Inc., 9 Sept. 1993.

58. Centers for Disease Control and Prevention. *Preventing Tobacco Use.* 214.

59. Association of State and Territorial Health Officials. *State Tobacco Prevention and Control Activities: Progress Report 1990 to 1992.* Washington, DC: ASTHO. May 1994. 69.

60. Congressional Budget Office. *Federal Taxation of Tobacco, Alcoholic Beverages, and Motor Fuels.* Washington, DC: U.S. Government Printing Office, August 1990. 25-37.

61. Townsend, Joy L. "Cigarette Tax, Economic Welfare and Social Class Patterns of Smoking." *Applied Economics* 19 (1987): 355-365.

62. Wasserman et al.

63. Federal Trade Commission. *Report to Congress for 1991 Pursuant to the Federal Cigarette Labeling and Advertising Act.* 1994. 14-15.

64. Herdman, Roger, Maria Hewitt, and Mary Laschober. Office of Technology Assessment. Smoking-Related Deaths and Financial Costs: Office of Technology Assessment Estimates for 1990. Before the Senate Special Committee on Aging. Preventive Health: An Ounce of Prevention Saves a Pound of Cure. 6 May 1993.

65. Sweanor and Warner.

66. Price Waterhouse. *The Economic Impact of the Tobacco Industry in the U.S. Economy.* Price Waterhouse, 1992.

67. Tobacco Institute. *Economic Losses from Increasing the Federal Excise Tax.* Washington, DC: Tobacco Institute, 1993.

68. Andersen, Arthur and Co., S.C. *Tobacco Industry Employment: A Review of the Price Waterhouse Economic Impact Report and Tobacco Institute Estimates of Economic Losses from Increasing the Federal Excise Tax.* Los Angeles, CA: Arthur Andersen Economic Consulting, 6 Oct. 1993.

69. Chase Econometrics. *The Impact of the Tobacco Industry on the United States Economy in 1983.* Balacynwood, PA: Chase Econometrics, 1985; and Warner, Kenneth E., and G. A. Fulton. "The Economic Implications of Tobacco Product Sales in a Nontobacco State." *Journal of the American Medical Association* 271:10 (1994): 771-776.

70. Andersen.

71. Sweanor et al., 1993; Perkurinen; and Laugesen, Murray. "Tobacco Advertising Restrictions, Price, Income, and Tobacco Consumption in OECD Countries." *British Journal of Addiction* 86 (1991): 1343-1354.

72. Toxic Substances Board. *Health or Tobacco: An End to Tobacco Advertising and Promotion.* Wellington, New Zealand: Department of Health, 1989.

73. Royal College of Physicians. *Smoking and the Young.* London: Royal College of Physicians, 1992.

74. Sweanor, David, S. Ballin, R. D. Corcoran, A. Davis, K. Deasy, R. G. Ferrence, R. Lahey, Lucido S., W. J. Nethery, and J. Wasserman. "Report of the Tobacco Policy Research Study Group on Tobacco Pricing and Taxation in the United States." *Tobacco Control* 1 (Suppl. 1992): S31-S36.

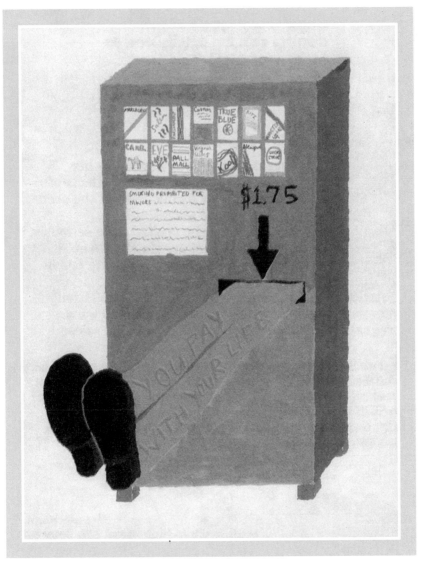

Cullen Duffy, Nightingale-Bamford School, Manhattan

CONTENTS

7 | YOUTH ACCESS TO TOBACCO PRODUCTS

At least 516 million packs of cigarettes per year are consumed by minors and at least half of those are illegally sold to minors.[1] The average age when people first try smoking a cigarette is 14.5 years, and 88% of persons who have ever tried a cigarette have done so by age 18. The average age when people become a *daily* smoker is 17.7 years; of those who have ever smoked daily, 71% have done so by age 18.[2] Few adults initiate tobacco use. Therefore, reducing youth access to tobacco products must be an essential component of any coherent strategy to prevent nicotine addiction in children and youths, and thereby to reduce the number of deaths from smoking-related diseases. In the United States, the law's potential for reducing access and consumption has not been realized. Although selling tobacco to minors is illegal in every state, these laws are widely unenforced. Youths easily acquire tobacco products. Furthermore, the lack of enforcement erodes the efforts of educators, parents, and health professionals to convince youths that they should not use tobacco products: the implied message is that the purpose and intent of the law are not to be taken seriously.

Fortunately, governments at all levels have begun to address the problem of youth access. Last year the Congress passed legislation, the Synar Amendment, that links ongoing program funding to control of youth access to tobacco. In addition, the surgeon general and the secretary of health and human services have focused attention on youth access as it relates to disease prevention and the nation's health objectives for the year 2000. Some states, such as Florida and Vermont, have already taken steps toward meaningful enforcement of their youth access laws.[3] Perhaps most important, in a growing number of localities, local governments, concerned citizens, advocacy groups, and health professionals are working together to implement new approaches to reducing youth access, often achieving significant success and providing the rest of the country with valuable insight and models. As the public's attitudes evolve toward a tobacco-free norm, most American citizens, including many tobacco users, widely favor measures to prohibit youth access to tobacco.[4] Yet, our national policy is lagging behind this emerging consensus regarding the public health importance of, and need for, meaningful restrictions on children's access to tobacco products. The time for effective action is at hand. We now know enough to design workable, effective legislation to curtail youth access without unduly burdening access to adults.

BACKGROUND OF YOUTH ACCESS MEASURES

A Brief History of the Emergence of Youth Access Measures

The curtailment of sales of tobacco products to minors has a long history in the United States. After the turn of the twentieth century, techniques enabling the mass production of cigarettes and the invention of the portable match contributed to a rapid increase in tobacco consumption. Reformers who associated tobacco use with social problems of the emerging large industrial cities were concerned about tobacco's demoralizing effects on young people. Because of these concerns, many states enacted laws limiting youth access to tobacco. These laws varied widely. Most laws prohibited tobacco sales to persons under 18 or 21, but some statutes did not specify an age. Penalties generally ranged from $0 to $100. Many of these early access laws were more concerned with cigarettes than with other forms of tobacco because the relative mildness of cigarettes was thought to present a special temptation to young people; therefore, lower minimum age limits for purchase, or no limitations at all, were set on the sale of cigars, pipes, and snuff.[5] A 1907 judicial decision, which upheld a regulatory distinction between cigarettes and other forms of tobacco, explained: "Before the day of the cigarette, mastery of the tobacco habit was obstructed by agonies of nausea usually sufficient to postpone it to a period of at least reasonable maturity."[6] In 1944, another court noted that Tom Sawyer's experience with the "wallop" from a cigar encouraged boys to take up cigarettes instead.[7] In part, youth access laws arose out of concerns about the health effects of tobacco use; many people associated tobacco use with heart disease and respiratory ailments. Often, these concerns were moralistic, intertwining the health effects of tobacco with arguments regarding the character of tobacco users.[8] In 1937, a federal court found that a local ban on cigarette vending machines was justified to prevent "the evil . . . of the purchase of cigarettes by immature minors."[9]

Although youth access legislation was adopted throughout the country, it was largely unenforced. The general disregard of these laws may have reflected a national ambivalence about tobacco. The federal government actively supported the tobacco industry, for example by providing free tobacco as a basic ration to U.S. soldiers. In 1942 Louisiana repealed its law prohibiting tobacco sales to minors because the law was unclear and unenforced. Wisconsin did the same in 1955 on the grounds that unenforced laws engendered disrespect for authority. Several other states rescinded their youth access laws during the 1960s as part of a general overhaul of juvenile codes.[10]

The approach to tobacco use as a public health issue began during the 1970s, but enforcement of youth access laws was still generally regarded as a low priority. In 1989, the surgeon general's report stated that in marked contrast to the trends in virtually all other areas of smoking control policy, the number of legal restrictions on children's access to tobacco products had actually decreased over the past quarter century. Studies indicated that vendor compliance with minimum-age-of-purchase laws was the exception rather than the rule.[11] Likewise, in 1990, the Office of the Inspector General reported that despite youth access laws in 44 states, no state was effectively enforcing its laws.[12]

National attention turned toward youth access during the late 1980s. Local pockets of successful enforcement of state and local access laws began to develop, resulting from the initiative of local leaders, often in partnership with academic researchers and health advocates. The surgeon general and the secretary of health and human services became interested in the problem, initiating studies and calling for legislative action.

Lack of Enforcement

Despite increased national interest in curtailing underage smoking, minors still have virtually unimpeded access to tobacco products. Although all states prohibit the sale of tobacco to minors, the inspector general of the Department of Health and Human Services found in 1992 that only two states were enforcing their access laws.[13] The secretary of health and human services estimates that three-fourths of the approximately one million tobacco outlets in the United States sell tobacco to minors, garnering over $1 billion in sales each year.[14] The University of Michigan's Monitoring the Future Study in 1993 found that 75% of eighth graders and 89% of tenth graders reported that cigarettes would be fairly easy or very easy to get.[15] Nearly all teen smokers have purchased a pack of cigarettes at least once.

Most minors who smoke purchase their own cigarettes. In a 1990 survey of ninth grade students, conducted as part of the National Cancer Institute's COMMIT trial, 67% of current smokers (those who had smoked at least once in the past month) reported that they usually bought their own cigarettes. Regular smokers (defined as smoking daily within the past month) were nearly twice as likely as occasional smokers to report buying their own cigarettes.[16] In a vending machine industry survey, 72% of teenage smokers reported that they purchased their own cigarettes.[17] In the COMMIT survey, 82% of ninth grade students said that it would be easy for them to obtain cigarettes.[18] The accuracy of this perception has been confirmed in numerous trials designed to measure the prevalence of retail sales of tobacco to minors.[19] The surgeon general recently summarized that in 13 studies of over-the-counter sales, the weighted average of the percentage of minors able to purchase tobacco was 67%, ranging from 32% to 87%. In studies including vending machine sales, the weighted average of successful purchase was 88%, ranging from 82% to 100%.[20] In general, girls are able to purchase cigarettes more easily than boys.[21] The most prevalent sources of cigarettes for underage buyers are small convenience stores and gas stations, followed by larger stores such as supermarkets.[22] Among the youngest group of adolescents, vending machines are a popular source.[23]

RECENT INITIATIVES

Local Initiatives

Since the late 1980s, communities around the country have shown a strong willingness to take action to limit youth access to tobacco, resulting in substantial progress in designing and enforcing local ordinances and in developing strategies to change merchant practices. These localities now have become models for other localities and serve as sources of information about what is effective. To date, various measures to reduce access have been implemented, including partial bans on vending machines, increased enforcement (including sting operations), merchant education, posting of warning signs, increased penalties, and increased sales prices. In 1992, 52 localities were actively enforcing state or local youth access laws.[24] In Minnesota, dozens of communities throughout the state have passed ordinances restricting minors' access to vending machines. Other pockets of enforcement include Minneapolis and White Bear Lake, Minnesota; Leominster and Brookline, Massachussets; King County, Washington; Allentown, Pennsylvania; Layton, Utah; and Marquette County, Michigan.

• One of the first (and now, the best known) community interventions occurred in Woodridge, Illinois. A systematic three-part program of establishing a retailer licensing system, using regular police stings, and imposing penalties for merchant sales violations reduced illegal sales to minors from 70% to less than 5% over a year and a half. A survey of seventh and eighth grade students before and after the intervention found that experimentation and regular tobacco use had decreased significantly, by over 50%.[25] The Woodridge approach was implemented by several neighboring communities, such as Bolingbrook, Illinois, where sales dropped from 90% to 23% after the adoption and active enforcement of a tobacco licensing law. Numerous communities around the country have also used the experience of Woodridge to adopt stronger laws and effective enforcement.[26]

The community of Santa Clara County, California, experimented with a comprehensive community education program to reduce tobacco sales to minors.

In January 1988, minors between 14 and 16 years of age visited over 400 tobacco outlets to ascertain accessibility of tobacco to minors. The minors were able to buy cigarettes at 74% of the retail stores. In July 1988, after an intensive intervention including community education, direct merchant education, contact with chief executive officers of chains and franchises, and grassroots work with community organizations, the underage buying rate decreased to 39%.[27] One year later, sales had rebounded considerably, suggesting that educational interventions alone may be insufficient to effect sustained reductions in youth access rates.[28]

In four suburban communities in Solano County, California, a comprehensive merchant and community education intervention was conducted from September 1988 through December 1988. In December 1988, after illegal tobacco sales to minors had decreased only slightly, a law enforcement intervention was introduced to supplement the ongoing educational campaign. Underage police cadets visited a total of 90 stores and issued citations to 34% of them. The three police departments involved spent about 8 hours each, including paperwork. In May 1990, illegal sales to minors decreased to 24%.[29]

Community action at the local and state levels is also increasing because of the National Cancer Institute's 17-state demonstration program called ASSIST— The American Stop Smoking Intervention Study. ASSIST, the largest and most comprehensive public-health-based smoking control project ever undertaken in the United States, was initiated in 1991 for a 7-year period. ASSIST is a coalition-based intervention that strategically uses the media to promote the adoption of tobacco control policies, and thereby to prevent tobacco use and to encourage cessation. ASSIST has made the issues surrounding youth access to tobacco a priority. Drawing upon ASSIST and other models, the Centers for Disease Control and Prevention recently funded non-ASSIST states to increase their capability for local smoking control efforts.

The Role of DHHS and the Model Law

Youth access to tobacco has aroused the attention of the U.S. Department of Health and Human Services (DHHS), which has taken a strong interest in assessing the problem and in providing information and guidance to state and local governments. In 1989, Dr. Louis Sullivan, then secretary of the DHHS, directed the Office of the Inspector General (OIG) to investigate how effectively states and localities were enforcing their laws prohibiting the sale of cigarettes to minors. In 1990, the OIG interviewed 1,200 health experts, students, parents, and vendors from 18 states and studied communities that were actively enforcing their youth access laws. The resulting report, *Youth Access to Cigarettes,* found that, despite laws in 45 states restricting sale of tobacco products to minors, state and local officials generally were not enforcing those laws.[30] The report suggested that state governments and most communities have not considered enforcement of youth access laws sufficiently important to warrant use of limited resources and funds.

On the basis of information from the OIG investigation, DHHS developed and distributed widely the "Model Sale of Tobacco Products to Minors Control Act: A Model Law Recommended for Adoption by States or Localities to Prevent the Sale of Tobacco Products to Minors."[31] The model law has the following features: (1) a retailer licensing system similar to the alcohol licensing system; (2) a graduated system of penalties, fines, and suspensions; (3) the required posting of warning signs at points of sale; (4) a designated state agency with primary responsibility for enforcement, supplemented by local efforts; (5) reliance on civil penalties to bypass overburdened court systems, but allowing the use of local courts to assess fines, similar to the traffic system; (6) a legal age of purchase set at 19; and (7) a ban on vending machines. The model law did not address penalties on possession by minors, the earmarking of revenues for enforcement, preemption of local ordinances, or the use of minors in compliance checks ("stings"). The model law attempted to minimize burdens on retailers, and emphasized that youth access can be reduced without significantly disrupting governments or the sales of tobacco to adults.

In 1992, the Office of the Secretary of Health and Human Services and the Congressional Subcommittee on Health and the Environment requested that the OIG update its survey of how effectively states and localities were enforcing laws limiting youth access to tobacco. The OIG found that little had changed. While all but three states had banned the sale of tobacco products to youths under 18, most states were not enforcing their laws and were in danger of failing to comply with provisions in the Alcohol, Drug Abuse, and Mental Health Agency Administration (ADAMHA) Reorganization Act requiring the enforcement of youth access laws (see below). Despite the lack of state efforts, the OIG reported, localities were demonstrating that effective enforcement is possible.[32]

The Synar Amendment and Regulations

A provision of the 1992 ADAHMA Reorganization Act (the "Synar Amendment") requires states to adopt laws prohibiting the sale and distribution of tobacco products to minors under age 18, to implement enforcement programs, and to provide annual reports to DHHS demonstrating that they have complied. If states fail to comply, they jeopardize state block grants for substance abuse prevention and treatment programs. States may lose up to 10% of federal funding for alcohol and drug programs in the first year of their failure to comply, 20% in the second year, 30% in the third year, and 40% in fourth and subsequent years.

The Synar Amendment did not provide details on how states are to implement the statutory requirements. Specific guidelines that were originally contained in the Synar Amendment, including a ban on free sampling, were dropped.

DHHS was given the responsibility to draft regulations for implementing the statute. During the months between the passage of the Synar Amendment and the release of the draft regulations, the tobacco industry pressed legislators to pass state tobacco control measures favorable to the industry.[33] These measures, while appearing to enact access restrictions, actually make them more difficult to enforce, typically by including preemption of local ordinances, weak restrictions on vending machines, prohibitions on youth possession, and prohibitions on youth sting operations unless supervised by sheriffs.

Draft regulations were released by DHHS on August 26, 1993. Public comments were solicited and considered in drafting the final rules for implementation of the statute. The following key provisions are included in the draft regulations:

> (1) The state must conduct annual, random, and targeted unannounced inspections of both over-the-counter and vending machine outlets. Random inspections must be "scientifically sound" in estimating the actual sales to minors.
> (2) To protect grant funding, states must demonstrate that underage sales rates (based on random inspections) do not exceed 50% in FY 1994, 40% in FY 1995, 30% in FY 1996, and 20% in FY 1997 and subsequent years.
> (3) The states must implement other "well-designed procedures" for reducing the likelihood or prevalence of violations, such as a tobacco sales licensing system similar to the alcohol licensing system, a graduated schedule of penalties for illegal sales culminating in loss of license, controls on tobacco vending machines, publication of the names of outlets making illegal sales, or use of local enforcement to supplement central enforcement.
> (4) The states may not use block grant program funds for enforcement activities, but may use block grant administrative funds.[34]

Comments to the proposed regulations covered three general areas. First, many focused on the methodology required for estimating sales to minors and therefore for assessing compliance. Some argued for a less demanding standard than "scientifically sound," while others recommended that DHHS prescribe a standard protocol. Second, a related concern was expressed regarding the states' conflict of interest in conducting compliance studies that determine whether they will continue to receive the federal block grant. Finally, attention was addressed to the cost of enforcement and the prohibition against using block grant funds for enforcement activities. Some commentators objected to an unfunded federal mandate. Comments were divided on whether DHHS had overestimated or underestimated the cost of enforcement.

THE BENEFITS OF REDUCING ACCESS

The Synar Amendment and the National Cancer Institute's ASSIST program signal a genuine commitment of the federal government to the goal of reducing access of tobacco products to minors. Important steps have already been taken in many states to revitalize the enforcement of longstanding, though moribund, legal access restrictions. Widespread public support for these efforts suggests that they will continue. It would be a mistake to assume, however, that the measures now being undertaken are uncontroversial or that public policy in this area is now settled. Hard questions remain: To what extent should adult purchasers be inconvenienced in the effort to prevent sales to minors? To what extent should efforts to reshape the market accommodate the vested interests of retailers in existing modes of commerce? These questions lead to a practical point: At what cost? How much should be spent by federal, state, and local governments to enforce youth access restrictions? More than nothing, to be sure, but how much more?

The answers to these difficult questions will turn in part on an assessment of the benefits of reducing access. For example, as a result of reduced access, will fewer children and adolescents experiment with tobacco products and become dependent on them? Even if underage access to tobacco products in commercial channels is significantly reduced, to what extent will underage consumers still be able to obtain tobacco products through other channels, for example, from older consumers or on a "gray" market?

The answers are not definitive at this time, but there are preliminary indications that making it more difficult for minors to purchase tobacco may substantially reduce consumption. In Woodridge, Illinois, 2 years after the passage of successfully enforced youth access legislation, the number of seventh and eighth grade students surveyed who reported having experimented with cigarettes had decreased from a pre-ordinance 46% to 23%. The number of students surveyed who described themselves as smokers had decreased from 16% to 5%.[35] In Leominster, Massachusetts, after active law enforcement of local age restrictions on tobacco sales, the number of students who identified themselves as smokers decreased from 22.8% at pre-test to 15.8% at post-test 2 years later.[36] A long-term follow-up survey has not yet been conducted to determine if these effects have persisted.

Despite this apparent success, caution about the potential effects of limiting access is warranted. Enforcement of youth access laws can be expected to have a significant direct effect on consumption only if, as in Woodridge and Leominster, the commercial accessibility of tobacco to minors is significantly reduced. Furthermore, the reductions in consumption witnessed in Woodridge and Leominster followed enforcement efforts whose intensity may be impossible to achieve in urban settings. The public health experience with restrictions on youth access to alcohol has had mixed results. Progress has been made, especially in reducing traffic fatalities, but alcohol remains widely available to underage youths, both through commercial sources and through parents, siblings, and friends.[37] In the University of Michigan's Monitoring the Future Study, findings for 1993 show that 74% of eighth graders and 89% of tenth graders say that alcohol is fairly easy or very easy to get.[38]

In the long run, the real public health benefit of a reinvigorated youth access policy lies not in its direct effect on consumer choices but rather in its declarative effects—that is, in its capacity to symbolize and reinforce an emerging social norm that disapproves of tobacco use. Legal restrictions often have important educative effects and thereby help to shape attitudes and beliefs.[39] They do this best when they are congruent with an emergent social norm accompanied by a strong social consensus, precisely the conditions that now exist in the context of tobacco control. The level of public support for youth access restrictions is high among youths as well as adults and among smokers as well as nonsmokers. This tobacco-free norm can be fostered through carefully coordinated, multidimensional programs as part of an integrated approach, both legal and nonlegal. Conversely, overt failure to implement the youth access restrictions actually undermines the tobacco-free norm; an unenforced restriction is probably worse than no restriction at all. Unenforced laws convey the message that the intent is not to be taken seriously and thereby undermine school and community attempts to educate youth regarding the serious health consequences of tobacco use. In the context of the emerging norm, contradictory messages should no longer be tolerated. Coupled with advertising images that convey the message that tobacco use is desirable, unenforced restrictions on sales to minors contribute to the web of psychosocial influences that lead children to begin using these products. The message should be strong and unequivocal that tobacco use is unhealthful and socially disapproved. Youth access laws are an essential part of that message.

DESIGNING A YOUTH ACCESS POLICY

Intergovernmental Roles

All three levels of government are now involved in the design and implementation of youth access policy. Without a common agenda and a proper allocation of prerogatives, however, the opportunity for a major advance in public health may be squandered. Thus, before outlining the essential elements of a youth access policy, it is important to outline a framework for intergovernmental cooperation.

In the present context, the federal role should be threefold: (1) to set the agenda and facilitate state and local efforts to effectuate the national public health goals; (2) to serve as a clearinghouse and resource center for information, models, and technical assistance for implementing access restriction programs; and (3) to use its spending power to induce states to adopt and implement state plans for tobacco control, including specific plans for enforcing access restrictions. In many respects, the Synar Amendment and its implementing regulations represent a valuable exercise of federal authority. The amendment signaled the need for public attention to an important public health issue, heightened the awareness and interest of state governments, and set goals and standards derived from recent innovations in Woodridge and other localities.

Unfortunately, however, several aspects of the Synar approach will be continuing sources of frustration to state and local governments and may ultimately undermine its overall effectiveness. First, the proposed regulations do not allow the states to use the substance abuse prevention and treatment monies to enforce youth access restriction. As a result, because the states need continued federal support for their substance abuse   programs, the Synar Amendment becomes equivalent to an unfunded federal mandate—and a costly one if the states take their obligations seriously. Yet the states are given considerable leeway in measuring their own success in reaching the Synar goals (that is, in documenting retailer compliance with youth access restrictions). Thus, a state inclined to cut corners could establish an inadequate system for implementing youth access restrictions without jeopardizing its substance abuse grants. This is a prescription for failure. In the Committee's view, it would be more sensible for Congress to disentangle the Synar mechanism from the substance abuse block grant. Instead, the obligation to enforce youth access restrictions should be tied to eligibility for CDC grants for tobacco control activities, and these grants should include sufficient funds to cover the costs of enforcement during the developmental phase of the new program. In addition, the states should be required to establish a mechanism for *independent assessment* of retailer compliance with youth access restrictions. The Committee recognizes that the opportunity to receive CDC grants might be ignored by states uninterested in tobacco control. However, the Committee believes that the growing grassroots political support for tobacco control will press otherwise reluctant states to apply for these CDC grants and to satisfy the necessary conditions for funding.

The relation between state and local authority is a second source of concern about the potential success of efforts to curtail youth access to tobacco products. The Synar Amendment properly locates ultimate responsibility for enacting and implementing youth access laws at the state level. The proposed regulations also properly allow the states considerable flexibility in allocating responsibility to state and local agencies. Unfortunately, however, enactment of a weak state law could undermine the entire effort if it preempts more aggressive local action. Whereas state governments have not yet proven themselves able to reduce youth access substantially or effectively, given shortages of resources and difficulties of scale, local governments have begun to play an important role. Local communities have implemented innovative programs, many of which have been evaluated by researchers. Local governments may be the best hope for effective enforcement of youth access laws. While state officials may have to be satisfied with moderate reductions in underage sales, local governments need not be. Local communities should be able to address their local health problems by enacting the measures they find necessary and feasible to protect their children. Their willingness to work with researchers and advocates to experiment with new approaches has produced results that should be shared with communities throughout the nation.

Localities should not lose the power to devise solutions with the speed and creativity possible only on the local level. Unfortunately, state legislatures sometimes unwisely preempt local initiatives. With preemption, localities lose their ability to be innovative and to mobilize the community. The communities lose control over their issues, and the tobacco industry gains the advantage at the state level where professional lobbyists enjoy access to state legislatures and where public health groups are not well organized.[40] Washington state is an instructive example. During the late 1980s, in response to national attention on the problem of youth access to tobacco, King County, Washington, passed some of the toughest youth access legislation in the country. The ordinance included a ban on free samples and mail-in coupons, restrictions on vending machines, and the requirement that merchants check identification of all customers. The King County Health Department actively enforced the law by educating retailers, using underage youth in "sting" operations, imposing fines on violators, and enlisting the media to increase public pressure on merchants. The underage buying rate, which had been measured at 79% before the law was enacted, plunged to a countywide rate of 7% in May of 1993. The King County program aroused the attention of other Washington counties and was expected to serve as a model for other local ordinances and to give momentum to state health department enforcement efforts. Those expectations were dashed, however, by a preemptive state law enacted in response to the Synar Amendment requirements. The Washington state legislature enacted legislation significantly weaker than the King County ordinances and, more importantly, prohibited localities from passing stricter laws. Those jurisdictions with tough laws already in place were permitted to keep them, but they lost the right to amend them and to use their own inspectors to enforce them. Instead, localities had to rely on the state liquor control board, thought to be understaffed for the task.[41]

Preemption is not always explicit. Even without specific preempting language, courts sometimes interpret state laws to have been intended by the legislature to be exclusive in the field and therefore to preempt localities from enacting stricter ordinances in that field. Recently, numerous vending machine companies have used this argument in lawsuits that challenge community ordinances on vending machines. In most cases, the courts have upheld the ordinances.[42] However, in some cases, communities have found their public health regulation efforts to control vending machines thwarted by interpretations of state laws with weaker provisions. For example, the Maryland Court of Appeals found that, although state laws did not explicitly address the placement of cigarette vending machines, state licensing and taxation of the vending machines preempted local ordinances restricting the location of vending machines.[43] Therefore, to protect the perogative of local communities to adopt more restrictive measures, state governments must be explicit regarding their intent not to preempt. In sum, the Committee recommends:

1. The federal government should set national goals for reducing youth access to tobacco and should provide resources and leadership to facilitate state and local efforts to effectuate those goals.

2. The federal government should use its spending power to induce states to adopt and implement state plans for tobacco control, including specific plans for enforcing access restrictions. The states' obligation to enforce youth access restrictions should be tied to eligibility for CDC grants for tobacco control activities, and these grants should include sufficient funds to cover the costs of enforcement during the developmental phase of the new program. In addition, the states should be required to establish a mechanism for independent assessment of retailer compliance with youth access restrictions.

3. A federal agency should serve as a clearinghouse and resource center for information, models, and technical assistance for implementing access restriction programs.

4. So that local communities may act as needed regarding local needs for tobacco control, states should adopt a youth access plan that does not preempt local governments from adopting stronger local initiatives.

Essential Components of a Reduced Access Plan

Implement a Retailer Licensing System

About three quarters of the approximately 1 million tobacco outlets in the United States currently sell tobacco products to minors.[44] Those outlets include grocery stores, convenience stores, newsstands, hotels, gas stations, and restaurants. They vary widely in size, in the types of products or services they offer, in their histories and business cultures, and in the types of people they serve and employ. In light of the number and variety of vendors, a tobacco retailer licensing program must be the cornerstone of any successful enforcement effort.

The licensing approach has been endorsed by the DHHS in its model law and by nearly every study that has examined youth access interventions. The aim of a tobacco retailer licensing program is to monitor compliance with restrictions on youth access without disrupting legitimate tobacco sales. Retailer licensing programs require a merchant to obtain a license to sell tobacco products, which may be suspended or revoked if the merchant sells tobacco to minors or violates other state and local laws designed to reduce youth access. Experience with licensing systems on the local level has demonstrated the effectiveness of this approach.[45] In the city of Woodridge, Illinois, the achievement of nearly complete compliance with youth access laws was attributed in part to an efficient licensing system, which took advantage of preexisting enforcement mechanisms.[46] Several surrounding communities followed Woodridge's example and adopted tobacco license laws as well. In one, Bolingbrook, sales to minors dropped from 90% to 23%.[47] As mentioned above, in King County, Washington, enactment of the licensing ordinance reduced sales to minors from 79% to 7% over a 4-year period.

Tobacco sales to minors are lucrative. Researchers have estimated that in 1991 children and youths in the United States used at least 516 million packs of cigarettes and 26 million containers of chewing tobacco, totaling sales of approximately one billion dollars.[48] Understandably, many merchants choose not to forego sales to minors. Merchants know that when restrictions on youth access are not enforced, if they refuse to sell cigarettes to a minor, the neighboring store or vending machine will do so.[49] Moreover, the fines of $100 to $500 imposed under most existing youth access laws do not approach the profit to be gained from selling to children and therefore may be considered a "cost of doing business." In contrast, licensing systems create a stronger economic disincentive for retailers to violate youth access laws by forcing them to weigh the profits from sales to minors against the threat of forfeiting the right to sell tobacco to adults. A licensing system not only gives merchants a stake in access enforcement, but also an incentive to monitor themselves.[50] Merchants are in the best position to implement company policies and train employees to prevent sales to minors. The licensing system also provides a mechanism that enables health departments or other law enforcement officials to support retailers' own efforts to comply with the law by setting standards, providing educational materials and assisting employee training programs. Authorities may also choose to promote merchant education and employee training through incentives such as lower licensing fees or penalties.

Ideally, responsibility for operating the licensing system should be assigned to a public health agency. As a practical matter, however, it may be sensible to build on an existing administrative foundation; and, in some states, this may mean that responsibility lies with the agency that licenses alcohol outlets. The only essential requirement is that the licensing authority and the control over licensing fees be joined in single agency, thereby assuring that these monies are available to support enforcement activities. Moreover, licensing fees should be set at a level high enough to cover the costs of enforcement. Retailers are likely to object to a significant fee. However, in exchange for the profitable opportunity to sell tobacco products, retailers should contribute to the cost of ensuring that those dangerous products are not purveyed to children.

In sum, the Committee recommends:

5. States should establish a licensing system requiring merchants to obtain a license to sell tobacco products, which may be suspended or revoked if the merchant sells tobacco to minors or violates other state and local laws designed to reduce youth access.

6. Licensing fees should be earmarked for the enforcement of youth access legislation and should be set high enough to cover those costs. If

possible, responsibility for operating the licensing system should be assigned to a public health agency. However, each state should assess existing regulatory structures to determine which agency is best able to administer effectively the licensing program. The agency selected should retain the authority both to administer the licensing program and to receive licensing fees.

Ban Tobacco Vending Machines

Minors rely on vending machines as a major source of tobacco products. In a mall-intercept survey commissioned by the vending machine industry, 24% of 13- to 17-year-olds who smoke reported that they purchased cigarettes from vending machines "often" or "occasionally."[51] Another study found that 38% of youths who smoke reported that they use vending machines "often" or "sometimes."[52] Younger children are most likely to rely on vending machines as a source of cigarettes. In the study commissioned by the vending machine industry, 11 times more 13-year-olds (22%) reported using a vending machine "often" than did 17-year-olds (2%). Another 14% of 13-year-olds and 12% of 17-year-olds use vending machines "occasionally."[53] A 1994 survey of secondary school students in Fond du Lac, Wisconsin, found that to 23% of eighth grade tobacco users "most often" obtain their tobacco from vending machines compared with 13% of tenth graders and 4% of twelfth graders.[54] For younger or less confident children, vending machines may provide a less intimidating avenue for purchasing tobacco than over-the-counter sales.

Statewide restrictions on tobacco vending machines are essential to buttress the enforcement of existing laws against over-the-counter sales. Indeed, plentiful and accessible vending machines may persuade retailers that it is pointless for them to refuse to sell tobacco to minors.[55] Unlike for over-the-counter sales, merchant education programs[56] and increased penalties do not appear to reduce vending machine sales to minors.[57]

Restrictions on vending machines are widely supported. According to a survey conducted by the American Cancer Society, a ban on cigarette vending machines is the most popular type of smoking restriction among American voters: 73% of voters, including 66% of all smokers, reported that they would favor banning cigarette vending machines because of concern with children's easy access to the machines.[58] Indeed, the recent OIG report on youth access laws points out that restrictions on vending machines are the most common youth access measures, adopted by 21 states and Washington, D.C.[59] As of July 1993, about 170 communities across the country have adopted ordinances eliminating or severely restricting cigarette vending machines. These ordinances are a step toward meeting the national Healthy People 2000 goals, which call for the elimination of vending machines to reduce the availability of tobacco products to children.

The only debatable issue relating to vending machine tobacco sales is whether any alternative less restrictive than a total ban on such sales is defensible. Two alternatives have been suggested: (1) requiring use of locking devices and (2) permitting use of vending machines in "adult-only" locations. Either of these approaches would be an acceptable alternative to a total ban *if* they could be successfully implemented. Although data are sparse, recent experience suggests that minors' use of the machines under either of these approaches could erode the effectiveness of the overall access strategy. This same concern led the drafters of the DHHS model law and the regulations implementing the Synar Amendment to recommend a total ban.

Locking Device Alternatives. Locking devices, which prevent purchase unless deactivated by an employee, do not effectively prevent youth access to vending machines.[60] Proponents of the use of locking devices argue that they render vending machine sales functionally equivalent to over-the-counter sales by requiring the assistance of a clerk. However, experience with locking devices has demonstrated that, although fewer cigarettes are sold to youths than where vending machines are completely unrestricted, businesses that installed locking devices on vending machines were still more likely to sell cigarettes to minors than businesses that used over-the-counter sales.[61]

Locking devices entail a greater enforcement burden than complete bans. Authorities must verify that the devices have been installed and are operating properly by inspecting all tobacco vending machine locations. Even when locking devices are installed and are working as intended, they are only as effective as the employees who operate them. Clerks must ask for identification and must refuse to deactivate the locking device when a minor attempts to make a purchase. A study in St. Paul, Minnesota, found that 1 year after a locking device ordinance was passed, the devices had still not been installed on 30% of the machines. Where locking devices were installed, they initially reduced the underage buying rate from 86% to about 30% 3 months after the law was enacted; however, compliance deteriorated to 48% after 1 year. Employees could not be relied on to refuse to sell cigarettes to minors. Employees allowed purchase 19% of the time at 3 months and 39% of the time at 1 year after the locking device ordinance was enacted. Locking devices are expensive to install and inconvenient for merchants; 25% of merchants in the St. Paul study decided to switch to over-the-counter sales or eliminate tobacco sales altogether rather than install the locking devices.[62]

Locational Restriction Alternatives. Nine states, the District of Columbia, and at least 95 U.S. cities have adopted locational restrictions in lieu of a total ban on vending machine sales of tobacco, allowing vending machines in locations from which minors are normally excluded, such as taverns and bars.[63] A partial ban has also been recently adopted in Canada. Partial bans mitigate the economic impact on the vending machine industry.

The issue is whether convenience to adult smokers can be achieved while access to minors is effectively limited. Youths do not now report "adult" locations as major sources of tobacco, but there is evidence that minors can often easily enter "adult" locations, and once inside, can easily buy tobacco products. In a University of Minnesota study, minors successfully purchased cigarettes from vending machines, even in "adult" establishments, 79% of the time.[64] A Fond du Lac, Wisconsin, study designed to measure the degree of retailer compliance with youth access laws found that underage buyers successfully purchased tobacco from vending machines in taverns 52% of the time, suggesting that bars could provide a source of tobacco to those young people bold enough to enter them.[65] In an Australian study, children were able to enter places traditionally restricted to adults, such as hotel bars, and were able to purchase tobacco without restriction on every occasion.[66] In a Springfield, Massachusetts, compliance check conducted by STAT (Stop Teenage Addiction to Tobacco), youths were able to buy cigarettes in all 13 (100%) of the bars they entered.[67]

If partial vending machine bans are to be effective, the statutes must define "adult" locations carefully and narrowly. For example, the bar area of a restaurant is not sufficiently inaccessible to minors to significantly deter their purchases. In a study commissioned by the vending machine industry, 47% of youths using tobacco vending machines reported that the machine was located in a restaurant or other eating establishment.[68] Many bars only restrict access to alcohol; they do not restrict entrance by age. Accordingly, if vending machines are permitted at all, they should be permitted only in locations to which minors may not be admitted. A partial ban should also require that merchants place cigarette vending machines no less than 25 feet from any entrance, to preclude the installation of vending machines in empty entrances where minors might enter unnoticed.

Enforcing a partial ban requires that the machines be licensed; that periodic compliance checks be conducted, as with over-the-counter sales; and that authorities verify that merchants have placed the machines at least 25 feet from any entrance.

The Committee recommends:

7. States should ban tobacco vending machines; less restrictive alternatives to a complete ban should be adopted only if shown to be effective.

Restrict Methods of Sale

Ban Self-Service Displays. Self-service displays allow underage customers to help themselves to tobacco products and present them to a clerk for purchase along with other items. Furthermore, self-service displays invite shoplifting, a method of obtaining tobacco products that may be expected to become more prevalent as sales to minors decrease. In a survey of 1,692 Georgia students in grades 7-12, about 5% reported shoplifting cigarettes within the preceding 12 months.[69] In a 1992 survey of 7,891 ninth grade students in Erie County, New York, 44% of daily smokers reported having shoplifted cigarettes.[70] A 1994 survey of secondary school students in Fond du Lac, Wisconsin, found that almost half of eighth and tenth grade tobacco users had shoplifted tobacco within the past year, and that 12% of them "most often" obtained their tobacco in this manner.[71]

A youth access plan should include a statewide ban on self-service displays to prevent purchasing and shoplifting of tobacco products by youths. If a youth must ask for tobacco products from a clerk, this direct interaction between clerk and customer increases the chance that a clerk will notice that the customer is underage and will refuse to conduct the sale. Younger or less confident children may be less likely to attempt a purchase in the first place if they must request the brand and type of product from the employee, rather than simply place a pack of cigarettes on the counter at checkout along with a soft drink and a pack of gum.

In addition, eliminating self-service displays may have two secondary effects. Placing the products out of reach reinforces the message that tobacco products are not in the same class as candy or potato chips. Placing the products behind the counter may also eliminate the accompanying tobacco advertising and promotional displays because of the limited space behind checkout counters or in locked cases. Point-of-sale advertising displays are often appealing to youths and tend to promote experimentation and impulse buying. Eliminating self-service displays may complement other advertising restrictions by reducing children's exposure to enticements to use tobacco.

Authorities can easily monitor bans on self-service displays during general compliance checks under the tobacco licensing system.

The Committee recommends:

8. States should prohibit the sale of tobacco products by self-service displays. During compliance checks, authorities should verify that tobacco is being sold only from behind the counter or from locked cases.

Ban Single Cigarette Sales. Despite the federal prohibition on selling tobacco products without the required warning label,[72] merchants sometimes remove cigarettes from the packages and sell them individually. The practice began during the early 1930s, when cigarette merchants offered single cigarettes, or "loosies," to Depression-Era customers who lacked enough money for an entire pack. When prosperity returned after World War II, many retailers continued to sell single cigarettes. In a recent study of convenience stores in a Southern California community, conducted after a statewide ban, 49% of stores were found to sell single cigarettes. The cigarettes were often kept behind the counter rather than displayed, and retailers were significantly more likely to sell the singles to minors than to adults. Retailers in neighborhoods of single ethnic groups were found to be more likely to sell cigarettes than in predominantly white or integrated neighborhoods.[73] The extent of this practice currently is unknown, but it can be expected to increase as the price of cigarettes continues to rise. At 15 to 20 cents each, single cigarettes remain attractive to children, the most price-sensitive group of tobacco buyers. For children who are considering experimenting with tobacco, buying single cigarettes may represent a less intimidating first step. Single cigarettes displayed in cups or trays may be easy to shoplift. The law should prohibit the sale of cigarettes that are not in a sealed package that conforms to the federal labeling requirements. Authorities who conduct compliance checks on the sale of tobacco products to minors under the tobacco retailer licensing system should verify that retailers are not offering single cigarettes for sale. Violations should be treated in the same manner as other sales of cigarettes to minors.

The Committee recommends:

9. Sale of single cigarettes, which violates federal tobacco labeling law, should also be banned by state youth access laws. During compliance checks, authorities should verify that retailers do not offer single cigarettes for sale, whether openly displayed or kept behind the counter.

Ban Free Distribution

Tobacco companies have increasingly shifted spending from traditional advertising to promotional activities. Among their most effective promotional tools is the distribution of free or heavily discounted tobacco products. The Federal Trade Commission reports that tobacco industry spending on coupons and retail value-added offers reached over $1 billion in 1990 and almost doubled to $1.9 billion in 1991; spending on distribution of free cigarette samples was up by 63% in 1990 but decreased in 1991 by 45%.[74]

Samples encourage experimentation by providing minors with a risk-free and cost-free way to satisfy their curiosity. Tobacco companies often distribute samples in places frequented by adolescents and children, such as rock concerts, shopping malls, sporting events, zoos, and fairs.[75] Sampling in these locations increases the likelihood that minors will obtain the tobacco products. In a survey of underage youths in Chicago, about half of the elementary and high school students and 28% of college students said they had witnessed the distribution of free tobacco products to minors; 14% of elementary and high school students reported that they had personally received free samples.[76]

Although most states prohibit the distribution of free samples to minors, monitoring the enforcement of these statutes presents practical difficulties for law enforcement officials, who may feel that their limited resources are better spent enforcing other laws. Nor is the tobacco industry's voluntary code effective. The code prohibits distribution to those under 21 years of age in sampling promotions, but distribution to minors appears to be nearly inevitable. Companies that conduct tobacco sampling contract with tobacco companies and agree to abide by the voluntary code. The sampling employees ("samplers") are instructed to ask for identification when they suspect that a potential recipient is under age; in addition, the samplers ask recipients a series of marketing information questions, such as whether they are smokers, what brand they now smoke, and what type of sample they prefer. Thus, samplers tend to be under pressure in crowded public places: "There is a significant time constraint in asking for proof of age from all young-looking individuals who solicit samples, not to mention the time required for the myriad of other questions which samplers are instructed to ask. Samplers are often surrounded on all sides by those soliciting samples and a dozen or more outstretched arms waiting (or grabbing) for samples."[77] Furthermore, samplers are often young people who may lack the skills to demand identification and refuse samples to their peers.[78] Samplers may also believe that it is futile to refuse samples to minors because under crowded and unstructured circumstances minors can easily recruit an adult to obtain the sample on their behalf.

The key to a successful youth access policy is a practical system of careful oversight and control of all outlets distributing tobacco products. The distribution of free tobacco samples in places accessible to the general public cannot be successfully monitored and should be banned entirely. Distribution of free samples through the mail should also be banned.

Public support is strong for bans on sampling and similar promotions. As of April 1993, about 74 communities and 3 states had adopted ordinances banning the distribution of tobacco samples. The Davis and Jason study found that 70% of college students who are smokers favored such an ordinance, even though they would lose an opportunity for occasional free cigarettes.[79] An American Cancer Society survey found that 58% of voters favor prohibiting tobacco companies from distributing free samples of their products.[80] Smokers may favor such a ban because of concern that samples encourage smoking by minors, increase the difficulty for smokers to quit, or undermine the resolve of former smokers.[81]

The Committee recommends:

10. Distribution of free tobacco products in public places or through the mail should be prohibited.

Foster Community Action to Monitor and Encourage Compliance

Develop Merchant Education Programs. The purpose of merchant education programs is to cultivate voluntary cooperation from retailers regarding enforcement of sales bans to minors. While educational interventions are a necessary first step, they tend not to be effective unless accompanied by the potential for legal enforcement.[82] Merchant education programs do increase business owners' and clerks' knowledge of the law, if not their compliance. A 1987 study in Massachusetts found that one-third of individuals selling cigarettes did not know the law, but that even among those informed of the law, compliance was poor. The study concluded that educating vendors is crucial to obtaining their cooperation, and that compliance was greatest in establishments where the law was posted.[83]

The most successful merchant education programs have involved multiple components, including repeated merchant contacts, mail or on-site visits, undercover buying operations, economic incentives and disincentives, community outreach, and media advocacy.[84] The Keay study demonstrated that an intensive educational campaign, in conjunction with a broadly based media campaign and community involvement, can reduce illegal cigarette sales in a variety of store types and in diverse communities, producing an overall sales rate decrease of about 54%.[85] An intensive, multifaceted approach may be the key to a successful merchant education program. This approach may not be feasible on a large, statewide scale, but may be a rewarding strategy for smaller communities. Also, cultural and ethnic population characteristics must be considered. For example, merchant education campaigns have been more effective in suburban communities than in urban communities,[86] and among Hispanics and whites than among African Americans.[87]

To be successful, a youth access program should attempt to improve not only retailers' awareness of the law, but also their understanding of the need to reduce youth access and the importance of their role in a coordinated effort to do so. A survey of executives of the U.S. companies that have the highest overall retail sales and that sell tobacco found that the executives tended to underestimate the extent of youth access.[88] Merchant education programs can make the requirements more palatable to retailers by facilitating their recognition that, as businesses dependent on the good will of the community, it is to their commercial advantage to support community goals to prevent nicotine addiction in children and youths. One community published a paid advertisement in the newspaper thanking retailers who did not sell to minors, a gesture that was well received by merchants.[89] A negative approach, in which violators are publicized in the media, might also provide further incentives for retailers to comply with the law.[90] If merchants do not voluntarily cooperate with the law, the community would likely support more active enforcement by law enforcement officials.[91]

Retailer education programs can be integrated with legal enforcement systems. The commitment of local officials and consistent media involvement were factors in the successful enforcement in Woodridge. Law enforcement compliance checks were accompanied by strong educational messages from police to merchants and community members. Police and city officials were able to promote positive police-merchant interaction and merchant-community ties.[92] Health officers may be another particularly effective avenue for providing retailer education because field staff already visit many retailers and have working relationships. Health officials are also viewed as authoritative by retailers because they can levy fines.[93] In conclusion, a comprehensive youth access plan should include a merchant education component that comprises information dissemination about the youth access laws, community pressure for compliance, and a legal enforcement capability. An ongoing educational program could be supported through vendor licensing fees.

The Committee recommends:

11. Education programs to increase merchants' awareness of and support for youth access laws should be fostered as a valuable complement to legal enforcement measures.

Promote Community Involvement. The greatest obstacle to enforcing access laws is public indifference. Sustained community action, including education campaigns, can counteract the public's failure to recognize the importance of curtailing sales of tobacco to minors. Community involvement can galvanize the interest and concern of community leaders.

A youth access plan should foster a community norm that disapproves of youth access to tobacco products. Such a norm can be communicated through mechanisms for community participation in enforcement. For example, a toll-free number could be posted on point-of-sale warning signs, inviting individuals to phone if they witness an apparent violation. Such reports ideally would trigger a series of targeted compliance checks by authorities. If the complaint is filed by a guardian or parent, the enforcement agency might be required to investigate the retailer's practices. Such measures would foster the idea that selling tobacco to minors is not a trivial infraction, and would demonstrate that preventing sales to minors could enhance the retailer's standing in the community.

Community approval may operate as an effective incentive for retailers to forego profits from illegal sales to minors and, conversely, loss of business from community members who disapprove of sales to minors may supplement legal penalties. However, in order to activate social pressure as a tool to induce merchant compliance, the local community must be educated and mobilized. In four Oregon cities, researchers galvanized public support by communicating extensively with local leaders, organizations, and businesses and by launching a community-wide publicity and education effort. Retail clerks who refused to sell to minors received material rewards and public recognition; clerks who were willing to sell received reminders about the law. Merchants were visited and provided information packets at the outset of the intervention and received feedback about their business's compliance. The interventions were accompanied by significant reductions in the proportion of retailers willing to sell tobacco to minors and increases in the proportion of stores that asked for identification.[94]

Community education campaigns aimed at retailers may have a number of positive spinoff effects. They may reduce the likelihood that parents, siblings, or other adults will give tobacco to minors or buy it for them. They may result in increased media pressure on police to enforce tobacco access laws.[95] They may also encourage community organizations to make tobacco access a focus of their activities. A survey of organizations conducting community-based anti-drug and anti-alcohol activities in the United States found that only 26% of responding organizations conduct extensive programs to prevent tobacco use.[96]

The Committee recommends:

12. The Centers for Disease Control and Prevention, through the Office on Smoking or Health, should provide technical assistance and resources to support states and localities wishing to implement youth access community education programs.

Actively Enforce Youth Access Legislation

The ultimate success of a youth access strategy lies in providing credible and effective mechanisms for enforcing the law. Community education and merchant education are important, but insufficient to reduce tobacco sales to minors. Active enforcement has been shown to be the most effective means to achieve long-term compliance with youth access restrictions.[97] For example, in the King County, Washington, study mentioned above two years after an ordinance was enacted requiring compliance checks of retailers the rate of successful purchase by underage buyers dropped to 7%. In contrast, Seattle (located within King County), which was exempt from inspections, had a sales success rate of 34%.[98]

As noted above, an enforcement plan should implement a graduated penalty system proportionate to the extent of the violation, beginning with fines for minor violations, and followed by stronger penalties (license suspension, then revocation) for serious and repeated infractions. Retailers should be held strictly liable—and subject to appropriate penalties—for any sale to an underaged purchaser unless the salesperson has taken reasonable steps, such as checking a driver's license, to verify that the purchaser is at least 18. This approach places the incentive on the retailer to seek evidence of majority in all cases involving young purchasers and is therefore preferable to the DHHS model law, and the laws of many states, which only penalize the retailer who "knowingly" sells tobacco to a minor. (Such a high standard of culpability would be appropriate only if the offense were punishable by criminal penalties. As will be explained below, however, criminal sanctions for selling tobacco to minors would be counterproductive and should be avoided.) Penalties should be imposed against the owners of businesses. If clerks are penalized and the fines are not reimbursed by the owners, there is no penalty to the store, and therefore no significant incentive to comply with the law. Owners who have the economic incentive to avoid violations are more likely to establish company-wide policies and to incorporate tobacco law instruction into new employee training. Businesses can teach clerks how to handle pressure from underage persons who want to purchase tobacco. Clerks should not be in the position of having to understand and follow the law without the support of company policies.

Compliance inspections, in the form of police observation, are not adequate to obtain accurate assessments of the law's overall effects. As the primary device for monitoring sales to minors and other violations of youth access legislation, the enforcement plan should utilize teens to conduct purchase attempts. Compliance checks should be conducted by teens at least 16 years old because 16- to 17-year-olds have the highest rates of tobacco use and tobacco purchases; use of younger minors may yield compliance rates that are artificially high. The minors should be representative of the ethnic makeup of the communities where the purchases are attempted. The minors should make no attempt to disguise their age, nor should they lie about their age if asked. An adult observer should be present.

A clearly designated enforcement agency is essential to an enforcement plan. Preferably, a single agency would administer the licensing system, collect licensing fees, monitor compliance, and administer civil penalties for violations. As a practical matter, however, it may be more efficient to allocate these responsibilities to existing agencies that already carry out similar duties. Many states currently use police officers, but studies have shown that law enforcement officials often view enforcement of youth access bans as a low priority. Other states, such as Florida, use the resources of the Division of Alcoholic Beverages and Tobacco. Ideally, unless a particular state's regulatory structure makes this infeasible, licensing and enforcement responsibility should be exercised by a public health agency. Public health agencies are likely to be more concerned and responsive.[99] Designating a health agency to enforce youth access bans also reinforces the message that youth access is a public health issue. Many retailers have established relationships with health officials in the field, enabling health officials to implement a merchant education program.

Historically, the most successful enforcement has occurred on the local level. However, by holding the states responsible for reducing tobacco sales to minors, the Synar Amendment prods the states to establish a centrally administered enforcement mechanism with a clearly designated enforcement agency at the state level. Central direction should not preclude the establishment of local ordinances and enforcement mechanisms or otherwise discourage local efforts. Indeed, the proposed regulations for the implementation of the Synar Amendment recommend the use of local enforcement to supplement centrally administered state enforcement.[100] Four states have specifically encouraged and provided resources for local enforcement. California, New Jersey, North Dakota, and Utah currently make funds available to localities to improve enforcement and otherwise take action to reduce sales to minors.[101] Also, local health and research institutions should be allowed to participate in the planning, conduct, and evaluation of compliance checks. They have played a vital role in bringing the low level of compliance to public attention and should be encouraged to remain in the field. Moreover, because states have a vested interest in documenting reduced sales to minors, independent inspections can provide an important verification of levels of compliance.

The Committee recommends:

13. Youth access laws should be effectively enforced. An enforcement plan should implement a graduated penalty system proportionate to the extent of the violation, beginning with fines for minor infractions and followed by stronger penalties (suspension, then revocation) for serious and repeated violations.

Retailers should be held strictly liable—and subject to appropriate penalties—for any sale to a minor unless the salesperson has taken reasonable steps, including checking a driver's license, to verify that the purchaser is at least 18. Penalties should be imposed against business owners, not against store clerks.

As the primary device for monitoring violations of youth access legislation, 16- and 17-year-olds should be utilized to conduct purchase attempts. The underage purchasers should be representative of the ethnic makeup of the community, should make no attempt to disguise their age, and should truthfully disclose their age if asked. An adult observer should be present.

A state agency should be clearly designated to enforce the youth access plan. Unless a state's regulatory structure makes it infeasible, the state public health agency should be given responsibility to administer the licensing system, collect fees, monitor compliance, and administer civil penalties for violations. State enforcement plans should maximize local participation.

Additional Considerations to Guide Youth Access Legislation

Many of the recommendations set forth above aim to increase the likelihood that those charged with enforcing the law will want to enforce it. A rational assumption is that sanctions that are too costly or that are perceived to be unfair or disproportionate to the seriousness of the offense will not be enforced or, if enforced, will be applied erratically and discriminatorily. From this viewpoint, three additional points should be kept in mind.

Youth access plans should not impose any legal penalties on youths who are able to obtain tobacco.

Imposing penalties on minors for buying, possessing, or using tobacco products is controversial. At least 21 states currently prohibit smoking and the use of tobacco products by minors. Proponents of these penalties argue that they may have some deterrent value, and that the failure to make possession illegal sends a mixed message, reinforcing the idea that tobacco use is a trivial infraction.[102] However, the Committee believes that penalizing minors is an unwise and ineffective strategy. Criminal sanctions or delinquency adjudications are grossly disproportionate to the seriousness of the offense and would not be sought by prosecutors or imposed by judges. Even if the offense were punishable with a civil fine, like a traffic ticket, the penalty would rarely be enforced. Because lack of enforcement would erode whatever deterrent effect the law might otherwise achieve, the only remaining rationale for such a prohibition is a symbolic one: the failure to make tobacco use an offense would somehow imply that tobacco use is not harmful or that it is socially acceptable. In the Committee's view, such speculative fears are groundless—social disapprobation is (or should be) strongly communicated by the laws on distribution, by warning labels, and by all of the other policies outlined in this report. Young people will not miss the point simply because their disapproved conduct is not against the law. Furthermore, purely symbolic prohibitions—laws that are not meant to be enforced—are harmful because they undermine respect for the law. Finally, imposing legal penalties on the underage purchaser also impedes the use of underage buyers to monitor retailer compliance with youth access restrictions. The need to obtain waivers unnecessarily increases the cost of enforcement.

The Committee recommends:

14. Legal penalties should not be imposed on youths who are able to obtain tobacco products; existing legal penalties on minors should be repealed.

Youth access plans should not impose criminal penalties on licensees who sell tobacco to minors.

Studies have shown that imposing criminal penalties on licensees who sell tobacco products to minors is not the best approach. First, enforcement is likely to be less effective. The criminal justice system is already overburdened and violations are unlikely to be treated as a priority. The public has been less supportive of criminal penalties, seeing them as being too harsh and diverting much-needed police attention.[103] Judges also tend to be unwilling to impose criminal penalties.[104] Administrative processing of civil penalties is less time-consuming and less costly. Efficient and credible enforcement of civil penalties and license revocation is a much more powerful deterrent than sporadically imposed criminal sanctions.

The Committee recommends:

15. Criminal penalties should not be imposed on licensees who sell tobacco to minors. Rather, appropriate civil penalties, including fines and tobacco license suspension or revocation, should be prescribed and enforced.

Youth access plans should not set excessively high age limits.

The presumptive age of adulthood in our society is 18. Exceptions have been made when compelling reasons arise. Teenagers younger than 18 are entitled to make their own medical decisions, reflecting constitutional respect for adolescent autonomy; but the minimum age for purchasing alcohol has been set at age 21, reflecting the government's compelling interest in reducing alcohol-related injuries and deaths on the nation's highways. In the present context, the Committee thinks that the presumptive age of adulthood should govern. From a public health standpoint, the primary focus of prevention is to reduce initiation by younger adolescents. The main argument for an age higher than 18 is to minimize spillover access to 16- to 17-year-olds; however, the Committee does not think that this argument is strong enough to overcome the presumptive case for an 18-year-old minimum age of purchase. Moreover, an unduly high age limit will be selectively ignored by retailers, thereby undermining respect for, and compliance with, the youth access ban. Although the model law recommends a minimum purchase age of 19, most states have wisely set the minimum age at 18, and the Synar Amendment also draws the line at 18.[105]

The Committee recommends:

16. Youth access plans should not set excessively high age limits; states should set the minimum age of purchase at age 18.

SUGGESTIONS FOR ADDITIONAL POLICY INITIATIVES AND RESEARCH

Further Initiatives

Limiting the number of licensed outlets for tobacco purchases would facilitate more efficient monitoring of retailer compliance with restrictions on purchases by minors and on other restrictions on tobacco sales and promotion. Regulatory experience with alcoholic beverages also suggests that the overall level of consumption is affected by the number and density of outlets.[106] However, because a substantial reduction in the number of outlets will inevitably curtail access of adults to tobacco products, such a strategy is not likely to be given serious consideration unless and until this country is ready to take the next major step on the road to a nation free of tobacco-related disease and death. Eventually, tobacco products should be available only through liquor stores or some equivalently restricted channel of distribution. In the meantime, however, two steps in the direction of outlet control would have special symbolic importance: banning tobacco sales within a prescribed distance of schools and banning sales in pharmacies would help to reinforce the changing normative climate toward tobacco use by young people.

Tobacco-Free Zones Near Schools

Convenient availability of tobacco products to children and youths has sent them mixed messages and has undermined health promotion efforts by schools and other youth leaders. A sound access policy should fortify the work of educators by eliminating the sale and promotion of tobacco within a reasonable distance of schools, one of the most important environments in a youth's life. Although the nature of such a ban is largely symbolic, removing tobacco sales from the immediate vicinity of schools might make it more difficult for students to obtain tobacco products during school breaks.

Bans on Pharmacy Sales

Eliminating the sale of tobacco products in pharmacies would send a strong message to youths that tobacco products are incompatible with health. This approach has begun to gain support. A coalition consisting of the Michigan Pharmacists' Association, the Michigan Academy of Family Physicians, Lederle Laboratories, and the Michigan Department of Public Health recently launched the "Tobacco-Free Pharmacy" campaign, which discourages pharmacists from selling tobacco and enlists their help in providing support and cessation counseling to their customers. As of October 1993, more than 60 pharmacies were participating in the program.[107] In Canada, health advocates have also had some success in convincing a number of pharmacies to stop selling tobacco and have lobbied colleges of pharmacy to preclude the sale of tobacco products in their ethical codes. The province of Ontario is considering legislation that would prohibit tobacco sales in pharmacies.

The Committee recommends:

17. States and localities should adopt long-term strategies for reducing the number of outlets licensed to sell tobacco products. Initial steps should include creation of tobacco-free zones around schools and bans of tobacco sales in pharmacies.

Restrict Mail-Order Distribution

Like the in-person distribution of tobacco samples, youth access through the distribution of tobacco products by mail cannot be meaningfully monitored. Signed statements that a purchaser meets the minimum age of purchase are not verifiable. The extent of mail-order purchase of tobacco products by minors is not known; however, it may be expected to become more prevalent as retail outlet sales to minors decrease. Recently, a survey of 12- to 17-year-olds found that 7.6% of the respondents were on tobacco company mailing lists.[108] The mailing lists, which furnish their recipients with coupons, samples, and promotional items, suggest that mail-order sales are a potential conduit between tobacco companies and youths. In a survey of ninth graders in Erie County, New York, 24% of the daily smokers reported having received free packs of cigarettes in the mail.[109]

Distribution of tobacco products through the mail raises complex regulatory questions. Although this type of distribution can undermine youth access restrictions, it provides a convenient method of promoting and distributing tobacco products (especially cigars and pipe tobacco) to adults. Moreover, mail-order distribution of alcohol and pornography illustrates that there is no regulatory precedent for sealing the gap in youth access restrictions created by mail-order purchases.

The Committee recommends:

18. As part of a long-term access strategy, Congress should enact a suitably limited federal ban on the distribution of tobacco products through the mail. At a minimum, the law should bar *free* distribution, as well as redemption of tobacco coupons, a promotional activity likely to be particularly attractive to children and youths.

The Committee has focused its attention here on coupons redeemable by mail for cigarettes because of the possibility that this practice will increase as retail outlets dry up. It should be noted, however, that coupons are usually redeemed at retail for tobacco products, and that retailer compliance with youth access restrictions can be monitored and enforced regardless of whether the distribution involves a coupon redemption or a cash purchase. By contrast, redemption of coupons through the mail typically involves promotional items such as t-shirts and other articles. These promotional practices do not undermine youth access restrictions, although they may be objectionable on other grounds.

The Committee notes, finally, that coupons and other types of direct price competition raise issues that go far beyond youth access policy because they can attenuate the consumption-reducing effects of a pricing policy. However, these practices are unavoidable in a competitive market and could be eliminated only under a very aggressive scheme of price regulation. In the analogous context of alcoholic beverage control regulation, the trend has been to loosen or remove these bans, and liquor couponing is now legal in most states.

Additional Research Needed

Innovations in youth access policy have been based on successful initiatives in a few localities. Little is known about the long-term effects of these initiatives or about their extension to more densely populated areas. It is therefore important to include in the programs now being developed in response to the Synar Amendment a component for evaluation research. In addition, the Centers for Disease Control and Prevention and other research sponsors should put in place ongoing information systems regarding the operation of the tobacco market in relation to youth access, especially as the market responds to restrictions on distribution in legal channels of commerce.

The Committee recommends:

19. Sponsors of research should support (a) studies of retailers' motivation for compliance or noncompliance; (b) studies of the cost-effectiveness of various enforcement approaches being developed in response to the Synar Amendment; and (c) most important, a surveillance system for monitoring the tobacco market in order to ascertain the sources (and cost) of tobacco products to youths, in both legal and illicit commerce.

REFERENCES

1. Cummings, K. Michael, Terry Pechacek, and Donald Shopland. "The Illegal Sale of Cigarettes to U.S. Minors: Estimates by State." *American Journal of Public Health* 84:2 (1994): 300-302.

2. Centers for Disease Control and Prevention. *Preventing Tobacco Use Among Young People. A Report of the Surgeon General.* S/N 0017-001-00491-0. Washington, DC: U.S. Government Printing Office, 1994. 67.

3. Office of the Inspector General. *Youth Access to Tobacco.* Department of Health and Human Services. OEI-02-92-00880. December 1992.

4. Marttila & Kiley, Inc. *Highlights from an American Cancer Society Survey of U.S. Voter Attitudes Toward Cigarette Smoking.* Boston: Sept. 1993.

5. Hawkins, Charles H. "Legal Restrictions on Minors' Smoking." *American Journal of Public Health* 54:10 (1964): 1741-44.

6. *Goodrich v. State.* 133 Wis 242, 113 N.W. 388, 1907.

7. *State v. Crabtree.* 218 Minn. 36, 15 N.W. 2d 98, 1944.

8. Brandt, Allan M. "The Cigarette, Risk, and American Culture." *Daedalus* 119:4 (1990): 155-176.

9. *Illinois Cigarette Service Co. v. City of Chicago.* 89 F. 2d 610 (7th Circuit), 1937.

10. Hawkins.

11. Centers for Disease Control. *Reducing the Health Consequences of Smoking: 25 Years of Progress. A Report of the Surgeon General.* DHHS Publication No. (CDC) 89-8411, 1989. 593.

12. Office of the Inspector General. *Youth Access to Cigarettes.* Department of Health and Human Services. OEI-02-90-02310. May 1990.

13. OIG, 1992.

14. U.S. Department of Health and Human Services. "Model Sale of Tobacco Products to Minors Control Act: A Model Law Recommended for Adoption by States or Localities to Prevent the Sale of Tobacco Products to Minors." May 24, 1990; and DiFranza, Joseph R., and Joe B. Tye. "Who Profits From Tobacco Sales to Children?" *Journal of the American Medical Association* 263:20 (1990): 2784-2787.

15. Johnston, L., J. Bachman, and P. O'Malley. "Monitoring the Future Study." Press release. The University of Michigan, Ann Arbor. January 27, 1994.

16. Cummings, K. Michael, Eva Sciandra, Terry F. Pechacek, Mario Orlandi, and William R. Lynn. For the COMMIT Research Group. "Where Teenagers Get Their Cigarettes: A Survey of the Purchasing Habits of 13-16 Year Olds in 12 U.S. Communities." *Tobacco Control* 1 (1992): 264-267.

17. Response Research, Inc. *Study of Teenage Cigarette Smoking and Purchase Behavior.* For the National Automatic Merchandising Association. Chicago: June/July 1989.

18. Cummings et al., 1992.

19. See for example: DiFranza, Joseph R., Billy D. Norwood, Donald W. Garner, and J. B. Tye. "Legislative Efforts to Protect Children from Tobacco." *Journal of the American Medical Association* 257:24 (1987): 3387-3389; DiFranza, Joseph R., Robert R. Carlson, and Ralph E. Caisse, Jr. "Reducing Youth Access to Tobacco." *Tobacco Control.* Letter to the Editor 1 (1992): 58; Centers for Disease Control and Prevention. "Accessability of Cigarettes to Youths Aged 12-17 Years—

United States, 1989." *Morbidity and Mortality Weekly Report* 41:27 (1992): 485-488; Hoppock, Kevin C., and Thomas P. Houston. "Availability of Tobacco Products to Minors." *Journal of Family Practice* 30:2 (1990): 174-176; Altman, David G., Valodi Foster, Lolly Rasenick-Douss, and Joe B. Tye. "Reducing the Illegal Sale of Cigarette to Minors." *Journal of the American Medical Association* 261:1 (1989): 80-83; Forster, Jean L., Mary E. Hourigan, and Paul McGovern. "Availability of Cigarettes to Underage Youth in Three Communities." *Preventive Medicine* 21:3 (1992): 320-328; and OIG, 1990.

20. Centers for Disease Control and Prevention, 1994. 249.

21. Altman et al., 1989; and Forster et al., "Availability," 1992.

22. Cummings et al., 1992, and Response Research.

23. Response Research.

24. OIG, 1992.

25. Jason, Leonard A., Peter Y. Ji, Michael D. Anes, and Scott H. Birkhead. "Active Enforcement of Cigarette Control Laws in the Prevention of Cigarette Sales to Minors." *Journal of the American Medical Association* 266:22 (11 Dec. 1991): 3159-3161.

26. Altman, David, Julia Carol, Christine Chalkley, Joe Cherner, Joseph DiFranza, Ellen Feighery, Jean Forster, Sunil Gupta, John Records, John Slade, Bruce Talbot, and Joe Tye. "Report of the Tobacco Policy Research Study Group on Access to Tobacco Products in the United States." *Tobacco Control* 1 (1992): S45-S51.

27. Altman et al., 1989.

28. Altman, D. G., L. Rasenick-Douss, V. Foster, and J. B. Tye. "Sustained Effects of an Educational Program to Reduce Sales of Cigarettes to Minors." *American Journal of Public Health* 81:7 (1991): 891-893.

29. Feighery, Ellen, David G. Altman, and Gregory Shaffer. "The Effects of Combining Education and Enforcement to Reduce Tobacco Sales to Minors: A Study of Four Northern California Communities." *Journal of the American Medical Association* 266 (1991): 3168-3171.

30. OIG, 1990.

31. USDHHS, 1990.

32. OIG, 1992.

33. Weisskopf, Michael. "Hill Bid to Curb Youth Tobacco Sales Falters." *The Washington Post* (10 July 1993): A10.

34. U.S. Department of Health and Human Services. "Substance Abuse Prevention and Treatment Block Grants." 45 CFR Part 96. *Federal Register* 58:164 (26 Aug. 1993): 45156-45174.

35. Jason et al.

36. DiFranza et al., 1992.

37. Wagenaar, Alexander C., John R. Finnegan, Mark Wolfson, Pamela S. Anstine, Carolyn L. Williams, and Cheryl L. Perry. "Where and How Adolescents Obtain Alcoholic Beverages." *Public Health Reports* 108:4 (July 1993): 459-464.

38. Johnston et al.

39. Bonnie, Richard J. "Discouraging the Use of Alcohol, Tobacco and Other Drugs: The Effects of Legal Controls and Restrictions." In Nancy Mello, ed. *Advances in Substance Abuse Research, Vol. II.* JAI Press, 1982. 145-184; and "The Efficacy of Law as a Paternalistic Instrument." In Gary Melton, ed. *Nebraska Symposium on Human Motivation, 1985.* Lincoln: University of Nebraska, 1986. 131-211.

40. Weisskopf.

41. Jaffe, Robert D., and Helene Starks. "Reducing Illegal Tobacco Sales to Minors." Unpublished manuscript on a 4-year evaluation in King County, by Washington DOC, 1993.

42. See for example: *CIC Corp. v. Township of New Brunswick.* 628 A.2d 753 (N.J. Super. Ct. App. Div.), 1993; *Bravo Vending v. City of Rancho Mirage.* 16 Calif App. 4th 383 (4th Dis.), 1993; and *Take Five Vending v. Town of Provincetown.* 615 N.E. 2d 576 (Mass.), 1993

43. *Allied Vending, Inc. v. City of Bowie.* 631 A.2d 77 (Md.), 1993.

44. USDHHS, 1990.

45. OIG, 1990.

46. Jason et al.

47. Altman et al., "Report," 1992.

48. Cummings et al., 1994; and DiFranza and Tye, 1990.

49. Altman et al., "Report," 1992.

50. Jason et al.

51. Response Research.

52. Cummings et al., 1992.

53. Response Research.

54. Cismoski, Joseph. *Fond du Lac School District Survey. Addendum to the Michigan Alcohol and Drug Survey.* Kercher Center for Social Research, Western Michigan University. Kalamazoo, MI: January 1994 (unpublished).

55. Altman et al., "Report," 1992.

56. Altman et al., 1989.

57. Forster et al., "Availability," 1992.

58. Marttila & Kiley, Inc.

59. OIG, 1992.

60. Feighery et al.

61. Forster, Jean L., Mary E. Hourigan, and S. Kelder. "Locking Devices on Cigarette Vending Machines: Evaluation of a City Ordinance." *American Journal of Public Health* 82:9 (1992): 1217-1219.

62. *Ibid.*

63. USDHHS, "Model Sale," 1990.

64. Forster et al., "Availability," 1992.

65. Cismoski, Joseph, and Marian Sheridan. "Availability of Cigarettes to Under-age Youth in Fond du Lac, Wisconsin." *Wisconsin Medical Journal* (Nov. 1993): 626-630.

66. Wakefield, Melanie, John Carrangis, David Wilson, and Christopher Reynolds. "Illegal Cigarette Sales to Children in South Australia." *Tobacco Control* 1 (1992): 114-117.

67. STAT. "Springfield Teen Tobacco Purchase Survey." News Release. November 11, 1993.

68. Response Research.

69. Cox, Dena, Anthony D. Cox, and George P. Moschis. "When Consumer Behavior Goes Bad: An Investigation of Adolescent Shoplifting." *Journal of Consumer Research* 17:2 (1990): 149-159.

70. Roswell Park Cancer Institute. *Survey of Alcohol, Tobacco and Drug Use: Ninth Grade Students in Erie County, 1992.* Buffalo, NY: Roswell Park Cancer Institute, Department of Cancer Control and Epidemiology, 1993.

71. Cismoski, 1994.

72. *Cigarette Labeling and Advertising Act.* P.L. No. 98-474, 98 Stat. 2201 (12 Oct. 1984) codified at 15 U.S.C. 1333 (a) (1986).

73. Klonoff, Elizabeth A., Jan M. Fritz, Hope Landrine, Richard W. Riddle, and Laurie Tully-Payne. "The Problem and Sociocultural Context of Single-Cigarette Sales." *Journal of the American Medical Association* 271:8 (23 Feb. 1994): 618-620.

74. Figures have been adjusted for inflation. Federal Trade Commission. *Federal Trade Commission Report to Congress for 1991. Pursuant to the Federal Cigarette Labeling and Advertising Act.* Washington, DC: Federal Trade Commission, 1994.

75. Davis, Ronald M., and Leonard A. Jason. "The Distribution of Free Cigarette Samples to Minors." *American Journal of Preventive Medicine* 4:1 (1988): 21-26.

76. *Ibid.*

77. *Ibid.*

78. *Ibid.*

79. *Ibid.*

80. Martilla & Kiley.

81. Davis and Jason.

82. Keay, Karen D., Susan I. Woodruff, Marianne B. Wildey, and Erin M. Kenney. "Effects of a Retailer Intervention on Cigarette Sales to Minors in San Diego County, California." *Tobacco Control* 2 (1993): 145-151. See also: Altman et al., 1991; and Feighery et al.

83. DiFranza et al., 1987.

84. Keay et al., and Altman et al., 1989.

85. Keay et al.

86. Feighery et al.

87. Keay et al.

88. Altman, David G., Juliette Linzer, Rick Kropp, Nancy Descheemaeker, Ellen Feighery, and Stephen P. Fortmann. "Policy Alternatives for Reducing Tobacco Sales to Minors: Results from a National Survey of Retail Chain and Franchise Stores." *Journal of Public Health Policy* 13:3 (1992): 318-331.

89. Keay et al.

90. Keay et al.

91. Feighery et al.

92. Jason et al.

93. Keay et al.

94. Biglan, Anthony, Jamye Henderson, Delaine Humphreys, Maija Yasui, Rebecca Whisman, Carol Black, and Lisa James. "Experimental Evaluation of a Community Intervention to Reduce Youth Access to Tobacco." Oregon Research Institute, 1993. Unpublished.

95. Feighery et al.

96. Join Together. *Community Leaders Speak Out Against Substance Abuse.* Boston: Join Together, 1993. 26.

97. Skretny, Michelle T., K. Michael Cummings, Russell Sciandra, and James Marshall. "An Intervention to Reduce the Sale of Cigarettes to Minors." *New York State Journal of Medicine* 90:2 (1990): 54-55. See also: Altman et al., 1991; Feighery et al.; and OIG, 1992.

98. Jaffe and Starks.

99. Chudy, N., R. Yoast, and P. Remington. "Child and Adolescent Smoking and Consumption." *Wisconsin Medical Journal* (Apr. 1993): 198-201. See also: Feighery et al.; and OIG, 1992.

100. USDHHS, "Substance Abuse," 1993.

101. OIG, 1992.

102. Jason et al., and DiFranza et al., 1987.

103. OIG, 1992.

104. Feighery et al.

105. USDHHS, "Substance Abuse," 1993.

106. Gruenewald, Paul J., William R. Ponicki, and Harold D. Holder. "The Relationship of Outlet Densities to Alcohol Consumption: A Time Series Cross-Sectional Analysis." *Alcoholism: Clinical and Experimental Research* 17:1 (Feb. 1993): 38-47.

107. U.S. Department of Health and Human Services. *Healthy People 2000: National Health Promotion and Disease Prevention Objectives Update.* Department of Health and Human Services. October/November 1993.

108. Slade, John. "Teenagers Participate in Tobacco Promotions." Abstract. Submitted to the 9th World Conference on Tobacco and Health (Paris), October 1994.

109. Roswell Park.

Ravi Blank, Abraham Lincoln High School, Brooklyn

CONTENTS

8 REGULATION OF THE LABELING, PACKAGING, AND CONTENTS OF TOBACCO PRODUCTS

TOBACCO: AN UNREGULATED HAZARD

Food products, bicycles, automobiles, matches and lighters, pharmaceuticals, and other consumer products are subject to a variety of federal regulatory statutes. These laws typically authorize administrative agencies to require manufacturers to reduce the risks associated with the use of the product or even to ban products that are unreasonably dangerous. Tobacco products, however, have been excluded from the coverage of these federal regulatory schemes, either by explicit statutory exemption or by agency practice. For example, the enabling legislation for the Consumer Product Safety Commission, the Consumer Product Safety Act of 1972 (CPSA), expressly excludes tobacco from its otherwise broad delegation of power to regulate consumer products that present an "unreasonable risk of injury." Shortly after a federal court ruled that the Consumer Product Safety Commission had jurisdiction to regulate high-tar tobacco products under the Federal Hazardous Substances Act, Congress amended that act to exclude tobacco from the definition of "hazardous substances."[1] Similarly, the Toxic Substances Control Act expressly exempts tobacco from regulation even though the constituents of tobacco smoke might otherwise be subject to regulation as "chemical substances which present unreasonable risk of impairing health," or as "mixtures of such substances."[2] Despite its addictiveness, tobacco is also specifically exempted from the Controlled Substances Act, which regulates the medical and scientific use of other psychoactive drugs and prohibits their distribution and use for nonmedical and nonscientific purposes.

It is not difficult to understand why Congress has excluded tobacco from

233

these regulatory schemes. If tobacco products were included, each of these statutes would require extensive regulation of tobacco products to reduce risks to the health and safety of users and nonusers, including changes in product design and mandatory disclosure of information regarding contents and hazards. Moreover, under most of these schemes, faithful adherence to the statutory criteria would authorize, or even require, the regulatory agencies to take tobacco products off the market. For example, the chronic risk of tobacco products is much greater than the hazards of other products that have been banned under the Consumer Product Safety Act, and the Consumer Product Safety Commission's priority-setting rule suggests that it would have no choice but to ban tobacco products as well.

An analogous problem arises under the Food, Drug, and Cosmetic Act (FDCA). The definition of "drug" in the FDCA includes "articles (other than food) intended to affect the structure or any function of the body of man." Although the act does not expressly exclude tobacco products from its coverage, the Food and Drug Administration (FDA) has long taken the position that tobacco products manufactured and sold to be used "for smoking pleasure" are not "drugs" under the FDCA and are not subject to regulation thereunder, in the absence of *intent* by the manufacturers or vendors of cigarettes to affect the structure or function of the body. This position was ratified by the courts and has become the settled understanding.[3]

The FDA has not declined to exercise jurisdiction over tobacco products in all cases. The FDCA's definition of drug also includes articles "intended for use in the cure, mitigation, or prevention of disease," and the FDA has asserted jurisdiction when manufacturers have expressly promoted cigarettes as beneficial to health. For example, during the 1950s, the agency took regulatory action against cigarettes advertised as effective in preventing respiratory and other diseases[4] and cigarettes promoted as weight-reducing aids.[5] The FDA has also exercised jurisdiction over cigarette additives promoted as mitigating disease and over nicotine delivery systems promoted as alternatives to conventional cigarette smoking or as aids to smoking cessation. In recent years, petitions have been filed seeking to invoke FDA jurisdiction over cigarettes promoted as being "light" or otherwise low in tar and nicotine on the basis that these assertions imply that the cigarettes are less dangerous than other cigarettes and less likely to result in dependence or disease. The FDA has not yet acted on these petitions.

On February 25, 1994, FDA Commissioner David Kessler indicated that the agency was reconsidering its traditional view that tobacco products are not "drugs" under the FDCA. In a letter to the Coalition for Smoking OR Health and in subsequent testimony on Capitol Hill, Dr. Kessler sought to focus attention on whether cigarettes and other tobacco products are marketed as "nicotine delivery systems" to satisfy the dependence of consumers on nicotine. In raising this question, Dr. Kessler referred to evidence that "manufacturers commonly add nicotine to cigarettes to deliver specific amounts of nicotine."[6] (As was subsequently discussed at hearings before the House Subcommittee on Health and the Environment, cigarette manufacturers remove nicotine and add it back, in the form of tobacco extract, in the manufacturing of cigaretttes with the desired level of nicotine.)[7] Although Dr. Kessler did not assert FDA jurisdiction, he stated that, in his view, a legal basis for regulation would be established by evidence proving that cigarette manufacturers intend that their products contain nicotine to satisfy an addiction on the part of some of their customers. At the same time, Dr. Kessler indicated that the agency was reluctant to move in this direction without explicit congressional authorization.

The FDA's longstanding reluctance to classify tobacco products as "drugs" under the FDCA is understandable. Under the regulatory logic of the FDCA, cigarettes (or other tobacco products) intended to produce or to satisfy nicotine dependence would have to be proven "safe and effective" in order to remain on the market. Tobacco products are demonstrably *un*safe. Thus, an inevitable effect of classifying nicotine-containing tobacco products as "drugs" would be to ban them. Yet, an agency ban under the FDCA arguably would be incompatible with a 30-year history of congressional action regulating the advertising and labeling of tobacco products while permitting their continued manufacture and use.

The net result of Congress' actions and inactions over the past 30 years is that tobacco products, as customarily manufactured, marketed, and consumed, are largely unregulated. The tendency of these products to produce addiction is currently without regulatory significance, notwithstanding extensive federal control over other dependence-producing drugs. In addition, the tendency of tobacco products to cause disease and premature death has no regulatory significance under any of the statutory schemes that regulate hazardous products, substances, or drugs. The only agency (FDA) with jurisdiction over any tobacco product now confines itself to peripheral situations in which a tobacco product is promoted as satisfying a desire for nicotine or as being effective in preventing or mitigating disease, and the agency is clearly reluctant to broaden its reach without explicit congressional direction.

The federal government's occasional regulatory initiatives have been severely circumscribed. Manufacturers of tobacco products are now required to provide a list of additives to the secretary of health and human services, but no agency has the authority to require disclosure of this information to consumers or to proscribe hazardous additives. (After a list of additives was obtained by the press in April 1994, the cigarette manufacturers jointly issued a combined list.) Although federal law requires that warnings about the health hazards of tobacco use be conveyed to purchasers on packaging and in advertising, no agency is directed by statute to monitor the efficacy of these warnings in discouraging youth initiation or other tobacco consumption, and no agency has the authority to require that the warnings be modified in light of advances in scientific and medical knowledge. Although the Department of Health and Human Services has adopted the reduction of tobacco use (and of tobacco-related morbidity and mortality) as major public health goals, no agency has the responsibility for determining whether the achievement of these goals could be promoted by regulating the constituents of tobacco products. (Indeed, as discussed below, no agency in the Department of Health and Human Services has clear-cut regulatory authority to coordinate the federal government's programmatic efforts to achieve this goal.)

Congress must rectify this massive regulatory default. A comprehensive national strategy of tobacco control must include a regulatory component. Specifically, **Congress should enact legislation that delegates to an appropriate agency the necessary authority to regulate tobacco products for the dual purposes of discouraging consumption and reducing the morbidity and mortality associated with use of tobacco products**. Although the Committee has not designed a detailed blueprint, the Committee has formulated a general outline of such a regulatory scheme, focusing on the ways in which such a plan would help reduce nicotine dependency among children and youths.

A comprehensive statutory scheme for regulating tobacco products should include at least two major components: regulation of product labeling and packaging and direct regulation of the product itself. In each context, the overall regulatory aim is twofold: to discourage people, especially children and youths, from using tobacco products, and to reduce the morbidity and mortality associated with use of tobacco products. Difficult questions of regulatory design must be addressed in each context. Two major issues are (1) which agency or agencies should be assigned regulatory responsibility and (2) what criteria or standards should guide the exercise of regulatory authority.

WARNINGS AND PACKAGING

Congress has enacted a series of laws specifying that warnings be placed on cigarette packages, first in 1965, again in 1969, and most recently in 1984. Also, in 1986 Congress enacted warning requirements for smokeless tobacco products. However, Congress has never delegated the authority to update these warnings, or to evaluate their effectiveness, to a regulatory agency. The adequacy of the current cigarette warnings has been repeatedly questioned by public health specialists. Moreover, in the Committee's view federal cigarette labeling legislation has reflected an unsatisfactory compromise between the public's health and the tobacco industry's desire to avoid concurrent state regulation and to reduce its exposure to tort liability. Negotiations in the legislative process have tended to favor the industry. Inevitably, congressionally prescribed warnings have reflected political trade-offs rather than an unequivocal goal of providing relevant and complete health information.

The inadequacy of current labeling policy is clearly revealed in the declaration of congressional purpose in the Comprehensive Smoking Education Act of 1984:

> It is the purpose of this Act to provide a new strategy of making Americans more aware of any adverse health effects of smoking, to assure the timely and widespread dissemination of research findings, and to enable individuals to make informed decisions about smoking.[8]

It is time to state, unequivocally, that the primary objective of tobacco regulation is not to promote informed choice, but rather to discourage consumption of tobacco products, especially by children and youths, as a means of reducing tobacco-related death and disease. Even though tobacco products are legally available to adults, the paramount public health aim is to reduce the number of people who use and become addicted to these products, through a focus on children and youths. The warnings must be designed to promote this objective. In the Committee's view, the current warnings are inadequate even when measured against an informed choice standard, but they are woefully deficient when evaluated in terms of proper public health criteria.

The History of Federal Action

The publication of the 1964 report of the Surgeon General's Advisory Committee on Smoking and Health, linking cigarette smoking to lung cancer, chronic bronchitis, and emphysema, marked the emergence of a public consensus and stimulated federal regulatory and legislative action. In response to the surgeon general's call for "appropriate remedial action," the Federal Trade Commission (FTC) proposed rules requiring that manufacturers disclose on all packaging and advertisements that "cigarette smoking is dangerous to health" and "may cause death from cancer and other diseases." Before taking effect, however, the FTC regulations were preempted by the Cigarette Labeling and Advertising Act of 1965. In their place, the act mandated a mild health warning on cigarette packaging without specific reference to the risk of death from cancer and other diseases:

> Caution: cigarette smoking may be hazardous to your health.[9]

Unlike the proposed FTC regulations, the 1965 act did not require warnings on product advertisements. The act also divested federal agencies and states of the authority to impose more stringent health warning requirements. In particular, the FTC was prohibited from requiring health warnings on tobacco advertising for four years, until July 1, 1969, although the FTC's authority to regulate unfair or deceptive advertising was left intact. Vesting nearly exclusive regulatory authority in the Congress, the Cigarette Labeling and Advertising Act freed the tobacco industry of the threat of bolder regulatory action and removed the debate to a forum where public health objectives shared the stage with economic concerns and other political pressures.

In 1967, the Federal Communications Commission (FCC) ruled that the "Fairness Doctrine," which required television stations to provide air time for alternate points of view on matters of public debate, applied to tobacco commercials. Broadcasters who carried cigarette commercials were required to provide free air time to health groups, whose imaginative and effective antismoking commercials contributed to a general decline in smoking rates.[10] In 1969, the FCC announced its intention to ban cigarette advertising on radio and television and the FTC proposed requiring health warnings on cigarette advertisements. As in 1964, those agency initiatives provoked congressional action.

The Public Health Cigarette Smoking Act of 1969 amended the original 1965 labeling act to require a slightly strengthened health warning:

> Warning: The Surgeon General Has Determined That Cigarette Smoking Is Dangerous to Your Health.[11]

Again, the congressionally mandated warning was milder than that recommended by the FTC and omitted specific reference to death, cancer, heart disease, chronic bronchitis, and emphysema. In addition, the act banned cigarette advertising on radio and television. Seeking to avoid the antismoking commercials mandated by the FCC's Fairness Doctrine, the tobacco industry staged little resistance to the broadcast ban. Again, Congress temporarily restricted the FTC from requiring manufacturers to include health warnings in print advertising until July 1, 1971. Congress also barred states from imposing "any requirement or prohibition based on smoking and health" on the advertising and promotion of cigarettes packaged with labels conforming to the statute. (The U.S. Supreme Court subsequently ruled in 1992 that this language not only preempted direct restrictions on advertising but also shielded the industry from liability in tort actions brought by or on behalf of injured smokers for failure to warn in advertising or promotion or for misrepresentation through overpromotion.)[12]

On March 30, 1972, the FTC and the cigarette companies agreed upon consent orders requiring all cigarette advertising to display, "clearly and conspicuously," the same warning required by Congress for cigarette purchases. The consent order specified the type size of the warnings in newspaper, magazine, and other periodical advertisements of various dimensions. The size of lettering was specified in inches for billboard advertisements.

In 1981, the FTC determined that the federally mandated health warnings had little impact on the public's level of knowledge and attitudes about smoking. In a staff report to Congress, the FTC concluded that the warning was "worn out," too abstract, difficult to remember, and not perceived as personally relevant.[13] The FTC report helped to spur Congress to enact the Comprehensive Smoking Education Act of 1984, which required four, more specific, rotating health warnings on all cigarette packages and advertisements:

> SURGEON GENERAL'S WARNING: Smoking Causes Lung Cancer, Heart Disease, Emphysema, and May Complicate Pregnancy.

SURGEON GENERAL'S WARNING: Quitting Smoking Now Greatly Reduces Serious Risks to Your Health.

SURGEON GENERAL'S WARNING: Smoking By Pregnant Women May Result in Fetal Injury, Premature Birth, and Low Birth Weight.

SURGEON GENERAL'S WARNING: Cigarette Smoke Contains Carbon Monoxide.[14]

Like the health warnings enacted by Congress in the past, the new warnings resulted from political compromises favorable to the tobacco industry, rather than from an unqualified effort to inform the public. The warnings retained the same rectangular format despite an FTC recommendation that a "circle-and-arrow" format would be more effective. The warnings contain no reference to addiction, miscarriage, or death and require no disclosure of tar, nicotine, and carbon monoxide yields.

Required warnings were extended to smokeless tobacco products by the 1986 Comprehensive Smokeless Tobacco Health Education Act. Under the act, three rotating warning labels must be displayed on smokeless tobacco packaging and advertising in the circle-and-arrow format that had been recommended by the FTC for cigarettes:

WARNING: This product may cause mouth cancer.

WARNING: This product may cause gum disease and tooth loss.

WARNING: This product is not a safe alternative to cigarettes.[15]

Federal agencies and state and local governments are preempted from imposing additional health warnings on smokeless tobacco products and advertisements.

The Importance of Warnings in Discouraging Use by Youths

In theory, tobacco health warnings are particularly relevant to persons who are experimenting with or deciding whether to use tobacco but who have not yet become regular users. Accordingly, since regular tobacco use is usually established before the age of 18, children and youths are an important target for health messages. Warnings that do no more than accomplish their original purpose—to promote informed choice—can increase the availability and salience of health risk information every time a young person decides whether to buy or use tobacco. However, tobacco health warnings should also aim to discourage tobacco use, not only by providing information regarding the harmful consequences of tobacco, but also by vitiating the appeal of advertising and promotion and by sending an unequivocal anti-tobacco message. In the Committee's view, strong health warnings, and accompanying package regulation, are an important component of a coordinated plan to reduce and prevent tobacco use by children and youths.

The Inadequacy of Existing Warnings

No published studies have directly evaluated the impact of the federally mandated tobacco health warnings on knowledge or behavior of adults or youths. Isolating the independent effects of the warnings themselves from the effects of other policies that discourage tobacco use and from the effects of other sources of information regarding smoking is a daunting, if not impossible, task. As the surgeon general recently stated, "there are no controlled studies that permit definitive assessment of the independent impact of cigarette warning labels on knowledge, beliefs, attitudes, or smoking behavior."[16] However, a body of indirect evidence suggests that the current warnings are probably not having the desired impact on knowledge or behavior, especially among youths.

It is clear, first of all, that adolescents continue to underestimate the adverse health consequences of tobacco use. Although they understand that smoking is hazardous and can associate smoking with particular health risks, adolescents underestimate the magnitude of the risks of regular smoking over the long term.[17] As discussed in chapter 1, adolescents do not appreciate the risk and consequences of becoming addicted. As a result, according to the University of Michigan's Monitoring the Future Study, *nearly half* (47%) of eighth graders in 1993 denied that there is "great risk" associated with smoking a pack of cigarettes per day. Even among high school seniors, more than 30% denied that there was a "great risk" associated with pack-a-day smoking. Only 35% of high school seniors reported believing that "great risk" was associated with regular use of smokeless tobacco.[18]

Steps must be taken to improve youngsters' awareness of the long-term dangers of tobacco use. The Committee is not suggesting that changes in warnings alone can produce the desired effects. Adolescents' deficient understanding of the adverse health consequences of tobacco can also be remedied by antitobacco media campaigns and by educational programs. Nonetheless, the potential contributions of improved warnings should not be ignored. The research literature strongly suggests that the desired impact of the current warnings is eroded by remediable deficiencies in format, composition, and content.

In a recent review of research on consumer response to labeling information, the 1994 report of the surgeon general concluded that two basic factors appear to influence the usefulness of warning labels:

> First, to have an impact on consumers, warning labels must be designed to take into account those factors that might influence consumer response (e.g., a consumer's previous experience with the product, previous knowledge of the risks associated with the product's use, and level of education or literacy). Second, the labels should be designed in an attention-getting format, and the information they bear should be specific rather than general and written in clear, nontechnical language.[19]

It appears to be generally agreed that the present cigarette warnings are easily and often overlooked, especially in contrast with the vibrant allure of tobacco packaging and advertising. Studies suggest that adolescents often do not notice or do not read the current warning labels.[20] The labels are small and inconspicuously located on the side of a package or in the lower corner of a print advertisement. They are often printed in colors that allow the warnings to blend in with packaging design or to be overwhelmed by the marketing imagery. Using an eye-tracking technique commonly used in market research, one study found that only 37% of adolescents viewing tobacco advertisements looked at the health warning long enough to read its words; 43.6% of the subjects did not look at the warning at all.[21] A similar response was found in a study of smokeless tobacco product packaging, in which only 43% of subjects noticed the warning label.[22]

Novel, eye-catching designs, such as the circle-and-arrow format recommended by the FTC and adopted by Congress for smokeless tobacco products, may increase noticeability.[23] The color and reflectiveness of the warning label in the context of the overall packaging or advertisement is also likely to affect noticeability. By requiring the warning to be printed in black and white, recent reform of tobacco labeling laws in Canada sought to prevent manufacturers from successfully blending the warning into the overall packaging. This concern is also addressed in H.R. 3614, introduced by Congressman Waxman in November 1993, which would require labels to be printed in white letters on a black background or black letters on a white background, whichever is more conspicuous, with the words "SURGEON GENERAL'S WARNING" printed in red and enclosed by a contrasting border.

To increase noticeability, Canada and Australia recently increased the size of warning labels, requiring the warning and its borders to occupy 30-40% of the display area of the package. The proposed H.R. 3614 also takes this approach, requiring the size of warning labels to occupy at least 25% of the side of the package on which they appear or 25% of the print advertisement. H.R. 3614 also would require the size, thickness, and typeface of the warning's lettering to be as "legible, prominent, and conspicuous" as any other lettering on the package or advertisement.

Studies also suggest that the current warnings are too small and too lengthy to be read in outdoor advertising media. A study of roadside billboards found that, under typical driving conditions, observers could read the entire warning message on only 5% of tobacco advertisements. Similarly, stationary observers were unable to read the health warnings in any of the tobacco ads on 100 New York taxicabs. In both media, however, observers were nearly always able to identify the brand name, advertising content, and imagery.[24] A study of the legibility of health warnings on cigarette billboards in Australia obtained similar results.[25]

Regulation of the other areas of the package can also help maximize the salience of the health warnings. One study found that existing tobacco packaging conjured specific brand images in the minds of adolescents, such as "rugged" or "classy." Large, clashing warning labels were found to vitiate the attractiveness of the pack images. In particular, "plain packaging," in which the brand name is presented on a plain, standardized background and all logos and identifying information other than the brand name are removed, was found to effectively destroy the positive images created by cigarette packaging (figure 8-1).[26]

Warnings are likely to become less effective with time as they become "worn out." An unchanging shape, size, and heading in the warning may discourage further exploration of the message. Novel formatting is more likely to capture attention.[27] The retention of the original rectangular shape of the pre-1985 warning may have diminished the potential communication effectiveness of the more explicit rotating warnings.[28] Periodically altering the format of the warnings may help to refresh their impact.[29]

Preliminary studies on the effects of labels on alcoholic beverage containers suggest that warnings on health risks are likely to be most effective in increasing awareness of the least-known risks. Although warnings can serve as a reminder of already known hazards (such as impaired driving), they might be more useful for conveying specific information that is not widely known. One study found that the most readily recalled portion of the alcohol label was the message about

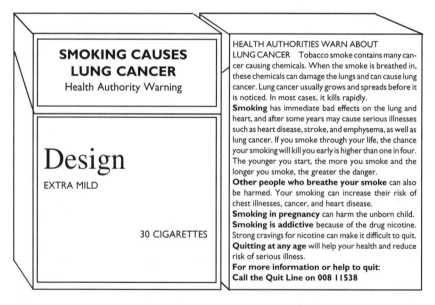

FIGURE 8-1 Proposed prototype of plain packaging for cigarettes in Australia. The per cigarette amounts of tar, nicotine, and carbon monoxide are listed and explained on the side panels.

birth defects.[30] Another found that, compared to baseline, there was no statistically significant change in knowledge of the health risks included in the labels but that awareness of two risks *not* included (risk of cancer and high blood pressure) declined from already low levels. These investigators concluded that it is "certainly plausible that rotating messages so as to keep them 'fresh' while increasing exposure to lesser known facts, could be a useful strategy to consider, and rigorously evaluate, in the future."[31]

Even when tobacco health warnings are noticeable and legible enough to be read, research suggests that the current warnings are not framed to be optimally understandable, believable, persuasive, and memorable.[32] In a recent study using standard market research techniques for evaluating advertisements, the congressionally mandated warnings performed poorly in communicating specific risk information. Although 79% of subjects exposed to the warnings reported the presence of a health message, only 15% reported the concept of the message and only 6% reported its exact content. On the other hand, the elements of the cigarette advertisements were frequently recalled: 97% of the subjects identified the brand of cigarettes being advertised.[33]

The impact of the current cigarette labels may be lessened by the fact that three of the four are framed in an impersonal manner. Readers are more likely to believe and heed warnings they perceive as personally relevant.[34] Using a larger number of rotating warnings is also more likely to provide a reader with one or several messages that will be perceived as personally relevant. H.R. 3614 proposes nine rotating warnings. Australia has chosen twelve rotating warnings and Canada has adopted eight. Using a larger number of rotating messages may also help to prevent the messages from becoming "worn-out" over time.

The power of the current warnings may also be diluted by wordiness and by combining several potential outcomes. One of the labels combines lung cancer, heart disease, emphysema, and pregnancy complications and another groups fetal injury, low birth weight, and premature birth. Short, concise, straightforward messages are thought to be the best vehicle for health warnings. For example, in a focus group study using adolescents to evaluate tobacco warnings labels, researchers found that the statement "Cigarettes kill. One in every 3 smokers will die from smoking." was perceived as direct and informative.[35] Lessons of this kind underlie one of the provisions of H.R. 3614, which would require shorter, more explicit statements than those currently used, including, "Cigarettes can kill you" and "Smoking during pregnancy can harm your baby."

Even if the current warnings were communicated effectively, they would fail to achieve Congress' stated purpose to "assure the timely and widespread dissemination of research findings" regarding the effects of smoking. The current warnings do not incorporate the substantial body of scientific knowledge that has accumulated since 1984 regarding the link between tobacco use and disease, the addictiveness of nicotine, the harmfulness of environmental tobacco smoke, and the dangers of chemical additives and byproducts. They omit any reference to death, addiction, miscarriage, stroke, infant mortality, and danger to nonsmokers. With regard to nearly all other consumer products, Congress has delegated power to federal agencies to allow flexible regulatory choices regarding the content of mandatory package warnings or package inserts. The legislative process is ill-suited to the task of evaluating the quality of health warnings in light of ongoing scientific advances.

In sum, studies on communication of health messages demonstrate that consumer response to warning labels depends on the format and presentation of the message, as well as on its content. The current tobacco health warnings are inadequate to attract attention or to communicate relevant and up-to-date information. For greater impact, the format and content of the warnings must be designed with the same communication techniques used to craft the pro-tobacco messages with which they must compete.

Recent Initiatives in Other Countries

Canada recently amended its Tobacco Products Control Act to require larger, more legible, and more potent health warnings. Under previous requirements that labels be in "contrasting colors," many manufacturers used color combinations that blended into the overall package design or that were highly reflective of light and thus difficult to read at the point of sale. The insufficiently noticeable and legible warnings were thought to undermine their overall credibility. In addition, surveys found that Canadians had only a superficial knowledge of the health effects of smoking, demonstrating that the then-required warning labels were not achieving their purpose of adequately informing the public. The amended law requires that all sides of tobacco packaging display one of eight rotating warnings, including messages about addiction, death, and passive smoking. The black-and-white warnings with their surrounding borders must occupy from 30% to 40% of the main display area of the package. Display of information regarding the toxic constituents present in cigarette smoke is also required.[36] Also, in Canada the Tobacco Products Control Act required outdoor billboards erected after January 1, 1991, to carry a health message equal to 20% of the top portion of the sign. Billboards began disappearing, as manufacturers were unwilling to risk the impact of large health warnings on sales.[37]

Australia has recently strengthened its regulation of tobacco warning labels and packaging. In 1992, the Ministerial Council on Drug Strategy agreed that states would adopt twelve rotating warning labels at the top and front of cigarette packages, including warnings stating: "Smoking kills" and "Smoking is addictive." The recommendations also call for display of information on tar, nicotine, and carbon monoxide yields on the side of the pack, and detailed health information about the hazards of smoking to appear on the entire back of the package. The back of the package also provides a "Quitline" telephone number to call for further information about health risks and help with quitting smoking.

Recommendations for Health Warnings and Packaging of Tobacco Products

Given the current lack of regulation of tobacco products and the inadequacy of current labeling requirements, the Committee makes the following recommendations:

1. Congress should take steps to strengthen the federally mandated warning labels for tobacco products. Health warning labels should be optimally noticeable, believable, and informative, especially to children and youths. The existing warnings fail to communicate current and comprehensive health risk information in an effective way.

2. Congress should take steps to increase the salience and effectiveness of health warnings on both advertising and packaging. This can be accomplished by regulating the format and design of the warning and the amount of area of the package devoted to the warning. "Plain packaging" should be considered.

3. Based on current knowledge, Congress should enact specific warning and format requirements now, and should delegate regulatory responsibility for future modifications to the secretary of health and human services. The secretary should ensure that ongoing research is conducted on the effectiveness of prescribed warnings. Congress lacks the institutional expertise and flexibility to monitor the efficacy of regulatory innovations and to respond to new information. Authority to amend the warnings should be delegated to an appropriate regulatory agency. **The secretary should be empowered to modify the format or content of existing warnings and to prescribe additional warnings, whenever such action is reasonably necessary to achieve effective communication of significant information regarding the health consequences of tobacco use or to discourage consumption of tobacco products.**

4. To the extent that promotional use of logos and trademarks of tobacco products is legally permitted, Congress should make accompanying health warnings mandatory. The tobacco industry has substantially increased its marketing budget for the sponsorship of public events and for promotional uses of non-tobacco products such as clothing, sports equipment, caps, and lighters. Trademarks and logos associated with tobacco products are pervasively displayed. Promotional items are often especially appealing to children and youths and project positive lifestyle images of the decision to use tobacco products without a counterbalancing health message. This is why Congress decided to require manufacturers of smokeless tobacco products to affix health warnings on promotional items using their insignia, logos, and trademarks. Unfortunately, Congress has not enacted parallel legislation for cigarettes, and this omission should be rectified as soon as possible. The data in the most recent FTC report on tobacco advertising indicate that there has been a shift from traditional mass media advertising to non-media promotions that are not required to carry health warnings.[38] Eventually, however, Congress should ban the promotional use of insignia, logos, and trademarks of all tobacco products, as recommended in chapter 4.

REGULATION OF CONSTITUENTS OF
TOBACCO PRODUCTS

A Unique Regulatory Challenge

A regulatory plan should be designed and implemented to discourage tobacco use, especially by children and youths, and to reduce the morbidity and mortality associated with tobacco use. A bill along those lines has been introduced in the House by Representative Synar and the Committee anticipates that an analogous bill will be introduced in the Senate by Senator Kennedy. Although the Synar bill would confer jurisdiction on the FDA, it recognizes that the regulatory regime already established by the Food, Drug, and Cosmetics Act is a poor fit for the regulation of tobacco products. As noted by Commissioner Kessler in his statement of March 25, 1994, to the House Subcommittee on Health and the Environment, if nicotine-containing cigarettes were regulated as drugs, "strict application of [the FDCA] could result in the removal from the market of tobacco products."[39] However fervently such a policy might be sought by public health advocates, the regulatory premise must be that tobacco products will remain lawfully available for adult consumption.

Once the continued lawfulness of tobacco products is acknowledged, legislative architects must confront a daunting challenge of regulatory design. As a nation, we have experience in designing and administering regulatory schemes under which dangerous products are not lawfully available outside tightly controlled channels of distribution. The Controlled Substances Act is illustrative. We also have experience in designing and administering regulatory schemes under which easily available consumer products are regulated to reduce the risks of injury or disease. Promulgation of safety standards for all-terrain vehicles and cigarette lighters under the Consumer Product Safety Act is illustrative. However, we have little experience with regulating dangerous products that are legally available but whose use is nonetheless discouraged. Even in the analogous contexts of alcohol and firearm regulation, the prevailing regulatory aim is to control the conditions and consequences of use, not to discourage it altogether.

For the foreseeable future, tobacco products will remain lawfully available for use by adults and will be accessible to minors as well, despite the prohibition on sales to youth. Therefore, the Committee recommends: **Congress should confer upon an administrative agency the authority to regulate the design** and constituents of tobacco products whenever it determines that such regulation would reduce the prevalence of dependence or disease associated with use of the product or would otherwise promote the public health. The agency should be specifically authorized to prescribe ceilings on the yields of tar, nicotine, or any other harmful constituent of a tobacco product.

The Regulatory Agency

Authority to regulate tobacco products should be exercised by a public health agency within the Department of Health and Human Services. Whether such authority should be delegated to the FDA or to a free-standing tobacco control agency requires careful study by the Secretary of HHS and by the Congress. The scientific expertise, independence, regulatory experience, and credibility of the FDA weigh in favor of a delegation to that agency. However, there are many countervailing concerns. The addition of a major new regulatory responsibility could impair the FDA's ability to carry out its many other important responsibilities. Moreover, part of the regulatory agenda—discouraging tobacco consumption—diverges considerably from the FDA's established mission of assuring the safety and efficacy of socially useful products. In carrying out its customary task of assuring the safety of food, cosmetics, pharmaceuticals, and medical devices, the agency's protective role serves the general interest of the regulated industries as well as that of the consumers; the relationship between FDA and the manufacturers therefore has a collaborative dimension. By contrast, regulation of tobacco would put the agency in an adversarial battle with the tobacco industry. For these reasons, this unique regulatory task might be accomplished more successfully, and at less risk, by an agency (a tobacco control administration) with a unitary mission.

The Committee has no strong views on the issue, although it does lean slightly in the direction of a separate agency. However, if authority were to be delegated to the FDA, the new responsibility should be assigned to a new bureau within FDA with a distinct budget, and should be accompanied by adequate resources to carry out the regulatory mission without impairing the agency's ability to fulfill its many other responsibilities.

Possible Regulatory Initiatives

The agency's regulatory attention should encompass nicotine, tar, and other dangerous constituents of tobacco products, including those added by the manufacturer or produced as byproducts of mainstream or sidestream smoke. The main focus of regulatory attention should be on tar and nicotine. However, the agency should also consider possible means of reducing the specific toxins in tobacco smoke, regardless of whether they are in gas or particulate phase.

A regulatory agenda relating to tar and nicotine cannot be formulated without confronting and resolving the ongoing debate about the possibility of a "less hazardous" cigarette. Most public health advocates are skeptical about the utility of efforts to shift smokers toward low-tar, low-nicotine brands in light of clear evidence that smokers compensate for the reduced nicotine content by inhaling more deeply and more frequently or by blocking vent holes in the filters. In fact, the industry has been criticized for promotional activity that allegedly implies, incorrectly, that "light," reduced tar and nicotine cigarettes are less hazardous. Tobacco control advocates have relied on these "implied health claims" to invoke FDA jurisdiction on the theory that those cigarettes are being promoted to prevent disease, and therefore are "drugs" for purposes of the FDCA.

The actual yield, that is, the amount taken in by people, from particular cigarettes, varies considerably among smokers. As discussed in chapter 2, this is because the standard yield is measured by a machine that smokes cigarettes in a mechanical and standardized way, whereas smokers can smoke their cigarettes with different numbers of puffs, different depths of inhalation, and the like. It is unknown whether there is a relationship between a person's smoking behavior (and therefore actual yields for particular cigarettes) and the person's degree of nicotine dependence or other individual factors. There is evidence that reduction of cigarette yields, particularly comparing the older unfiltered cigarettes to the modern filtered ones, has somewhat reduced the risks of lung cancer and chronic lung disease, although not the risk of coronary heart disease, caused by cigarette smoking.[40] It is unknown if different brands of modern filtered cigarettes with different yields of tar and nicotine produce different risk levels for disease. In any case, it is possible that products with particularly low yields, if the yields are confirmed to be low by measurements in human smokers, would have some advantage in public health terms for smokers who are unable to quit. Satisfactory information for addressing the comparative harmfulness of tobacco products will be available only if a methodology is developed for ascertaining actual yields in human consumers; only then will there be a scientific basis for deciding whether or not to develop a regulatory program centered on reducing yields of tar or nicotine.

Thus, **the regulatory agency, as its first step, should develop a sound methodology for ascertaining the actual yields of nicotine, tar, or any other constituents of tobacco products, based on human consumption.** Human exposure to some constituents of tobacco smoke can be assessed by use of biochemical markers of exposure to those constituents, although at present this methodology is technically difficult and still imprecise; however, it is likely that better exposure measures will be developed in the future. In any case, even the currently available measures of human exposure are likely to provide a better indicator of relative risk than do the standard cigarette smoking machine yields. At a minimum, the smoking machine tests can be modified to reflect the range of ways in which people actually smoke, including numbers of puffs and blocking of ventilation holes, to determine likely *ranges* of delivery. In addition, the manufacturers of tobacco products could be directed to submit information to the regulatory agency regarding the actual yields of their products in humans for particular brands of tobacco products, based on use of prescribed protocols.

A variety of regulatory initiatives relating to tar and nicotine yields can be envisioned. **At a minimum, the regulatory agency should take steps to inform consumers about the meaning of statements regarding tar and nicotine yields, and particularly about the behavioral influences on intake, and the relative importance of the characteristics of the cigarette and the way it is smoked.**[41] The agency might also require that tar and nicotine yields be presented in a standard format, such as absolute content together with a statement of the range of expected systemic yield determined according to number of puffs or other behavioral factors. Currently, marketed cigarettes typically *contain* 8-9 mg nicotine in the tobacco rod, and have an expected actual yield to the smoker of 0.5-3.0 mg nicotine. Stating the nicotine content of the tobacco contained in the cigarettes is important because the content reflects the maximum possible yield, and reduction of content would be expected to result in a reduction in actual yield. Manufacturers might be required to convey this information on the package or through package inserts. In order to avoid misunderstanding, the agency might require consumers to be told that small differences in nominal yield do not reflect significant differences in health risks. Regulations of this nature will improve risk perception among consumers, and will correct any misleading impression about the relative hazards of cigarettes with different levels of tar and nicotine.[42] From the same perspective, the agency should be authorized to ban or regulate use of misleading terms (such as "light") in advertising or on packaging, and should be authorized to require the use of standard terms.

If the regulatory agency finds that reduction of tar and/or nicotine yields would reduce morbidity or mortality associated with use of tobacco products, it should be authorized to prescribe ceilings of tar and/or nicotine yields and to develop a regulatory program of phased reductions in those ceilings over time.

Tar and nicotine yields are closely linked in cigarette smoke. However, it is possible for the manufacturer to unlink them and, as noted earlier, there is evidence that cigarette manufacturers currently manipulate the nicotine yield. The possibility of unlinking tar and nicotine yields has led researchers and public health officials to consider a variety of regulatory strategies. One possibility is a low-tar cigarette that would reduce health risks while providing satisfactory levels of nicotine sought by addicted users. Although this strategy is inherently limited by the fact that the taste of cigarettes is associated with the constituent toxins, it should be explored by the regulatory agency. The potential for reduced levels of tobacco toxins independent of changes in nicotine may be greater for smokeless tobacco.

Another possibility would be to focus directly on reducing the nicotine content as a strategy for reducing addiction and therefore, ultimately, for reducing exposure to the harmful effects of tobacco products. A coordinated strategy of reducing tar and nicotine yields in tandem could also be envisioned.

Public health officials in the United States have heretofore been reluctant to pursue a policy of reducing the tar and nicotine content of tobacco products because of concern about misleading consumers or potential consumers into thinking that tobacco use can be safe. However, international health officials and policymakers in other countries have endorsed and implemented such policies.

International support has been growing for ceilings on tar content. The World Health Organization and the International Union Against Cancer (UICC) have endorsed a goal of reducing tar content of cigarettes to 15 mg. The UICC recommends a progressive eradication of high-tar brands from the market, starting with brands over 25 mg, then 20 mg, and then 15. The European Community has issued a directive requiring its member states to set an upper limit to 15 mg, falling to 12 mg in 1995.

FDA Commissioner Kessler has recently initiated public discussion of nicotine regulation as a primary regulatory strategy. One possible goal of a nicotine reduction strategy might be to reduce the nicotine content below the level that is likely to produce addiction. Based on the intake of cigarette smokers who appear not to be addicted (that is, who smoke less than five cigarettes per day), Benowitz and Henningfield have estimated that "5 mg of nicotine per day is a threshold level of nicotine that would readily establish addiction."[43] Extrapolating from this figure, they calculate that a maximum yield of 0.25 mg of nicotine per cigarette (considering the possible effects of compensatory increases in the intensity of puffing) might be adequate to prevent the development of addiction in most individuals. If the regulatory agency were to use a threshold concept of addiction as a basis for regulatory action, it might gradually depress the ceiling of allowable nicotine yield toward that threshold over a 10- to 15-year period.

A series of reductions in tar and/or nicotine yields would have to be carefully planned and gradually implemented. Imposition of such ceilings could result in the development of a black market in unregulated tobacco products, grown domestically or imported. There could also be substitution effects with different tobacco products or other nicotine delivery systems. It is also conceivable that a regulatory initiative favoring less hazardous tobacco products could lead to increased initiation, which could offset the public health gains among smokers. Thus, complex regulatory judgments will be required. It will also be necessary for the agency to monitor the effects of its regulatory policies in order to ensure that they promote the public health and that the benefits exceed the costs.

In conclusion, this is an important, complex regulatory agenda. It should be implemented with caution, but the complexity of the effort does not justify continuing refusal to undertake it. It is time for Congress to act.

A final caveat is in order. Recent discussions of the possibility of FDA regulation have focused on nicotine. According to the emerging regulatory vo-cabulary, cigarettes and other tobacco products are "nicotine delivery systems." This new vocabulary is useful because it heightens public awareness of the ad-dictive properties of tobacco products and reinforces the premise of this report—that preventing nicotine dependence among children and youths is an essential component of a coherent strategy for reducing the social burden of disease and death associated with smoking and chewing of tobacco.

It must also be remembered, however, that the social burdens of tobacco use are not associated with nicotine *per se*. Nicotine dependence is problematic because it causes use of tobacco, which in turn causes disease and dysfunction, and the nation's regulatory strategy must ultimately maintain a clear focus on the *adverse health effects of using tobacco*. Preventing nicotine dependence among children and youths is a means of protecting the public health, not an end in itself. As the nation moves along the path toward regulation of tobacco prod-ucts, the focus should be on reducing harm related to use of tobacco. Similarly, classification of tobacco products as "nicotine delivery systems" should be de-scribed as a regulatory strategy for promoting the public health, not for winning a "war" against nicotine.

REFERENCES

1. O'Reilly, James T. "A Consistent Ethic of Safety Regulation: The Case for Improving Regu-lation of Tobacco Products." *Administrative Law Journal* 3 (1989): 235-250.

2. *Ibid.*

3. *Action on Smoking and Health v. Harris.* 655 F. 2d 236 (D.C. Cir. 1980).

4. *United States v. 46 Cartons, More or Less, Containing Fairfax Cigarettes.* 113 F. Supp 336 (D. N.J., 1953).

5. *United States v. 354 Bulk Cartons Trim Reducing-Aid Cigarettes.* 178 F. Supp. 847 (D. N.J., 1959).

6. Kessler, David A. Letter to Scott Balin, Coalition on Smoking OR Health. 25 Feb. 1994.

7. Hilts, Philip. "Tobacco Chiefs Say Cigarettes Aren't Addictive." *New York Times* (15 Apr. 1994): A1.

8. *Comprehensive Smoking Education Act of 1984.* P.L. 98-474. Section 2. 12 Oct. 1984.

9. *Cigarette and Labeling Advertising Act of 1965.*

10. Warner, Kenneth E. "Clearing the Airwaves: The Cigarette Ban Revisited." *Policy Analysis* 5:4 (1979): 435-450.

11. *Public Health Cigarette Smoking Act of 1969.*

12. *Cipollone v. Ligget Group, Inc.* 112 S. Ct. 2608 (1992).

13. Myers, M. L., C. Jennings, W. Lenox, E. Minsky, and A. Sachs. "Federal Trade Commission Staff Report on the Cigarette Advertising Investigation." *Federal Trade Commission Report* (May 1981).

14. *Comprehensive Smoking Education Act*, Sec. 4.

15. *Comprehensive Smokeless Tobacco Health Education Act of 1986.* P.L. 99-252. Section 3. 27 Feb. 1986.

16. Centers for Disease Control and Prevention. *Preventing Tobacco Use Among Young People: A Report of the Surgeon General.* S/N 017-001-004901-0. Washington, DC: U.S. Government Printing Office, 1994. 262.

17. Levanthal, Howard, Kathleen Glynn, and Raymond Fleming. "Is the Smoking Decision an 'Informed Choice'? Effect of Smoking Risk Factors on Smoking Beliefs." *Journal of the American Medical Association* 257:24 (26 June 1987): 3373-3376.

18. Johnston, L., J. Bachman, and P. O'Malley. "Monitoring the Future Study." Press release. The University of Michigan, Ann Arbor. January 27, 1994.

19. Centers for Disease Control and Prevention. *Preventing Tobacco Use*, 262.

20. Fischer, Paul M., John W. Richards, Earl F. Berman, and Dean M. Krugman. "Recall and Eye Tracking Study of Adolescents Viewing Tobacco Advertisements." *Journal of the American Medical Association* 261 (1989): 84-89.

21. *Ibid.*

22. Brubaker R. G., and S. K. Mirby. "Health-Risk Warning Labels on Smokeless Tobacco Products: Are They Effective?" *Addictive Behavior* 15 (1990): 115-118.

23. Myers et al.

24. Davis, Ronald M., and Juliette S. Kendrick. "The Surgeon General's Warnings in Outdoor Cigarette Advertising: Are They Readable?" *Journal of the American Medical Association* 261 (1989): 90-94.

25. Cullingford, R., L. Da Cruz, S. Webb, R. Shean, and K. Jamrozik. "Legibility of Health Warnings on Billboards that Advertise Cigarettes." *Medical Journal of Australia* 148 (1988): 336-338.

26. Centre for Behavioral Research in Cancer. *Health Warnings and Contents Labelling on Tobacco Products.* For Ministerial Council on Drug Strategy, Tobacco Task Force on Tobacco Health Warnings. Anti-Cancer Council of Victoria, Australia. 1992. 9-20, 31, 85-131.

27. Cohen, J., and T. Srull. *Information Processing Issues Involved in the Communication and Retrieval of Cigarette Warning Information. Report to the Federal Trade Commission.* Center for Consumer Research: University of Florida, 1980.

28. Bhalla, G., and J. L. Lastovicka. "The Impact of Changing Cigarette Warning Message Content and Format." *Advances in Consumer Research* 11 (1984): 305-310. Cited in Kaiserman, Murray. "The Effectiveness of Health Warning Messages." *Tobacco Control* 2 (1993): 267-269.

29. Myers et al.

30. Mayer, Robert N., Ken R. Smith, and Debra L. Scammon. "Evaluating the Impact of Alcohol Warning Labels." *Advances in Consumer Research* 18 (1991): 713.

31. Kaskutas, Lee, and Thomas K. Greenfield. "First Effects of Warning Labels on Alcoholic Beverage Containers." *Drug and Alcohol Dependence* 31 (1992): 1-14.

32. Beltramini, Richard F. "Perceived Believability of Warning Label Information Presented in Cigarette Advertising." *Journal of Advertising* 17:1 (1988): 26-32.

33. Fischer, Paul M., Dean M. Krugman, James E. Fletcher, Richard J. Fox, and Tina H. Rojas. "An Evaluation of Health Warnings in Cigarette Adverstisements Using Standard Market Research Methods: What Does It Mean to Warn?" *Tobacco Control* 2 (1993): 279-285.

34. Myers et al.

35. Fischer et al.

36. *Tobacco Products Control Act 1993*. P.C. 1993-1542. 21 July 1993. In *Canada Gazette Part II.* 127:16 (8 Nov. 1993): 3277ff.

37. Kaiserman, Murray. "The Effectiveness of Health Warning Messages." *Tobacco Control* 2 (1993): 267-269.

38. Federal Trade Commission. *Report to Congress for 1991. Pursuant to the Federal Cigarette Labeling and Advertising Act.* 1994. 15.

39. Kessler, David A. "Statement on Nicotine-Containing Cigarettes." To the House Subcommittee on Health and the Environment, U.S. Congress. 25 March 1994.

40. Benowitz, Neal L. "Health and Public Policy Implications of the 'Low Yield' Cigarette." *New England Journal of Medicine* 320:24 (15 June 1989): 1619-1621.

41. See for example: Kozlowski, Lynn. *Low Tar Cigarettes Are Hazardous to Your Health.* Toronto: Alcohol and Drug Addiction Research Foundation, 1993.

42. Viscusi, W. Kipp. *Smoking: Making the Risky Decision.* New York: Oxford Univerity Press, 1992.

43. Benowitz, Neal L., and Jack E. Henningfield. "Establishing a Nicotine Threshold for Addiction." *New England Journal of Medicine* 331:2 (1994): 123-125.

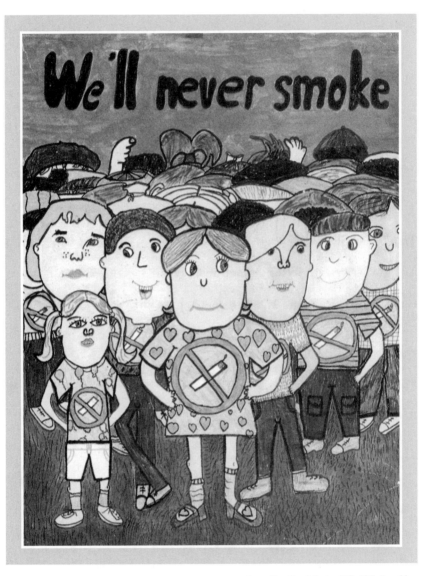

Amarilys Candelaria, P.S. 124, Brooklyn

CONTENTS

9 | COORDINATION OF POLICIES AND RESEARCH

Recent data show that progress has stalled toward achieving the Healthy People 2000 goal of reducing, by half, smoking initiation among youths. Preventing smoking initiation by youths is the most efficient means of reducing long-term morbidity and mortality from heart disease, cancer, chronic lung disease, and other tobacco-related disorders.

In recent years, the emphasis of tobacco control has been shifting from interventions aimed at individual smokers to those intended to change the social environment in which tobacco use takes root. The most effective preventive measures are likely to be universal interventions that reduce youth access to tobacco products and that promote and reinforce a tobacco-free social norm. These measures generally fall in the realm of social policy—taxation of tobacco products, enforcement of youth access laws, constraints on advertising and promotion, regulation of tobacco products, and tobacco control advocacy for tobacco-free environments.

Previous chapters have dealt with the addictive process, promotion of a tobacco-free social norm, preventive and cessation interventions, advertising and promotion of tobacco, pricing and taxation, youth access, and regulation of tobacco products. The potential policies are numerous and diverse, but the Committee has made specific recommendations in those chapters for policy measures it believes will achieve the greatest reduction in tobacco use in the shortest time. Those recommendations will not be repeated or summarized here. This chapter focuses on the coordination of policy and research on the implementation of comprehensive approaches to tobacco control.

257

THE ROLE OF THE FEDERAL GOVERNMENT

Leadership

The most important role of the federal government is to provide leadership for the nation in a comprehensive multi-pronged effort to achieve a society free of tobacco-related disease and death. This responsibility requires the setting of goals, together with a visible and emphatic commitment to achieve those goals. As discussed below, this does not mean that the federal government should try to manage or direct state and local initiatives or those of the private sector. The nation does not need a "czar" of tobacco control. However, the federal government must commit *itself* to the effort and, by its own actions, lead the way. Until now, this has not been the case.

There are important signs of change. The General Services Administration has established a smoke-free policy for federal buildings. The Occupational Safety and Health Administration (OSHA) has initiated a rule-making process that could require smoke-free policies for all workplaces covered by OSHA. The Department of Defense has implemented a smoke-free workplace policy. The Food and Drug Administration has initiated an important discussion regarding the need for regulation of tobacco products. The surgeon general's 1994 report on smoking and health was devoted to children and youths and, upon its release, Surgeon General Elders called for restriction on advertising and promotion of tobacco products.

Since 1964, the surgeon general has provided the most consistent and most authoritative federal voice on tobacco control. The annual reports on smoking and health have documented the health consequences of tobacco use and disseminated new research findings to broad public and scientific audiences, and substantial progress in reducing smoking prevalence has been achieved over the past three decades, since Surgeon General Luther Terry issued the federal government's first comprehensive report on the devastating health toll caused by smoking. However, the surgeon general has no direct-line authority to regulate tobacco products, provide technical assistance to states, monitor public health, conduct research, or provide service. Nor does the surgeon general have the authority to manage or coordinate these activities, which are spread throughout the Public Health Service. In the Committee's view, however, the problem of coordination, which will be addressed below, is separate from the issue of leadership.

Federal leadership requires an unequivocal commitment to tobacco control, and specifically to a youth-centered tobacco control policy, that is acknowledged and vigorously pursued by all agencies of the federal government. This means that the goal of preventing nicotine addiction must be enunciated clearly and that the specific objectives of *Healthy People 2000* (and successor documents) should set the template for all federal activities. The commitment must be unequivocal and visible throughout the Executive Branch and in Congress.

Regulation of the Tobacco Industry

The most evident failure of federal leadership has been in Congress. In some instances, legislative action has actually retarded progress toward tobacco control. Many of the major recommendations in this report are directed to Congress, including those that have the highest priority in the Committee's view. Specifically, Congress should enact a major increase in tobacco excise taxes to discourage consumption as well as raise revenues. Congress should repeal the law that preempts state and local regulation of advertising and promotion occurring exclusively within the state's boundaries, and should also enact comprehensive restrictions on advertising and promotion of tobacco products. Congress should also rectify its massive regulatory default by enacting a comprehensive scheme for regulating the labeling, packaging, and constituents of tobacco products, and by conferring regulatory authority on FDA or a separate tobacco control agency.

Some federal regulatory initiatives can be undertaken without congressional action. The Food and Drug Administration could use its existing authority to regulate tobacco products and labeling. The Federal Trade Commission could take a more active role in assuring that advertising and promotion of tobacco complies with existing statutory requirements. The Environmental Protection Agency has stepped forward in recent years to review the effects of environmental tobacco smoke, and OSHA is considering regulations restricting smoking in the workplace. The Department of Transportation has promulgated regulations that ban smoking on domestic airline flights. An active, multi-pronged regulatory effort at the federal level can set the tone for analogous actions at the state and local levels.

Monitoring Public Health and Providing Technical Assistance to States

One of the most promising federal initiatives in recent years has been community mobilization efforts for state-level tobacco control. This effort evolved from research and is developing into a technical assistance function that the federal government provides to the states. The movement was pioneered by the National Cancer Institute (NCI) through its American Stop Smoking Intervention Study (ASSIST), which concentrates on building a statewide infrastructure through a state's department of health and through local coalitions. The coalitions mobilize the community to conduct policy and media advocacy activities. The idea for the ASSIST program grew out of decades of work at NCI, particularly strategic planning by the Smoking and Tobacco Control Program.[1]

In 1991, NCI funded 17 states to participate in the ASSIST program, which encompasses 2 years of assessment, analysis, and planning, and 5 years of program implementation. During that time, states will attempt to build permanent capabilities for continuing tobacco control activities when federal funding ceases. In 1993, in its IMPACT Project, CDC initiated cooperative agreements with the non-ASSIST states to help them develop tobacco control efforts. Similarly, through the SmokeLess States program, the Robert Wood Johnson Foundation has funded 10 states to enhance their efforts.

The Committee commends the National Cancer Institute, the Centers for Disease Control and Prevention, and the Robert Wood Johnson Foundation for these important programs, but has several concerns about their future. As initially planned, the ASSIST program is time-limited. ASSIST is a demonstration program, a culmination of a research approach; in time, the emphasis should shift from demonstration to permanent program operation and support. To expedite the progress of state-based policy efforts, the CDC IMPACT states, which currently receive an average of $211,000 per year (for core states) and $74,000 per year (for states in the planning phase), should be funded to an amount commensurate with their task. The ASSIST states receive an average of $900,000 per year. **Funding to the non-ASSIST states should be increased to a level commensurate with ASSIST states.** This could be accomplished by expanding the current ASSIST project to non-ASSIST states with an expectation of long-term support, or by increasing CDC's IMPACT program to increase the funding per state to ASSIST levels and expanding the program to include ASSIST states as NCI funding terminates. The NIH Revitalization Act of 1993 opted to increase the set-aside of annual NCI cancer control activities and exhorted NCI "to assume increasing leadership in the demonstration, implementation, and operation of programs to reduce or control the incidence of cancer" and specifically to use the increased funds "to fully fund each of the existing 17 ASSIST states and support related programs of the 33 states without ASSIST programs" (Report of the Conference Committee on S.1, *Congressional Record* 139:72 [May 20, 1993]: H2648).

The Committee believes that state-based efforts along the line of the ASSIST and IMPACT programs are among the most promising policy initiatives. For effective continuation, these programs will require either a commitment to practical operation of a non-research effort at NCI until states develop the requisite infrastructure, a significantly increased funding and staffing of the IMPACT program at CDC, or a combination of the two options. The level of federal funding should depend on whether the states have successfully established the infrastructure required to sustain the tobacco control effort over the long term. The federal funding role is not envisioned to be a permanent one. How long it will be necessary remains to be seen.

The program of technical assistance to states is but one of the promising avenues pursued by the Office on Smoking and Health (OSH), whose budget rose from $3.5 million in 1984 to $20 million in 1994.[2] CDC is also the nation's preeminent public health monitoring agency, with a series of health-reporting structures and periodic national data-gathering surveys. Tracking statistics on smoking, use of smokeless tobacco, and health outcomes such as the morbidity and mortality caused by tobacco-related diseases will be an essential feature of national tobacco control policy. Gathering those data is one of CDC's main functions.

In addition to CDC, the Office of the Assistant Secretary for Health and the Inspector General's Office of the Department of Health and Human Services have important public health monitoring functions. The inspector general monitors the functioning of the agencies with the department, and has issued reports on various aspects of tobacco control. The Office of the Assistant Secretary for Health administrator, the Public Health Service, and its Office on Health Promotion and Disease Prevention coordinate prevention activities throughout the Public Health Service, including progress toward achieving the goals set forth in *Healthy People 2000*.

Support of Research

The federal government has traditionally carried the major responsibility for funding tobacco-related research. In recent years, other sponsors, such as the California Tobacco-Related Disease Research Program, funded under Proposition 99, and the Robert Wood Johnson Foundation, have underwritten important investigations. Even with diversification of support, however, the federal government will continue to play a central role. In so doing, federal agencies should coordinate their efforts in order to ensure that research support is available for all aspects of tobacco-related research. The research strategy should be rooted in a comprehensive public health model of nicotine addiction, one that encompasses environment, agent, host, and vector. ("Vector" refers, in this paradigm, to the industry.)

Specifically, further research is needed to elucidate the basic biology of addiction and how tobacco use results in adverse health outcomes. Such research is needed to provide valuable clues about how better to prevent nicotine addiction and to avoid specific diseases associated with tobacco use. Simultaneously with a basic and clinical research agenda, a complementary agenda should be supported to conduct epidemiologic studies to identify the characteristics of children and youths most at risk for initiating tobacco use, behavioral research to test prevention programs, sociocultural research to elucidate differences in risk and responsiveness to prevention interventions among various ethnic and racial groups, and surveillance to monitor the trends in tobacco use. Epidemiologic research should include nationally representative samples, preadolescents at the beginning of longitudinal investigations, and multiple levels of risk factors, including larger social-environmental factors (such as price, exposure to advertising, and promotional activities). Such studies would necessitate large sample sizes and careful selection of proximal to distal factors but might provide a more complete explanation of etiology than that which is currently available. Particular attention should be paid to further understanding some of the well-known risk factors and correlates of tobacco use, such as low socioeconomic status, and psychosocial characteristics, such as sensation-seeking.

Knowledge about health interventions and the system of care is needed in addition to understanding the biology of addiction and the mechanisms of tobacco-related disease. The Agency for Health Care Policy and Research (AHCPR) is the part of the federal Public Health Service responsible for carrying out health services research. This includes the study of health outcome measures, clinical practice guidelines, quality assurance, and system performance indicators. AHCPR has, for example, focused on clinical use of nicotine patches in the treatment of nicotine addiction. AHCPR could, in addition, become the home for policy-relevant research focused on the health care system.

A Multicultural Research Agenda

The marked divergence in smoking prevalence between African-American teens and white teens over the past decade, for example, is clear in multiple data sets, but its underlying cause is unknown. Some attribute the disparities to reporting bias, that is, they believe that African-American youths report lower than actual use. To explain the differences in the data, this reporting bias would have to be selective for African-American youths compared with other groups, and would also have to differ consistently between younger and older African Americans. If there is consistent bias, it may be that the survey instruments used to gather the data are culturally biased and need to be improved. If, on the other hand, the results reflect a real trend, the implications are intriguing and important. It could be that progress in tobacco control among African-American youths is a success story revealing a stronger tobacco-free norm, or a failure of tobacco advertising to reach this market segment. If the norm was created by a specific intervention of, for example, churches, or by cultural consensus against youth tobacco use, then efforts to pursue similar measures for other populations might be productive; if the reductions stem from lack of attention from advertisers, or inadvertent alienation of African-American youths from advertising messages, then it could be highly instructive to learn how these processes worked, in hopes of devising effective measures for other groups.

The United States comprises an immense diversity of subcultures, both rural and urban, within this multiethnic, multiracial population. The Committee has also repeatedly observed in reports from national data and small pilot studies, and in focus groups conducted by Committee members, that tobacco use varies regionally and among ethnic and social groups and even within these groups. Hence, underlying the aggregate statistics that describe large-scale trends over time is a multitude of differences in norms and behaviors regarding tobacco use. Elucidating those differences requires social science research. Much more work is needed to elucidate the etiologic factors that affect prevalence of tobacco use among different cultural groups and to understand how environmental and cultural influences interact with biological factors. The public health goal of reducing tobacco use is clear, but the appropriate approach to achieving that goal is certain to depend critically on social organization and cultural norms. **Social science research should be conducted to enhance understanding of how norms are formed and transmitted, and of the regional and cultural differences in the acceptability of tobacco use.**

A Youth-Centered Research Agenda

The Committee requested descriptive abstracts of research studies and funding amounts from all federal agencies known to have research programs related to youth tobacco use and control, and from private foundations and large state efforts. Our analysis of data obtained from the CRISP system (Computer Retrieval of Information on Scientific Projects) shows that total funding for research grants from 1990 to 1993 on issues related to tobacco use by children and youths was approximately $119 million. Of this amount, about $47.5 million (less than half) supported primary research efforts, that is, studies that identified youth tobacco issues as the principal subject of investigation. The remainder of related research funding went to studies that included youth tobacco issues as incidental (secondary) to the investigation. It is important to note that not all primary studies directly or specifically targeted issues related to youth tobacco use. Primary studies included research that looked at all related issues, such as the effects of environmental tobacco smoke exposure on respiratory control in infants, the effects of *in utero* exposure to the components of tobacco on fetal growth and development, the effects of cigarette smoke constituents on the immune system, smoking cessation programs for pregnant women, and so on. Funding for primary research that directly and specifically targets tobacco use in children and youths represents approximately 25% ($30 million) of the total for those years.

Breaking the research into categories by type, in addition to principal focus (primary versus secondary), reveals a clearer picture of public health funding for research on tobacco use in children and youths. For the purposes of this report, research was placed in one of five categories for analysis: basic science, epidemiology, prevention, cessation, and psychosocial factors.

Basic Science (biophysiologic, pharmacologic, technologic, and/or training studies): Primary studies were funded for around $3.5 million; however, no research dollars were reported on basic research specifically relating nicotine addiction or the biological consequences of tobacco use to children and youths.

Epidemiology (prevalence, relation to disease, and/or risk factor studies): Primary epidemiologic research directly targeted to tobacco use in children and youths (2 studies) accounted for a little over $500,000, or around 10% of all dollars spent on primary epidemiologic research.

Prevention (school-based, community-based, and skills training projects, policy studies, and/or education through the media): Twenty primary research studies on prevention of initiation were targeted directly to children and youths, representing just over half ($22.5 million) of total grant monies allocated for prevention studies. While proportionately more funding went to prevention research, this amount is still less than one-fifth of all research dollars allocated for youth tobacco-related research for the period.

Cessation (school-based, community-based, and skills training projects, policy studies, and/or education through the media): Studies directly targeted to cessation of tobacco use in children and youths (5 studies) accounted for almost $6 million of about 13.5 million primary cessation dollars allocated.

Psychosocial (theoretical models of behavior change, social factors or predictors of tobacco use, and/or development of assessment tools): Primary psychosocial research received just under $3 million in funding, of which about half ($1.4 million) was specifically directed to tobacco use by youths (5 studies).

In all five categories of primary research, 32 of the 62 funded studies directly targeted tobacco use in children and youths. Of these 32 studies, 8 addressed culturally specific populations (1 study looked at Hispanic, African American, and non-Hispanic white teens, one at Hispanic teens only, 4 at American Indian teens only, and 2 at African American teens only). Of these 8 studies, 6 were prevention studies and 2 were epidemiologic studies. One primary study directly targeted to children and youths addressed policy. This was one prevention study that looked at local policy change to reduce tobacco availability. Four studies looked specifically at preventing the use of smokeless tobacco by youths, while an additional 8 studies included smokeless tobacco use in conjunction with smoking prevention.

After reviewing these data, the Committee concluded that the focus of the research effort relative to youths and tobacco use has been preventive interventions, especially school-based interventions. These interventions have achieved some success, and such efforts should continue to be an element in a youth-centered tobacco control policy. Unfortunately, few if any of these studies explored in a culturally appropriate way the group-specific characteristics of tobacco use among members of the major ethnic groups in the United States. Apart from the preventive intervention research, however, the research base is weak. For example, despite intriguing and potentially important insights about ethnic differences in youth smoking that have been widening for two decades, there are only two epidemiologic studies for a total of $500,000 focused on youth. The Committee did not find quantitative or qualitative sociological or anthropological studies that might test the validity of the reported ethnic differences, or elucidate the mechanisms if they are indeed valid. Only 5 studies address the wealth of social and interpersonal influences that the Committee believes are central to youth initiation. And the federal support for policy studies is extremely weak with only a single study, except to the extent that youth smoking is made part of NCI's ASSIST, CDC's states initiative, and the general service programs of the Center for Substance Abuse Prevention (CSAP).

The budgets for research on the diseases caused by tobacco use—such as cancer, heart disease, and lung disease—are considerably larger than the amounts devoted to direct study of the cause—tobacco use. The NCI budget for tobacco research and control was $47 million in 1991 and $60 million in 1993.[3,4] Smoking accounts for an estimated 30% of deaths from cancer, for example, but tobacco control accounts for only about 3% of the National Cancer Institute's $2 billion budget. Tobacco use is linked to 20% of deaths from heart disease and is the main cause of chronic lung disease,[5] but tobacco-related research accounts for only $24 million of the National Heart, Lung, and Blood Institute budget, and only $122 million of the total NIH budget.[6] Nicotine is the most prevalent addiction, and the health toll from tobacco is vastly greater than that for illicit substances, and yet relatively little nicotine research is supported by the National Institute on Drug Abuse. While the disability caused by tobacco use should not necessarily bear a linear relationship to the research effort at the federal research institutes, the Committee nonetheless believes that nicotine addiction and the health effects of other tobacco constituents merit greater emphasis.

The Committee concludes that initiation of tobacco use by youths is a critical event in the causation of a large number of severely disabling and deadly conditions. **Federal agencies that sponsor tobacco-related research should increase the resources devoted to understanding and preventing initiation of tobacco use by children and youths.** In particular, attention should be given to the factors that predict tobacco use initiation among members of the major ethnic groups in the United States. The critical problem of youth initiation has received inadequate research support, and studies that explicitly attend to youth should be given high program priority. As background for this effort, Congress might request that the relevant federal agencies (1) prepare a baseline report on their specific research activities aimed at preventing initiation of youth tobacco use during the past 5 years, and (2) use that foundation as a starting point for developing long- and short-term research plans, with funding needs and allocations specified. Congress should require a tracking of progress, possibly by requesting the federal agencies to prepare annual reports summarizing program announcements, requests for applications, targeted training grants, relevant program project and center grants, and other relevant activities.

A Policy-Oriented Research Agenda

In its review, the Committee was constrained by the dearth of policy research on tobacco control. Policy research, both empirical and theoretical, is conducted to generate information useful in making and implementing policy choices by local, state, and federal governments and by the private sector. Policy research is usually interdisciplinary, involving the social sciences and other fields. It includes, for example, studies of how excise taxes decrease consumption, how community organization affects the effectiveness of tobacco control measures, how enforcement of youth access laws can reduce illicit sales, the impact of "tombstone" advertising on sales and use rates, and similar studies.

In particular, policy research that distinguishes what is effective for youths is lacking. If tobacco control policies come to focus on prevention of youth initiation, determining what works for youths, regardless of its effectiveness for adults, will be important. For example, policy studies support the concept of an increase in the excise tax (and hence price) as a means of reducing purchases (and presumably use) among youths. As discussed in chapter 6, data indicated that youths are sensitive to price; smoking prevalence declines among youths when the price of cigarettes increases. Evidence from California also support this price-sensitivity hypothesis for the general population.[7] Determining the effect of price on the purchasing behavior of youths is a central question in tobacco control. This is but one example of important unanswered questions amenable to research which, if answered, could lead to effective policy and program choices for preventing nicotine addiction in children and youths. Recently, general policy initiatives have been introduced. The Robert Wood Johnson Foundation (RWJF) initiated a tobacco policy research program in 1991, and renewed that effort in 1993; the National Cancer Institute began a $1 million policy research effort in 1993. The California and Massachusetts programs have also included a component of policy research. **Federal agencies should give special attention to research on the efficacy of policies aiming to prevent initiation of tobacco use by youths.**

Services

Several agencies of the federal government provide or fund services relevant to youth tobacco use. The Health Resources and Services Administration funds grants and demonstrations for health programs, primarily through block grants. The Center for Substance Abuse Prevention also funds block grants, but its mission is focused as its name implies. CSAP's mandate was expanded in 1993 to include nicotine addiction, and recent grants have reflected this change. Services for treatment are federally funded through the Center for Substance Abuse Treatment, a sister agency to CSAP. In addition to their block grant authority, the Health Resources and Services Administration, the Center for Substance Abuse Prevention, and the Center for Substance Abuse Treatment also have technical assistance mandates. CSAP, for example, has established a clearinghouse for substance abuse prevention programs, which will be a national clearinghouse and technical assistance center. It will include tobacco products under its purview, although it will also address alcohol and illicit drugs.

In addition to the agencies that fund primarily through block grants, several federal agencies provide direct services. The Department of Defense provides health services for those in the military and their dependents. It also manages commissaries, post exchanges, and other tobacco outlets, and controls policies over tobacco use on its bases and in its facilities. The Indian Health Service (IHS), part of the Public Health Service, provides services to American-Indian populations throughout the nation. Because of its expertise and access to American-Indian populations, IHS is ideally suited to address the distinctive tobacco use issues among the various tribes, for example, the high rates of use of smokeless tobacco by boys and girls in some tribes. The Department of Education prepares curriculum aids for health education to assist teachers throughout the nation; these can incorporate a focus on the use and harmful effects of tobacco products. This mechanism has been used to produce programs on drug abuse, and could be similarly used in the education of youths about tobacco use. Some ASSIST states have included educational materials that could be used as models.

THE ROLE OF STATE AND LOCAL GOVERNMENTS

Much of the leadership on tobacco control has come from states and local governments. In 1988, California passed Proposition 99, which increased the state excise tax by $0.25 per pack and devoted a fraction of those revenues to support education (20% was stipulated by law, but the actual figure has never matched this) and research (5%). In 1992, Massachusetts also passed a comprehensive tobacco control package. In 1993, 23 states passed 37 less comprehensive tobacco control laws, including excise tax increases, youth access restrictions, vending machine restrictions, indoor air controls, public smoking bans, and other measures—many of which will have an impact on youth tobacco use. This state initiative is similar to NCI's ASSIST program, CDC's initiative to bolster state public health departments, and the RWJF SmokeLess States initiative.

Local governments have passed a multitude of ordinances against smoking in public places and workplaces, restricting vending machines, and establishing licensing procedures. By May 1993, NCI found that there were more than 700 such ordinances nationwide.[8] In tobacco control, the federal government has lagged well behind the more venturesome states and local governments.

One feature of Proposition 99 that most appealed to voters was the direct linkage between the new excise tax and expenditures on tobacco control (education and research). A similar measure would have been unlikely to emerge from the legislative process, because it crosses the jurisdictional boundaries of committees. (One committee controls tax collection and finances, and other committees control expenditures.) By linking taxes collected to tobacco control measures, Proposition 99 created a tax that, if successful in reducing tobacco use, also reduces public expenditures toward that end. This has already begun to happen in California. In addition to this self-regulating feature, however, the linkage between levying a tax and using it to promote a directly related public health goal helps focus political accountability. Unfortunately, that same linkage has made the program a continuing source of political wrangling, as the tobacco industry confronts the tobacco control features. The educational and research elements funded by Proposition 99 have, therefore, gone through many fits and starts in their short and tempestuous history.

In addition to the dedicated tobacco control programs that have emerged in a few states, all states also maintain a capacity to monitor public health, provide services, and regulate products—functions parallel to those discussed above for the federal government. The exact configuration of these functions varies widely, but all states have some public health capacity that can incorporate tobacco control policies. Most states do not sustain a large research capacity, unlike the federal government, although California has been an exception in this regard: the Tobacco-Related Diseases Research Program is larger than its counterparts in federal agencies, remarkable given its origin in a single state. Much work of national importance is thus being supported by this one state's research program. The nation would benefit if other states were also to contribute to research as they become more engaged in tobacco control.

Discussions on the tobacco excise tax at the federal level have to date focused on generating revenue for health care reform and other programs, not on the public health goal of reducing use of tobacco products. There has been little discussion of replicating this feature of the California tobacco control program. The Committee acknowledges that an exactly parallel program at the federal level is politically and practically infeasible. Making a tax policy serve the purposes of public health cuts across jurisdictions among congressional committees, making it difficult to develop a coherent policy. Furthermore, many executive branch agencies already have a role in tobacco control, a situation more complex than in many states where tobacco control is being developed. And there is no federal counterpart to citizen-initiated ballot initiatives such as Proposition 99. For these reasons, the states are likely to provide the policy leadership and models for the federal government rather than the reverse.

THE ROLE OF PRIVATE SECTOR ORGANIZATIONS

Tobacco control policy has largely grown from the bottom up; private organizations have been crucial to the policy successes that have been achieved. Many corporations, labor unions, religious organizations, and other groups have taken steps on their own, without government pressure, to discourage tobacco use. Their actions have served as models for other organizations. Private voluntary health organizations such as the American Cancer Society (ACS), the American Heart Association (AHA), and the American Lung Association (ALA) have also played crucial roles. Those three groups took a further significant step in 1981 by forming the Coalition for Smoking OR Health. The coalition invites participation from other groups, but the three private voluntaries have been its stalwart supporters.

The Advocacy Institute in Washington, D.C., has become a clearinghouse for tobacco control information, offering the Smoking Control Advocacy Resource Center Network (SCARCNet), an on-line source of information contributed by members throughout the country. Dozens of advocacy organizations have emerged throughout the nation to promote tobacco control policies. Prominent among these grassroots organizations are Americans for Nonsmokers' Rights (ANR) (which started as Californians for Nonsmokers' Rights), Doctors Ought to Care (DOC), Stop Teenage Addiction to Tobacco (STAT), Action on Smoking and Health (ASH), and the Tobacco Products Liability Project. Among these, STAT is the major national advocacy group primarily concerned with youth tobacco use. There are also several regional groups that have effected local policy change, such as Smokefree Educational Services in New York City and Stop Tobacco Access for Minors (STAMP) in Northern California. Joseph DiFranza edits *Tobacco Access Law News,* a bimonthly newsletter disseminated to tobacco control advocates.

The Robert Wood Johnson Foundation has emerged as the leading source of foundation support for tobacco control, as a prominent part of its work against substance abuse. Many other foundations have supported projects from time to time, particularly foundations that support local activities throughout the nation, but RWJF alone has channeled a part of its substantial funding resources into tobacco control. Its attention to policy research, beginning in 1991, has been a major factor, as well as its support for most of the nationally and regionally prominent advocacy organizations, including all those mentioned above. (See table 9-1 for a list of organizational roles in tobacco control.)

LINKAGE BETWEEN EXCISE TAX REVENUES AND TOBACCO CONTROL PROGRAM FUNDING

Some of the policy proposals made in this report can be effected with little expenditure of public funds or loss of revenues. Bans on advertising and vending machines, for example, or restrictions on promotional activities require only modest resources for enforcement. Some items are moderate in cost, such as increased budgets for research and coordination. Some options are costly: for example, creation of a regulatory regime for tobacco products will require a moderate increase in public funding for tobacco control. Expansion of

TABLE 9-1   Functions and organizations concerned with preventing tobacco use among children and youths

Function	Organization	Specific roles
Regulation	Food and Drug Administration	Possible role regarding tobacco products as drug delivery devices
	Federal Trade Commission	Enforce truth in advertising, possible role in regulating promotions
	Environmental Protection Agency	Environmental tobacco smoke standard
	Consumer Product Safety Commission	Tobacco currently exempted
	State and local governments	Enforcement of youth access laws; vending machine standards; licensing of sales outlets; advertising restrictions
Public health monitoring	Centers for Disease Control and Prevention (esp. Office on Smoking and Health and National Center for Health Statistics)	Office on Smoking and Health; prepare surgeon general's reports; staff Interagency Committee on Smoking and Health; coordinate federal public health efforts; monitor smoking rates; gather national health statistics; liaison with state health and substance abuse offices
	Office of the Inspector General, Department of Health and Human Services	Reports on youth access, spit tobacco, public health agencies' tobacco control measures
	Office of the Assistant Secretary for Health	Healthy People 2000 objectives; coordination of Public Health Service agencies
	State offices for substance abuse and health	Gather state health statistics, liaison with CDC, coordinate with local governments
	Association of State and Territorial Health Officials	Annual report on state tobacco control efforts

TABLE 9-1 *Continued*

Function	Organization	Specific roles
Research	National Institute on Drug Abuse	Basic, clinical, and preventive intervention research on addiction
	National Cancer Institute	Basic, clinical, and preventive intervention research on cancer; ASSIST program; COMMIT program; new program on policy research
	National Heart, Lung, and Blood Institute	Basic, clinical, and preventive intervention research on pulmonary and cardiovascular disorders
	National Institute on Child Health and Human Development	Basic, clinical, and preventive intervention research on childhood disorders
	Agency for Health Care Policy and Research	Health outcomes, quality assurance, clinical practice guidelines, system performance measures, and health policy research
	Tobacco-Related Diseases Research Program	California state-funded research program: basic, clinical, prevention, and policy research
Services	Health Resources and Services Administration	Federal funding to state block grants for health; limited direct grants for health services; health professional training; program evaluation
	Substance Abuse and Mental Health Services Administration (esp. Center for Substance Abuse Prevention)	Federal funding to state block grants for substance abuse; technical assistance for state and local government; program evaluation

continued on next page

TABLE 9-1 *Continued*

Function	Organization	Specific roles
Services—*continued*	State offices for substance abuse and health; county and local governments	Direct funding of special programs; some states have dedicated tobacco control efforts; education through university system
	Indian Health Service	American-Indian health services
	Department of Defense	Tobacco use in military facilities; health services for military personnel and their dependents
	Department of Education	Materials and technical assistance for schools
Private research and professional organizations	American Heart Association	Cardiovascular research; Coalition on Smoking OR Health
	American Lung Association	Lung research; Coalition on Smoking OR Health
	American Cancer Society	Cancer research; Coalition on Smoking OR Health
	American Medical Association	SmokeLess States
Advocacy	Advocacy Institute	National advocacy
	Coalition on Smoking OR Health	National advocacy organization, funded by ACS, ALA, AHA and joined by many professional and private voluntary health organizations
	Stop Teenage Addiction to Tobacco (STAT)	National volunteer organization
	Doctors Ought to Care (DOC)	National physician and health professional advocacy organization
	Americans for Nonsmokers' Rights	National advocacy organization
	Join Together	Advocacy resource center

TABLE 9-1 *Continued*

Function	Organization	Specific roles
Private foundation	Robert Wood Johnson Foundation	Support for research, demonstrations, policy, and advocacy on substance abuse

programs for anti-tobacco media campaigns and assistance to state public health offices for tobacco control would entail substantial budget commitments. It is essential that agencies to which Congress and state governments delegate responsibility for tobacco control measures be given sufficient resources to accomplish their tasks. This was a theme that recurred often in interviews with government officials, advocates, and academic experts.

The most sensible models have been established in California, Michigan, and Massachusetts, and should be adopted in other states. At the federal level, if an increase in excise tax on tobacco products is contemplated by Congress in the near future, as part of health care reform or other legislation, **Congress should ensure that some fraction of revenues raised by the federal excise tax on tobacco products be devoted to a credible tobacco control effort.** This may be difficult, as the revenues and expenditures may derive from separate pieces of legislation, but to the extent possible, the Committee encourages a linkage between new taxes and an energetic federal tobacco control program.

OPTIONS AND RECOMMENDATIONS FOR COORDINATION

The reduced rates in adult smoking have been achieved without a centralized and strongly coordinated national tobacco control policy. The Committee debated at some length the desirability and feasibility of a more centralized and planned effort. It considered the virtues of a federal tobacco control administration that could be held accountable for progress in dealing with the nation's most prominent public health problem. The functions of such an agency, however, would span a very wide range—from monitoring advertising and ensuring its accuracy, to measuring nicotine and tar levels in cigarettes, to public education efforts and public health monitoring. An effective tobacco control administration would require consolidation of functions currently performed in different departments, and in different parts of the Public Health Service. Such an institutional arrangement would face immense political obstacles, not only by forcing a new structure on existing functions, but also by perturbing long-standing congressional committee jurisdictions. Thus, despite the temptation to craft a clear organizational chart linking multiple government functions, the Committee concluded that progress would be realized more quickly, and forward movement was far more likely, if its recommendations built on existing structures that could accommodate new tobacco control efforts by incremental expansion.

The programs that promise to have a strong impact on tobacco use—such as those in Canada, California, and Massachusetts—have arisen from grassroots anti-smoking movements that produced new programs, rather than evolving out of a large federal bureaucracy with numerous agencies. Several parts of the federal government already have missions related to tobacco control, although none has it as a central objective.

The Center for Substance Abuse Prevention has initiated a major effort to gather information about, and provide technical assistance for, preventive services. The Committee commends CSAP for this action, for taking steps to fill a critical gap, and notes the usefulness of including tobacco in drug abuse prevention programs. The tobacco control effort extends well beyond preventive interventions, however, and the Committee believes that similar efforts are needed at the federal level on tax policy, youth access, licensing, advertising and promotion, regulation, and other public policy domains. Monitoring of state and local tobacco control efforts can build on the excellent annual surveys of the Association of State and Territorial Health Officials.

The incremental, multi-agency approach endorsed by the Committee does not solve an underlying problem—tobacco control is a small part of many agencies, but central to none. Experience in California, Massachusetts, and Canada reveals strong public support for tobacco control measures when voters are presented with direct choices. That type of public mandate—and the possibility of accountability that it entails—are sorely lacking at the federal level. Tobacco control at the federal level has consistently been marginal to the missions of multiple agencies, and this is also true of most private sector organizations.

Michael Pertschuk, executive director of the Advocacy Institute and a longtime tobacco control advocate, recently observed, "while we have many able and talented and committed leaders, that leadership is fragmented. The limited financial resources committed by both government and non-government funders are, too often, mis-directed. We still lack the structures and capacity for overall priority setting, strategic planning, tactical coordination, and effective coordination."[9] The ACS, AHA, and ALA founded the Coalition on Smoking OR Health as a means of coordinating efforts and supplementing their public education approaches. The coalition has played a major role in several prominent successes, but the supporting agencies have numerous other priorities as well. The Advocacy Institute is well positioned, but can make only "indirect contributions to the movement's strategic cohesion."[10] The many grassroots organizations— such as ANR, DOC, STAT, and others—have enormous energy, but they also have specific focuses.

In the Committee's judgment, this lack of coherent organization and strategic planning may well have hampered tobacco control efforts to date. The Committee invited numerous policymakers and tobacco control advocates to discuss their concepts for a leadership structure. An option that the Committee finds appealing is a "Tobacco Control Institute in the private sector to function as an authoritative policy development and analysis center."[11] It is difficult to determine, however, to whom this recommendation should be directed or how such a center would function in the absence of government authority and substantial resources. Nevertheless, it would seem appropriate for voluntary health agencies, professional associations, advocacy groups, and foundations to consider the concept. The major groups funding tobacco control efforts at the national level have in the past included the federal government, the Robert Wood Johnson Foundation, and the private voluntary health organizations noted above. A Tobacco Policy Coordinating Committee functioned for several years, bringing these groups together, and despite repeated and ample discussion about the advantages of a coherent policy leader, that committee did not evolve into an institute.

The base of support for tobacco control must surely be broadened, but new players are unlikely to have resources equal to or larger than those already involved. The major potential funding organizations have historically decided not to establish a central policy institute, despite ample opportunities to do so. The Committee consulted with several individuals in government and private health organizations, and sees little prospect of their coming together to support a national tobacco control institute. Over time, one of the major academic centers might evolve into a national policy analysis center. The more likely scenario seems to be a policy analysis capacity distributed among many academic centers, government agencies, and private sector organizations. As a long-term goal, the Committee believes that prospects for a more coherent and accountable national tobacco control policy would be brighter if the various government and private organizations concerned with tobacco use pooled their resources to create such a national resource in the private sector. Regardless of whether a central policy analysis institute is possible or desirable, it will be important to broaden the base of support for tobacco control efforts at all levels, and to exhort federal, state, and local governments, private voluntary health organizations, and advocacy groups to collaborate.

In recent years, responsibility for coordinating federal activities has been delegated mainly to the Office on Smoking and Health of the Centers for Disease Control and Prevention. OSH staffs an Interagency Committee on Smoking and Health that brings together most, but not all, of the federal agencies concerned with tobacco control. (The Bureau on Alcohol, Tobacco, and Firearms, for example, is not included.) The Interagency Committee on Smoking and Health has the potential to enhance coordination at the federal level. It held meetings on youth tobacco use in December 1992 and April 1994, for example, that highlighted innovative programs from throughout the country and the findings of the 1994 surgeon general's report. In general, however, the Interagency Committee has not been a major policy force in tobacco control. This conclusion was corroborated in interviews with officials of Public Health Service agencies, advocates, academic researchers, and private sector organizations. The IOM Committee believes that the unique complexity of tobacco-related politics makes true leadership within the federal government difficult, and this complicates interagency coordination. However, the task of coordination can be simplified if the participating agencies coalesce around a single priority. The need to focus on youths seems to be a recognized priority in all the relevant agencies. Therefore, the Committee recommends that **the Interagency Committee on Smoking and Health should set as its highest priority the achievement of the Healthy People 2000 goal for youth smoking and use of smokeless tobacco.**

The Office on Smoking and Health also generally takes the lead in preparing the surgeon general's report. In 1978 the National Clearinghouse for Smoking and Health was renamed the Office on Smoking and Health, was transferred from Atlanta to Washington, D.C., and was given expanded responsibilities to coordinate federal smoking and health activities. It was then moved structurally to the CDC, but remained in Washington. In 1991, the OSH moved to Atlanta, to CDC headquarters. This location has the advantage of bringing OSH closer to the core public health activities of CDC, including many programs that involve working with state health departments, but it has the disadvantage of being remote from the nation's political center; thus, CDC has retained a small liaison office in Washington for OSH.

The Committee believes that OSH is an appropriate choice to coordinate efforts to reduce tobacco use among youth. This should not be construed as calling for consolidation of functions, along the lines of a tobacco control administration as outlined above, but rather for better linkage of activities in various federal agencies, in states, and in private sector organizations. It will probably fall short of the mission of even a tobacco control institute, as discussed above, which would be a national resource for policy analysis and planning (but without implementing authority for research, public health monitoring, regulation, and services). Where the office is located is less important than that it command sufficient resources to monitor policy initiatives at all levels and disseminate that information. This clearinghouse and technical assistance function would be a laudable, if incremental, advance in tobacco control at the federal level. **CDC's Office on Smoking and Health should be given the responsibility for coordinating federal tobacco control initiatives, with a focus on reducing initiation of smoking and use of smokeless tobacco by children and youths, and should be given additional resources for this purpose.**

Funding needs cannot be predicted with any certainty, as they will depend on the degree to which states pursue tobacco control policy. So much activity is taking place at the state and local levels that funding needs may well increase dramatically in the near future. At a minimum, however, the Committee believes that the infrastructure for tobacco control in each state should resemble that which has been established in the current 17 ASSIST states, implying a need for additional resources for the vast majority of non-ASSIST state programs.

The nature of OSH's function will also vary according to state. California, Massachusetts, and Michigan are likely to be sources of expertise and information useful to other states, and their function in this regard will be to transfer knowledge, using the federal government as a clearinghouse. In other states where tobacco control is rudimentary, federal support can be a major impetus for reducing initiation of youth smoking. These incremental funds will be needed even more if federal activity is increased (for example in the Food and Drug Administration, if Congress gives it regulatory authority, or in the Federal Trade Commission, in connection with advertising and promotion constraints).

EPILOGUE

This Committee's work began in May 1993 and was completed in 10 months. During this brief period, the weight of public opinion seems to have shifted decidedly in the direction of reducing tobacco use in the United States. Actions and initiatives on Capitol Hill and in a variety of federal agencies, ranging from the Department of Defense to the Food and Drug Administration, have given an historic burst of political energy to the cause of tobacco control. The public health appears ascendant in what has been a 30-year struggle to modify social norms favorable to tobacco use.

The stage is now set for aggressive action to reduce tobacco use by children and youths as a central feature of the nation's tobacco control efforts. The initiatives recommended in this report, which seemed so remote only a few years ago, are strongly justified and have broad public support. They should be undertaken with dispatch.

Nascent optimism among advocates for tobacco control must be coupled with resolve. If the necessary initiatives are not taken, the political momentum could be lost and the tobacco epidemic could take a new turn for the worse. The recent reversal of the nation's success in tuberculosis (TB) control provides a sobering lesson in the need for forceful efforts even when the prospects for success seem most bright. At the turn of the twentieth century, TB was the chief single cause of death in the United States and millions of Americans suffered from chronic illness and disability related to TB. In an extraordinary public health achievement, the rate of TB declined markedly throughout the century until, in the early 1980s, it seemed that the disease could be eradicated early in the twenty-first century. Unfortunately, however, the downward trend was suddenly halted in 1985, and the incidence of TB has risen every year since 1986. Even more alarming has been the appearance of a new drug-resistant strain of the disease.

Complacency is always dangerous in public health. Notwithstanding significant changes in predominant social attitudes toward tobacco, smoking continues to be associated with a variety of positive images, especially for children and youths. Notwithstanding recent political setbacks, the tobacco industry remains economically powerful and continues to spend more than $4 billion every year to promote and advertise its products. The prices of tobacco products continue to drop in real terms as the industry responds to a shrinking market, making tobacco products more affordable to children and youths. The prevalence of tobacco use now appears to be *increasing* among children and youths.

The nation must commit itself to a vigorous public health initiative in tobacco control. The CDC recently responded to the upsurge in TB by formulating a new strategic plan for the elimination of tuberculosis in the United States by the year 2010.[12] The nation cannot reasonably expect to eliminate tobacco-related disease and death by 2010. However, by putting a youth-centered prevention strategy at the center of tobacco control efforts, and by implementing the initiatives proposed in this report, the nation can take a firm and resolute step on that path.

REFERENCES

1. National Cancer Institute. *Strategies to Control Tobacco Use in the United States: A Blueprint for Public Health Action in the 1990's. Smoking and Tobacco Control Monograph No. 1.* NIH Pub. No. 92-3316. Washington, DC: U.S. Department of Health and Human Services, 1991: ix-xii.

2. Walter, Gailya P., Program Officer, National Center for Chronic Disease Prevention and Health Promotion, Office on Smoking and Health. Personal communication. April 22, 1994.

3. Shopland, D. R. "Smoking Control in the 1990s: A National Cancer Institute Model for Change." *American Journal of Public Health* 83:9 (1993): 1208-1210.

4. National Cancer Institute.

5. Herdman, Roger, Maria Hewitt, and Mary Laschober. *Preventive Health: An Ounce of Prevention Saves a Pound of Cure.* Testimony before the Senate Special Committee on Aging. Hearing on *Smoking-Related Deaths and Financial Costs: Office of Technology Assessments Estimates for 1990.* 6 May 1993. 2, 4.

6. National Heart, Lung, and Blood Institute. Data supplied by the Information Center of the NHLBI, 1994.

7. Hu, Teh-wei. "The Economic Effects of California Cigarette Taxation." Abstract in *Annual Report from the University of California to the State of California Legislature* Tobacco-Related Disease Research Program (1993): 74.

8. National Cancer Institute. *Major Local Tobacco Control Ordinances in the United States. Smoking and Tobacco Control Monograph No. 3.* NIH Pub. No. 93-3532. Washington, DC: U.S. Department of Health and Human Services, March 1993: ix-xii.

9. Pertschuk, Michael. Advocacy Institute. "Opportunity Knocks; Will We Open the Door?" In *Tobacco Use: An American Crisis. Final Report of the Conference.* January 9-12, 1993: 8.

10. *Ibid.*, 9.

11. Slade, John. Letter to Paul Torrens, Chair, Committee on Preventing Nicotine Addiction in Children and Youths. 12 Sept. 1993.

12. Rieder, Hans L., George M. Cauthen, Gloria D. Kelly, Alan B. Bloch, and Dixie E. Snider. "Tuberculosis in the United States." *Journal of the American Medical Association* 262:3 (21 July 1989): 385.

APPENDIXES

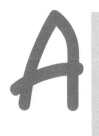

SPECIFIC RECOMMENDATIONS, BY CHAPTER

Chapter 2: The Nature of Nicotine Addiction

1. Research should be conducted to determine individual susceptibility to nicotine addiction.

2. For all forms of tobacco products, research should be conducted on the characteristics of nicotine addiction in the early stages, that is, in the first few years during which the transition between experimental and addictive nicotine use occurs.

3. Research should be conducted on the relationship between the characteristics of tobacco products and addiction.

Chapter 3: Social Norms and the Acceptability of Tobacco

1. Public education programs and messages should be increased and implemented on a continuous basis to (a) inform the public about the hazards of tobacco use and of environmental tobacco smoke and (b) promote a tobacco-free environment. In particular, mass media campaigns, including paid counter-to-bacco advertisements, should be intensified to reverse the image appeal of pro-tobacco messages, especially those that appeal to children and youths.

2. Tobacco-free policies should be adopted and enforced in all public locations, especially in those that cater to or are frequented by children and youths, including all educational institutions, sports arenas, cultural facilities, shopping malls, fast-food restaurants, and transit systems.

3. All levels of government should adopt tobacco-free policies in public

buildings. The Department of Defense should continue its aggressive efforts to adopt tobacco-free policies in all military services.

4. All workplaces should adopt tobacco-free policies.

5. All organizations involved with youths should adopt tobacco-free policies that apply to all persons attending or participating in all events sponsored by the organizations, and should actively promote a tobacco-free norm.

6. Parents should clearly and unequivocally express disapproval of tobacco use to their children, and, if smokers themselves, should quit smoking.

7. Research should be conducted to determine the factors influencing the substantial decline in tobacco use by African-American youths, with particular attention to the role of social norms.

8. Youths should be involved in the development of research questions and approaches and in designing and evaluating health messages and programs.

Chapter 4: Tobacco Advertising and Promotion

1. Congress should repeal the federal law preempting state regulation of tobacco promotion and advertising that occurs entirely within the states' borders.

2. After state regulatory authority has been clarified and restored, states and localities should severely restrict the advertising and promotion of tobacco products on billboards and other outdoor media, on vehicles, in facilities of public transportation, in public arenas and sports facilities, and at the point of sale.

3. Congress should enact comprehensive legislation establishing a timetable for gradual implementation of a plan for restricting tobacco advertising and promotion in interstate commerce. Essential components of this plan, which should become fully effective by the year 2000, include:

(a) restricting to a tombstone format the advertising of tobacco products in print media, including magazines and newspapers, or in other visual media, including videotape, videodisc, video arcade game, or film;

(b) banning the commercial use of the registered brand name of a tobacco product, trademark, or logo, or other recognizable symbol for such a product in any movie, music video, television show, play, video arcade game, or other form of entertainment, or on any other product; and

(c) banning the use of the registered brand name of a tobacco product, a trademark or logo, or other recognizable symbol for such a product, in any public place, or in any medium of mass communication for the purpose of publicizing, revealing, or documenting sponsorship of, or contribution to, any athletic, artistic, or other public event.

4. Research should be conducted that attends to ethnic, gender, and social class differences; that is sensitive to youths' responses to advertising and promotional messages; and that assesses the success as well as the failure of advertising campaigns.

Chapter 5: Prevention and Cessation of Tobacco Use:
Research-Based Programs

1. Under federal leadership, the United States should develop a national child health policy that gives high priority to the prevention of tobacco use by youths.

2. All schools should adopt and implement the CDC guidelines to prevent tobacco use and addiction.

3. Already proven models of school-based prevention programs should be systematically integrated into a comprehensive approach to reducing tobacco use by children and youths.

4. Tobacco prevention should be integrated into any drug prevention program aimed at youth.

5. Systematic research should be conducted on the optimal way to disseminate and implement tobacco use prevention programs on a large scale.

6. Research should be conducted on the development and evaluation of programs to help children and youths who are regular tobacco users to quit their habitual use of cigarettes, snuff, or chew.

7. Research should be conducted to identify the need for, and to develop and evaluate, prevention programs aimed at reducing tobacco use among specific ethnic groups.

Chapter 6: Tobacco Taxation in the United States

1. Tobacco tax policies at the federal and state levels should be linked to the national objectives for reducing tobacco use. In other words, government policymakers should use tobacco taxes as an intervention to accomplish these health goals.

2. The excise tax on cigarettes should be increased to a level comparable with that in other major industrialized countries. A reasonable target would be to increase the federal cigarette tax by $2 by 1995. Accomplishing this objective would also have the added benefit of reducing illegal smuggling of tobacco products between Canada and the United States.

3. All tobacco products should be taxed on an equivalent basis. For example, when cigarette taxes are increased, taxes on non-cigarette tobacco products should also be increased on an equivalent basis to discourage substitution of one harmful form of tobacco for another (such as smokeless tobacco).

4. The real value of tobacco taxes should be maintained to account for inflation over time. Optimally, tobacco tax policy should take into consideration the affordability of tobacco products to prevent tobacco from becoming more affordable.

5. Tobacco products in U.S. military stores should be priced at the same rate that exists in the surrounding community. This policy change would have

an effect on the smoking behavior of military personnel, many of whom are young adults. Also by eliminating the price differential between military and nonmilitary retail outlets, the incentive for illegal smuggling of tobacco products out of military bases would be eliminated.

Chapter 7: Youth Access to Tobacco

1. The federal government should set national goals for reducing youth access to tobacco and should provide resources and leadership to facilitate state and local efforts to effectuate those goals.

2. The federal government should use its spending power to induce states to adopt and implement state plans for tobacco control, including specific plans for enforcing access restrictions. The states' obligation to enforce youth access restrictions should be tied to eligibility for CDC grants for tobacco control activities, and these grants should include sufficient funds to cover the costs of enforcement during the developmental phase of the new program. In addition, the states should be required to establish a mechanism for independent assessment of retailer compliance with youth access restrictions.

3. A federal agency should serve as a clearinghouse and resource center for information, models, and technical assistance for implementing access restriction programs.

4. So that local communities may act as needed regarding local needs for tobacco control, states should adopt a youth access plan that does not preempt local governments from adopting stronger local initiatives.

5. States should establish a licensing system requiring merchants to obtain a license to sell tobacco products, which may be suspended or revoked if the merchant sells tobacco to minors or violates other state and local laws designed to reduce youth access.

6. Licensing fees should be earmarked for the enforcement of youth access legislation and should be set high enough to cover those costs. If possible, responsibility for operating the licensing system should be assigned to a public health agency. However, each state should assess existing regulatory structures to determine which agency is best able to administer effectively the licensing program. The agency selected should retain the authority both to administer the licensing program and to receive licensing fees.

7. States should ban tobacco vending machines; less restrictive alternatives to a complete ban should be adopted only if shown to be effective.

8. States should prohibit the sale of tobacco products by self-service displays. During compliance checks, authorities should verify that tobacco is being sold only from behind the counter or from locked cases.

9. Sale of single cigarettes, which violates federal tobacco labeling law, should also be banned by state youth access laws. During compliance checks,

authorities should verify that retailers do not offer single cigarettes for sale, whether openly displayed or from behind the counter.

10. Distribution of free tobacco products in public places or through the mail should be prohibited.

11. Education programs to increase merchants' awareness of and support for youth access laws should be fostered as a valuable complement to legal enforcement measures.

12. CDC, through the Office on Smoking and Health, should provide technical assistance and resources to support states and localities wishing to implement youth access community education programs.

13. Youth access laws should be effectively enforced. An enforcement plan should implement a graduated penalty system proportionate to the extent of the violation, beginning with fines for minor infractions and followed by stronger penalties (suspension, then revocation) for serious and repeated violations.

14. Legal penalties should not be imposed on youths who are able to obtain tobacco products; existing legal penalties on minors should be repealed.

15. Criminal penalties should not be imposed on licensees who sell tobacco to minors. Rather, appropriate civil penalties, including fines and tobacco license suspension or revocation, should be prescribed and enforced.

16. Youth access plans should not set excessively high age limits; states should set the minimum age of purchase at age 18.

17. States and localities should adopt long-term strategies for reducing the number of outlets licensed to sell tobacco products. Initial steps should include creation of tobacco-free zones around schools and bans of tobacco sales in pharmacies.

18. As part of a long-term access strategy, Congress should enact a suitably limited federal ban on the distribution of tobacco products through the mail. At a minimum, the law should bar *free* distribution, as well as redemption of tobacco coupons, a promotional activity likely to be particularly attractive to children and youths.

19. Sponsors of research should support (a) studies of retailers regarding their motivation for compliance for noncompliance; (b) studies of the cost-effectiveness of various enforcement approaches being developed in response to the Synar Amendment; and (c) most important, a surveillance system for monitoring the tobacco market in order to ascertain the sources (and cost) of tobacco products to youths, in both legal and illicit commerce.

Chapter 8: Regulation of the Labeling, Packaging, and Contents of Tobacco Products

1. Congress should enact legislation that delegates to an appropriate agency the necessary authority to regulate tobacco products for the dual purposes of

discouraging consumption and reducing the morbidity and mortality associated with use of tobacco products.

2. Congress should take steps to strengthen the federally mandated warning labels for tobacco products.

3. Congress should take steps to increase the salience and effectiveness of health warnings on both advertising and packaging.

4. Based on current knowledge, Congress should enact specific warning and format requirements now, and should delegate regulatory responsibility for future modifications to the secretary of health and human services. The secretary should ensure that ongoing research is conducted on the effectiveness of prescribed warnings.

5. To the extent that promotional use of logos and trademarks of tobacco products is legally permitted, Congress should make accompanying health warnings mandatory.

6. Congress should confer upon an administrative agency the authority to regulate the design and constituents of tobacco products whenever it determines that such regulation would reduce the prevalence of dependence or disease associated with use of the product or would otherwise promote the public health. The agency should be specifically authorized to prescribe ceilings on the yields of tar, nicotine, or any other harmful constituent of a tobacco product.

7. The regulatory agency, as its first step, should develop a sound methodology for ascertaining the actual yields of nicotine, tar, or any other constituents of tobacco products, based on human consumption.

8. At a minimum, the regulatory agency should take steps to inform consumers about the meaning of statements regarding tar and nicotine yields, and particularly about the behavioral influences on intake, and the relative importance of the characteristics of the cigarette and the way it is smoked.

9. If the regulatory agency finds that reduction of tar and/or nicotine yields would reduce morbidity or mortality associated with use of tobacco products, it should be authorized to prescribe ceilings of tar and/or nicotine yields and to develop a regulatory program of phased reductions in those ceilings over time.

Chapter 9: Coordination of Policies and Research

1. Funding to the non-ASSIST states should be increased to a level commensurate with ASSIST states.

2. Social science research should be conducted to enhance understanding of how norms are formed and transmitted, and of the regional and cultural differences in the acceptability of tobacco use.

3. Federal agencies that sponsor tobacco-related research should increase the resources devoted to understanding and preventing initiation of tobacco use by children and youths.

4. Federal agencies should give special attention to research on the efficacy of policies aiming to prevent initiation of tobacco use by youths.

5. Congress should ensure that some fraction of revenues raised by the federal excise tax on tobacco products be devoted to a credible tobacco control effort.

6. The Interagency Committee on Smoking and Health should set as its highest priority the achievement of the Healthy People 2000 goal for youth smoking and use of smokeless tobacco.

7. CDC's Office on Smoking and Health should be given the responsibility for coordinating federal tobacco control initiatives, with a focus on reducing initiation of smoking and use of smokeless tobacco by children and youths, and should be given additional resources for this purpose.

COMMITTEE BIOGRAPHIES

Paul R. Torrens, M.D., M.P.H. (*Chair*), is professor of health services administration at the University of California, Los Angeles, School of Public Health. He received his M.D. degree from Georgetown University School of Medicine in 1958 and his M.P.H. degree from the Harvard University School of Public Health in 1962. From October 1989 to October 1990, Dr. Torrens was the Founding Director of the Tobacco Disease Research Program within the Office of the President of the University of California. This $72 million program was supported by the new California state tax on tobacco products; its purpose was to sponsor research on all aspects of tobacco-related diseases in California. Dr. Torrens has 12 years of experience as a health care manager in hospitals and health maintenance organizations. He has been a consultant for 15 years for a major national accounting/management consulting firm as a consultant for 15 years and has accumulated 31 service-years of membership on governing boards or boards of directors of hospitals, health care systems, and health maintenance organizations. He has served in a wide variety of health policy advisory and consulting capacities to governmental and nongovernmental organizations in all parts of the United States and in 13 foreign countries. His range of governmental experiences in the United States includes local and state government agencies as well as various branches of the federal government. Dr. Torrens is a fellow of the American Board of Preventive Medicine, the American College of Preventive Medicine, and the American Public Health Association.

Albert Bandura, Ph.D., is David Starr Jordan Professor of Social Science in Psychology, Stanford University. He received his Ph.D. degree from the Uni-

289

versity of Iowa in 1952. Dr. Bandura has expertise in social psychology, including the psychological determinants of smoking behavior, the psychological mechanisms through which change is achieved, and the effects of programs to prevent smoking among children. He is a member of the Institute of Medicine (IOM) and serves on IOM's Board on Biobehavioral Sciences and Mental Disorders. Dr. Bandura is the author of 8 books on social behavior, is currently on the editorial board of 16 journals or serial volumes, and has received 7 honorary degrees in addition to his many scientific awards. He is a past president of the American Psychological Association (APA) and the Western Psychological Association (WPA), and past chair of the boards of directors of the APA and the WPA; he has served on various other boards, councils, and committees of the APA.

Neal Benowitz, M.D., is professor and chief, Division of Clinical Pharmacology, Departments of Medicine, Pharmacy, and Psychiatry at the School of Medicine of the University of California at San Francisco. He received his M.D. with distinction at the University of Rochester School of Medicine in 1969 and was an intern and resident at the Bronx Municipal Hospital Center in the Bronx, New York, from 1969 to 1971. Dr. Benowitz is a recognized authority on clinical pharmacology and experimental therapeutics and counts among his publications over 140 original articles and 40 book chapters in such areas as pharmacology, toxicology, substance abuse, and, specifically, nicotine use and addiction. Among his many professional activities, Dr. Benowitz was scientific editor for the *U.S. Surgeon General's Report on the Health Consequences of Smoking: Nicotine Addiction*, 1988; member, Clove Cigarette Scientific Advisory Board to the Department of Health for the State of California, 1986-1987; technical consultant and chapter author for the *U.S. Surgeon General's Advisory Committee Report on the Health Consequences of Smokeless Tobacco;* and contributing author for the *U.S. Surgeon General's Report on Health Consequences of Cigarette Smoking: Health Effects of Involuntary Smoking*, 1986. He is on the editorial boards of *The Journal of Smoking-Related Disorders*; *Cardiovascular Drugs and Therapy*; *Archives of Environmental Health*; *Drug Safety*; and *Drug Therapy*.

Richard J. Bonnie, LL.B., is the John S. Battle Professor of Law at the University of Virginia School of Law and director of the Institute of Law, Psychiatry and Public Policy at the University of Virginia. He received his LL.B. in 1969 from the University of Virginia. Mr. Bonnie is a member of the Institute of Medicine, a member of the Institute's Board of Biobehavioral Sciences and Mental Disorders, a charter fellow of the College on the Problems of Drug Dependence, and was secretary of the National Advisory Council on Drug Abuse from 1975 to 1980. His expertise is in the broad area of substance abuse and legal approaches to discouraging substance abuse, with a specific focus of the efficacy of public health law. Mr. Bonnie is the author of numerous articles and book chapters, some of which are *Legal Aspects of Drug Dependence*; "Discouraging the Use of Alcohol, Tobacco, and Other Drugs: The Effects of Legal Controls and Restrictions" (book chapter); "Regulation of Alcohol, Tobacco and Other Drugs: The Agenda for Law Reform" (book chapter); "Discouraging Unhealthy Personal Choices Through Government Regulation: Some Thoughts About the Minimum Drinking Age" (book chapter); "Law and the Discouragement of Unhealthy Personal Choices" (book chapter); "The Efficacy of Law as a Paternalistic Instrument" (book chapter); and "Regulating Conditions of Alcohol Availability: Possible Effects on Highway Safety" (article).

K. Michael Cummings, Ph.D., M.P.H., is director of the Smoking Control Program, and Cancer Research Scientist in the Department of Cancer Control and Epidemiology at the Roswell Park Cancer Institute in Buffalo, New York. He also holds two positions at the State University of New York at Buffalo: associate research professor in the Department of Experimental Pathology and Epidemiology and assistant clinical professor in the Department of Social and Preventive Medicine in the School of Medicine. Dr. Cummings received his M.P.H. degree in health behavior from the University of Michigan in 1977 and his Ph.D. in health behavior from the University of Michigan in 1980. He has published over 100 articles on such topics as the behavior and withdrawal symptoms of recent ex-smokers, factors influencing health behavior and changes in health behavior, cigarette advertising strategies, race-linked differences in cigarette brand preference, awareness and implementation of laws banning the sale of tobacco to minors, and Native American health. He has also conducted a number of smoking-related studies for the National Institutes of Health. Dr. Cummings also authored "Smoking Education and Cessation Activities," a chapter in the *U.S. Surgeon General's Report on Reducing the Health Consequences of Smoking: 25 Years of Progress*, 1989, and "Public Opinion and Changing Patterns of Tobacco Use," a chapter in *Strategies to Control Tobacco Use in the United States: A Blueprint for Public Health Action in the 1990's*, 1991. He is on the editorial boards of *Tobacco Control: An International Journal, Cancer Epidemiology, Biomarkers and Prevention*, and *Health Education Quarterly*.

Donald Dexter, Jr., D.M.D., received his D.M.D. degree from the Oregon Health Sciences University School of Dentistry in 1987 and is a member of the Klamath Tribes. Dr. Dexter is executive director, Klamath Tribal Health and Family Services, in Klamath Falls, Oregon. The $2.8 million program is responsible for the delivery and management of health services for the Klamath Tribal members in Klamath County. Although primarily a clinician, Dr. Dexter has an active commitment to reducing rates of tobacco use among young Native Americans, whose rate of use is one of the highest in the nation. From 1986 to 1987 he was the primary investigator of "Use of Smokeless Tobacco Among NW

Native Youth," a research project funded by the IHS and published in the *American Journal of Public Health*. From 1988 to 1991 he was a member of the Oregon Tobacco Free Coalition. In 1991 Dr. Dexter was a member of the Youth Tobacco Task Force of the Alcohol and Substance Abuse Branch of the IHS and served on the Oral Cancer Subcommittee, Tobacco Advisory Group, of the IHS Oral Health Promotion/Disease Prevention Program. In 1992 he was the key source of information for *Spit Tobacco and Youth*, published by the Office of the Inspector General, Department of Health and Human Services. Dr. Dexter is currently working on a tobacco education video and curriculum directed at children in grades three through six.

Ellen Ruth Gritz, Ph.D., is professor and chair of the Department of Behavioral Science, M. D. Anderson Cancer Center, University of Texas, Houston. Dr. Gritz is also a psychologist who specializes in the psychotherapeutic needs of cancer patients and their families and in smoking cessation. In addition to her expertise in psychology and clinical psychology, Dr. Gritz has broad experience in issues concerning the pharmacology, treatment, prevention, and cessation of smoking, particularly for women. She is currently studying smoking cessation among Hispanic and African-American women. From 1980 to 1986 Dr. Gritz was an expert consultant in the Office on Smoking and Health, Office of the Assistant Secretary for Health, Department of Health and Human Services. In this role she served as behavioral editor for the *U.S. Surgeon General's Annual Report on Smoking and Health*. From 1982 to 1985, she was a member of the Board of Scientific Counselors to the Addiction Research Unit at the National Institute on Drug Abuse. From 1984 to 1987 Dr. Gritz served on the Interdepartmental Committee on a Smoke-Free Society in the Year 2000 of the national office of the American Cancer Society. During 1985-1986 she was on the technical advisory committee to Lester Breslow for "Setting Goals for Cancer Control in California for the Year 2000." From 1984 to 1990 Dr. Gritz was a member of the research advisory committee of the Institute for the Study of Smoking Behavior and Policy at Harvard University's John F. Kennedy School of Government. Dr. Gritz is an associate editor of *Cancer Epidemiology, Biomarkers and Prevention*; consulting editor of *Health Psychology*; and a member of the editorial advisory boards of *Quality of Life Research*; *Tobacco Control*; and the *Journal of Women's Health*. She is also a senior reviewer of the *U.S. Surgeon General's Annual Report on Smoking and Health*. Dr. Gritz has over 100 publications to her credit.

Gerardo Marín, Ph.D., is professor of psychology and associate dean for academic affairs, College of Arts and Sciences, at the University of San Francisco. Dr. Marin received his Ph.D. degree in social psychology from DePaul University in 1979. He has published internationally in the fields of psychology and sociology and has particular expertise in intercultural psychosocial issues. In the field of nicotine use he is conducting two studies among Hispanics: "A Smoking Cessation Intervention with Hispanics" through the decade 1985-1995 (supported by the National Cancer Institute) and "Tobacco Control Strategies for Hispanics and Network on Hispanic Tobacco Control," 1991-1994 (supported by the Tobacco Control Section of the California Department of Health Services). Dr. Marín has also conducted major studies on drug use among high school students and social factors in the acquisition of new behaviors (e.g., abuse of drugs, use of condoms). He has over 90 publications in the areas of psychology and sociology and 9 years' experience in tobacco-use issues within the Hispanic communities of California. He is associate editor of the *Hispanic Journal of Behavioral Sciences* and is a member of the editorial boards of *The InterAmerican Journal of Psychology*; *Revista de la Asociacion Latinoamericana de Psicología Social*; *Jornal de Psicología*; *Comportamiento*; *Revista de Psicología Social*; *Journal of Cross-Cultural Psychology*; and *Revista Intercontinental de Psicología y Educación*.

Mark A. Nichter, Ph.D., M.P.H., is a professor in the Departments of Anthropology and of Family and Community Medicine, University of Arizona. He received his Ph.D. in social anthropology from the University of Edinburgh in 1977 and his M.P.H. in international health from the Johns Hopkins University School of Hygiene and Public Health in 1978. Dr. Nichter is conducting, for the National Institute on Child Health and Development, a major study of "Adolescent Smoking and Dietary Behavior." He has done extensive anthropological fieldwork, particularly in the areas of medical anthropology, culture and the individual, and South Asian ethnography. In the area of medical anthropology Dr. Nichter has focused on cross-cultural study of the body, health, and illness-related behavior; ethnomedicine; comparative medical systems; medicine, power, and the production of knowledge; and international health development and anthropology. His training in medical anthropology and international health is complemented by a two-year residency in psychiatry. He received the Margaret Mead Award in 1989 and a Fulbright Professorship in Health Education and the Anthropology of Health (in Sri Lanka) in 1983-1984. He recently was awarded Rockefeller Foundation Grants for sabbatical research (1991-1992) and for acting as coordinator of a "Small Grants Scheme for Third World Health Social Scientists" (1992). In 1990, the National Science Foundation made Dr. Nichter a Field Methods Training Camp Grantee. He is editor of *Anthropological Approaches to the Study of Ethnomedicine* (1992) and associate editor of the journal *Medical Anthropology*.

Peggy O'Hara, Ph.D., is associate professor and director of Graduate Studies in the Department of Epidemiology and Public Health, the University of Miami School of Medicine. She received her Ph.D. degree in education from the University of Pittsburgh in 1981. Dr. O'Hara has crosscutting expertise in study design and clinical, educational, and epidemiological arenas. In addition to her doctorate in education, Dr. O'Hara has nine years of experience teaching children in the public school systems of Pittsburgh. Her research has focused on physical factors such as exercise, weight gain, and menstrual cycles in relation to cessation and relapse of smoking. From 1987 to 1990 she was principal investigator on "Influences of Menstrual Cycle Changes on Smoking Relapse," 1987-1990 (supported by the National Institute on Drug Abuse) and from 1984 to 1990 was co-investigator on the "Lung Health Study" (National Heart, Lung, and Blood Institute). She has also been on the National Steering Committee of the National Heart, Lung, and Blood Institute's Lung Health Study since 1986; a member of the American Cancer Society's Lung Cancer Prevention Task Force since 1991; and from 1986 to 1989 served as Director of the Smoking Program for Women at the Western Psychiatric Institute and Clinic of the University of Pittsburgh. Dr. O'Hara's book chapters include "Relapse Prevention" in *The Clinical Management of Nicotine Dependence* (1991); "Smoking" in *Behavioral Medicine for Women* (1988); and "Nicotine Dependence" in *Adult Behavior Therapy Casebook* (in press). Her publications examine the use of nicotine gum, and age and gender differences in such use; physical activity and continued smoking cessation; whether low tar and nicotine cigarettes decrease nicotine dependence and cardiovascular risk; smoking-induced lung diseases; and interventions for high-risk smokers. As a consultant, she has developed employee smoking cessation programs for a number of businesses (Mellon Bank, PPG Industries, Gulf Oil Corporation, Mobay Chemical Corporation, Merrell Dow Pharmaceuticals, U.S. Steel Corporation, Society of Automotive Engineers, and DeLuxe Check Printers, Inc.).

Cheryl L. Perry, Ph.D., is professor, Division of Epidemiology, and co-director of the Doctoral and Post-Doctoral Training Program on the Behavioral Aspects of Cardiovascular Disease, Division of Epidemiology, at the University of Minnesota. She received her Ph.D. degree in education from Stanford University in 1980. Dr. Perry's expertise is in the areas of child and adolescent health and development; prevention of substance abuse by children and adolescents; community models of intervention; and psychosocial aspects of health promotion and disease prevention. She has published over 80 articles and was senior scientific editor of the 1994 *Surgeon General's Report on Preventing Tobacco Use Among Young People.* Dr. Perry has also been principal investigator or co-principal investigator of 18 grants, including "Project CLASP: Peer Leadership for Smoking Prevention," 1978-1979 (supported by the National Interagency Council on Smoking and Health); "A Developmental Approach to Drug Abuse Prevention," 1982-1985 (National Institute on Drug Abuse); "Tailoring Drug Abuse Prevention Programs to the School Environment," 1983-1986 (National Institute on Drug Abuse); and the Young Adult Lifestyles Study: A Longitudinal Follow-up of Smoking Behavior in Young Adulthood," 1984-1989 (National Cancer Institute).

Thomas C. Schelling, Ph.D., is Distinguished Professor of Economics and Public Affairs, University of Maryland, and Lucius N. Littauer Professor of Political Economy, emeritus, Harvard University. He received his Ph.D. degree in economics from Harvard University in 1951. From 1983 to 1989 Dr. Schelling headed the Institute for Smoking Behavior and Policy at Harvard University; he has expertise in addictive behavior and issues of self-control in cessation and relapse of nicotine use. He is a member of the Institute of Medicine and of the National Academy of Sciences. He is also a fellow of the American Association for the Advancement of Science, the Association for Public Policy Analysis and Management, and the American Academy of Arts and Sciences. Dr. Schelling was elected President of the American Economic Association for 1991, was named a distinguished fellow of the association in 1987, and received the Frank E. Seidman Distinguished Award in Political Economy in 1977. He has twice served as chairman of the Research Advisory Board of the Committee for Economic Development and is a trustee of the Aerospace Corporation. Dr. Schelling served in the U.S. Bureau of the Budget from 1945 to 1946, the Economic Cooperation Administration in Europe from 1948 to 1950, and the White House and the Executive Office of the President from 1951 to 1953. He joined the Department of Economics at Yale University in 1953 and was appointed professor of Economics at Harvard in 1958. During 1958-1959 he was on the staff of the RAND Corporation. Dr. Schelling has been a consultant to the Departments of State and Defense, the Arms Control and Disarmament Agency, and the Central Intelligence Agency and has been a member of the Defense Science Board and the Scientific Advisory Board of the U.S. Air Force. He has frequently lectured at the Foreign Service Institute and the several U.S. war colleges. Dr. Schelling has published articles on tobacco and drug policy and is the author of *Choice and Consequence*, 1984; *Micromotives and Macrobehavior*, 1978; and six other books on such topics as international economics, arms control, and energy and environmental policy.

Herbert H. Severson, Ph.D., is research scientist, Oregon Research Institute; associate professor of educational psychology, University of Oregon; and a clinical psychologist in private practice. He also provides consultant services, such as to the National Training Network in Colorado about systematic screening for behavior disorders for identifying at-risk students in grades one through five. He received his Ph.D. in educational psychology from the University of Wisconsin, Madison, in 1973. In addition to his research and expertise in adolescent psychology, Dr. Severson has hands-on experience as a school psychologist in public schools. He has also developed many educational and evaluative products including: *Big Dipper* (1985), a videotape on the risks of smokeless tobacco use by teens; *Up to Snuff: A Comprehensive Manual on Smokeless Tobacco* (1987); *Making a Difference: Counseling Patients to Quit Smoking* (1990), a videotape funded by the National Heart, Lung, and Blood Institute that is used in medical schools to train physicians to counsel patients to quit smoking; *A Healthy Start: Smoke Free Babies* (1990), a videotape funded by the National Heart, Lung, and Blood Institute to be shown to smoking mothers when they come to pediatric offices for well-baby care; *Enough Snuff: A Guide to Quitting Smokeless Tobacco on Your Own* (1992); *Systematic Archival Record Search* (1991), a procedure for systematically assessing at-risk students using school record information; and *Preschool Screening for Behavioral Problems* (1993). Dr. Severson has expertise in the prevention of substance abuse in schools, child health psychology, refusal skills training, and systematic screening for health risks or behavioral disorders. He has been the principal investigator or co-investigator on 16 studies.

Sarah Moody Thomas, Ph.D., is associate director for Community Education and Applications at the Stanley S. Scott Cancer Center, Louisiana State University Medical Center. She is also clinical professor in the Department of Psychology, University of New Orleans. Dr. Thomas received her Ph.D. degree in clinical psychology, with a co-major in public administration from the University of Georgia in 1978. Her areas of expertise are factors influencing adolescent behavior; the health behaviors of adolescents, particularly African-American youths; and smoking prevention. Her clinical experience includes a study of smoking prevention among 970 black urban adolescents in 14 Orleans Parish schools from 1987 to 1989. The intervention was a 7-day teacher-led program in social skills and health information for ninth graders; follow-up after one year indicated that only 7% of the students had smoked in the past month. She has also examined parental involvement in the program (1988-1990) and adolescents' concerns about their parents who smoke. In addition, Dr. Thomas has worked with the Louisiana Tobacco Task Force to develop a statewide cancer control plan.

Robert Mullan Cook-Deegan, M.D., is the director of the Division of Biobehavioral Sciences and Mental Disorders at the Institute of Medicine. He was previously an expert (consultant advisor) to the National Center for Human Genome Research at the National Institutes of Health. Dr. Cook-Deegan served as the acting executive director of the Biomedical Ethics Advisory Committee of the U.S. Congress from December 1988 to October 1989. Before that, he was a senior associate at the Office of Technology Assessment (OTA) of the U.S. Congress for six years. While at OTA, he directed a project entitled *Mapping Our Genes—Genome Projects: How Big? How Fast?* and subsequently obtained awards from the Alfred P. Sloan Foundation to write a book on the science and politics of the human genome and from the National Science Foundation to establish an archive and oral history resource on the same topic. He is a senior research fellow at the Kennedy Institute of Ethics (Georgetown University), an associate in the Department of Health Policy and Management in the School of Hygiene and Public Health at the Johns Hopkins University, and a fellow of the American Association for the Advancement of Science. He now serves or has recently served on national advisory boards to the National Institutes of Health, UNESCO, the Health Care Financing Administration, the Robert Wood Johnson Foundation, and the Alzheimer's Association. He is a member of the Board of Directors, Physicians for Human Rights, and of the national steering committee for the Health Professional Network of Amnesty International, USA. His background included two years of postdoctoral basic research on the molecular biology of oncogenes with Lasker Award scientist Raymond L. Erikson. This followed clinical training at the University of Colorado, where he completed his internship and two years of residency in pathology. He received his M.D. degree from the University of Colorado in 1979.

Barbara S. Lynch, Ph.D., is study director for the study on preventing nicotine dependency in children and youths. Dr. Lynch has a broad range of interrelated professional experiences in program design, development, and implementation; training and teaching; publications development, writing, and photography; and analytic research and synthesis. Her audiences—through programs, training, and publications—have included the general public, policymakers, federal agency personnel, public school personnel, university students, and the multiple constituents of the health care and health promotion fields: biomedical researchers, physicians, nurses and allied health professionals, health management personnel, epidemiologists, and health and medical educators. She has worked with federal agencies, with contractors and grantees, with voluntary health organizations, and with committees, national commissions, and advisory boards. She has been on the faculties of Louisiana State University at New Orleans, Louisiana State Medical School, and the University of Maryland, where she taught writing and literature, science writing, and health communications. As a consultant, her activities have spanned research, applications, and technology transfer related to communications, health education, specific diseases, women's health, and smoking and health.

INDEX

A

Accessibility of tobacco, 19, 199–200, 201
  national reduction goals, 19, 210, 284
  and price-sensitivity of adolescents, 17, 19, 108, 187–191, 266
  surveillance systems, 19, 227, 285
  through adults, 206, 246
Acetylcholine, 34, 35
Addiction. *See* Nicotine addiction/dependence
Adult tobacco use, 5–6, 7, 8, 11, 23, 63
  perceived prevalence of, 14, 18, 21, 77, 78, 79
Advertising and promotions, 11, 105–114
  African Americans, 112, 114
  appeal to children and youths, 18, 106, 116–122, 130–131, 245
  expenditures, 11, 105, 107–108, 109, 278
  impacts on child and youth tobacco use, 18, 55, 124, 131
  market segmentation, 115–116
  non-media promotional items, 80, 108, 110, 245–246
  Old Joe Camel campaign, 116–117, 120, 129
  promotional allowances, 110–111
  recall studies, 123–124
  research needs, 18, 133–134, 282
  value-added promotions, 108, 110
  women as targets, 116

Advertising restrictions, 18, 131, 132, 133
  constitutional challenges to, 133
  effects on smoking prevalence, 124–128
  federal, 21–22, 133, 282
  health warnings, 245
  industry voluntary code, 128–130
  insignia, logos, trademarks, 133, 245–246, 282
  interstate, 18, 133, 282
  on misleading terms, 249
  preemption law, 17, 132, 282
  public support for, 12
  smokeless tobacco promotions, 245
  by states, 12, 17, 18, 21, 131–132, 133, 259, 283
  total ban, 128, 133
  transportation systems, 132, 282
  See also Tombstone advertising formats
Advocacy Institute, 269, 274
Advocacy organizations for tobacco control, 93–97, 268–269, 274–275
  health professions, 94–95
  local coalitions, 12, 17, 21, 93, 94
  youth involvement, 96–97
Affective education model, 145
Affordability of tobacco products
  relation to consumption, 192
  and tax policy, 17, 180–182, 192, 193, 283